Manual of Retinal Diseases

Carlos A. Medina • Justin H. Townsend
Arun D. Singh
Editors

Manual of Retinal Diseases

A Guide to Diagnosis and Management

Springer

Editors
Carlos A. Medina
Bascom Palmer Eye Institute
Miami, FL
USA

Justin H. Townsend
Bascom Palmer Eye Institute
Miami, FL
USA

Arun D. Singh
Cleveland Clinic Foundation
Cole Eye Institute
Cleveland, OH
USA

ISBN 978-3-319-20459-8 ISBN 978-3-319-20460-4 (eBook)
DOI 10.1007/978-3-319-20460-4

Printed on acid-free paper

This Springer imprint is published by Springer Nature
The registered company is Springer International Publishing AG Switzerland

Contents

Section Editors

Section I. Ocular Trauma: Jonathan H. Tzu: Department of Ophthalmology, Bascom Palmer Eye Institute, University of Miami, 900 NW 17th St., Miami, FL, 33136, USA

Section II. Pediatric Retinal Diseases: Ryan C. Young: Bascom Palmer Eye Institute, University of Miami, 900 NW 17th, St. Miami, FL, 33136, USA

Section III. Retinal Dystrophies: Veeral Shah: Department of Ophthalmology, Baylor College of Medicine, Texas Children's Hospital, Houston, TX, USA

Section IV. Disorders of the Vitreous and Vitreo-Retinal Interface: Carlos A. Medina: Department of Ophthalmology, Bascom Palmer Eye Institute, University of Miami, 900 NW 17th Street, Miami, FL, 33136, USA

Section V. Uveal Tumors and Associated Conditions: Mary Beth Aronow: Wilmer Eye Institute, Johns Hopkins University School of Medicine, 600 N Wolfe Street, Baltimore, MD 21287-9277, USA

Section VI. Abdul Hassan Aziz: Department of Ophthalmic Oncology, Cole Eye Institute, Cleveland Clinic, Cleveland, Ohio, USA

Section VII. Retinal Detachments and Associated Diseases: Christopher R. Henry: Department of Ophthalmology, Bascom Palmer Eye Institute, University of Miami Miller School of Medicine, 900 NW 17th Street, Miami, FL 33136, USA

Section VIII. Diabetic Retinopathy: John E. Legarreta: Department of Ophthalmology, Bascom Palmer Eye Institute, University of Miami, 900 NW 17th St., Miami, FL 33136, USA

Section IX. Retinal Vascular Diseases: Amir Mohsenin: Bascom Palmer Eye Institute, University of Miami, 900 NW 17th St., Miami, FL 33136, USA

Section X. Age Related Macular Degeneration: John E. Legarreta: Department of Ophthalmology, Bascom Palmer Eye Institute, University of Miami, 900 NW 17th St., Miami, FL 33136, USA

Section XI. Macular Diseases: Royce W. S. Chen: Department of Ophthalmology, Edward S. Harkness Eye Institute, Columbia University College of Physicians and Surgeons, 635 W. 165th Street, Box 104, New York, NY 10032, USA

Section XII. Toxic Maculopathy: Carlos A. Medina: Department of Ophthalmology, Bascom Palmer Eye Institute, University of Miami, 900 NW 17th Street, Miami, FL, 33136, USA

Section XIII. Uveitis: White Dot Syndromes: Jared Knickelbein: Laboratory of Immunology, National Eye Institute, National Institutes of Health, 10 Center Dr., Bldg. 10, Room 10D45, Bethesda, MD 20892, USA

Section XIV. Uveitis: Non White Dot Syndromes: Jared Knickelbein: Laboratory of Immunology, National Eye Institute, National Institutes of Health, 10 Center Dr., Bldg. 10, Room 10D45, Bethesda, MD 20892, USA

Section XV. Infectious Diseases: Department of Ophthalmology, Bascom Palmer Eye Institute, University of Miami, 900 NW 17th Street, Miami, FL 33136, USA

Section XVI. Endophthalmitis: Ajay E. Kuriyan: Bascom Palmer Eye Institute, University of Miami, 900 NW 17th Street, Miami, FL 33136, USA

Section XVII. Systemic Disease and Associated Retinal Disease: Marco A. Gonzalez: Department of Ophthalmology, University of Miami, Bascom Palmer Eye Institute, 900 NW 17th St., Miami, FL 33136, USA

Section I
Ocular Trauma

Jonathan H. Tzu

Chapter 1
Classification of Open Globe Injuries

Andrew J. McClellan

1.1 Definitions

- Eye wall-sclera and cornea
- Open globe injury-full-thickness wound of the eye wall
- Penetration-when a projectile enters a target without passing through it
- Perforation-when the projectile completely passes through the target
- OTS: ocular trauma score

1.2 Symptoms

- Decreased vision
- Pain
- Bleeding
- Red eye
- Periorbital bruising
- Periorbital swelling

1.3 Signs

- Corectopia
- Seidel-positive laceration

A.J. McClellan, MD
Department of Ophthalmology, Bascom Palmer Eye Institute, University of Miami,
900 NW 17th St., Miami, FL 33136, USA
e-mail: andrew.mcclellan@med.miami.edu

C.A. Medina et al. (eds.), *Manual of Retinal Diseases: A Guide to Diagnosis and Management*, DOI 10.1007/978-3-319-20460-4_1

- Uveal prolapse
- Vitreous prolapse
- Intraocular foreign body
- Lenticular capsular rupture
- Retinal detachment
- Vitreous hemorrhage
- Hyphema

1.4 Epidemiology

- ~200,000/year worldwide
- ~10,000/year USA
- Male predominance
- 3rd–5th decade of life

1.5 Differential Diagnosis

- Subconjunctival hemorrhage
- Partial-thickness laceration
- Commotio retinae
- Traumatic iritis
- Lens dislocation
- Hyphema
- Traumatic posterior vitreous detachment

1.6 Ocular Trauma Classification System (OTCS)

A. Type (Mechanism)

   1. Rupture-open globe injury caused by blunt-force trauma
   2. Penetration-entrance wound with no exit wound
   3. Intraocular foreign body
   4. Perforation-entrance wound and exit wound
   5. Mixed

B. Grade (Visual Acuity)

   1. ≥20/40
   2. 20/50 – 20/100

3. 19/100 – 5/200
4. 4/200 – light perception
5. No light perception

C. Pupil: presence or absence of an afferent pupillary defect
D. Zone (most posterior aspect of wound)

1. Cornea (including limbus)
2. Within 5 mm of limbus (pars plana)
3. Posterior to 5 mm from limbus

1.7 Ocular Trauma Score (OTS)

Initial visual acuity	
No light perception	60
Light perception – hand motion	70
1/200 – 19/200	80
20/200 – 20/50	90
<20/40	100
Characteristics	
Rupture	−23
Endophthalmitis	−17
Perforation	−14
Retinal detachment	−11
Afferent pupillary defect	−10

1.8 Prognosis and Management

The presence of an afferent pupillary defect, the initial entering acuity, and the OTS have been shown to carry the highest prognostic value.

All open globe injuries warrant surgical exploration to confirm the magnitude of the wound as an important part of not only the treatment but also the diagnosis of the injury, as the full extent of many wounds may be hidden by chemosis or hematoma.

Primary closure is typically offered to nearly all patients in the acute setting, regardless of the visual prognosis, to restore the normal anatomy as much as possible. Lensectomy and pars plana vitrectomy are often deferred to allow for inflammation to subside and some healing of the primary wound.

Presence of an intraocular foreign body, however, may necessitate that these procedures be performed at the time of primary closure. Enucleation, whether primary or secondary, is usually only offered to patients with complete extrusion of intraocular contents on initial presentation.

1.9 Follow-Up

Postoperative patients should be seen 1 day, week, and month after closure for the least severe of injuries. More extensive injuries may require more frequent examination.

References and Suggested Reading

1. Fabian ID, Eliashiv S, Moisseiev J, Tryfonides C, Alhalel A. Prognostic factors and visual outcomes of ruptured and lacerated globe injuries. Eur J Ophthalmol. 2014;24(2):273–8.
2. Kuhn F, Maisiak R, Mann L, Mester V, Morris R, Witherspoon CD. The ocular trauma score (OTS). Ophthalmol Clin North Am. 2002;15(2):163–5, vi.
3. Kuhn F, Morris R, Witherspoon CD, Heimann K, Jeffers JB, Treister G. A standardized classification of ocular trauma. Ophthalmology. 1996;103(2):240–3.
4. McGwin Jr G, Xie A, Owsley C. Rate of eye injury in the United States. Arch Ophthalmol. 2005;123(7):970–6.
5. Negrel AD, Thylefors B. The global impact of eye injuries. Ophthalmic Epidemiol. 1998;5(3):143–69.
6. Pieramici DJ, Au Eong KG, Sternberg Jr P, Marsh MJ. The prognostic significance of a system for classifying mechanical injuries of the eye (globe) in open-globe injuries. J Trauma. 2003;54(4):750–4.
7. Pieramici DJ, Sternberg P, Aaberg TM, et al. A system for classifying mechanical injuries of the eye (globe). Am J Ophthalmol. 1997;123(6):820–31.

Chapter 2
Principles of Globe Repair

Jonathan H. Tzu

2.1 Preoperative Evaluation and Preparation

- History/mechanism of trauma
- Gentle pressure on globe to avoid further prolapse of intraocular contents
- May need exam under anesthesia/exploration if history and findings are suggestive of a penetrating injury
- Determine extent of injury, cornea, corneoscleral, scleral, and extraocular tissues
- Computed tomography (CT, thin cuts) to evaluate for intraocular foreign body
- Occult rupture: findings include SCH, low IOP, and vitreous strands directed toward one direction
- Ultrasound may be helpful in cases of occult rupture/IOFB
- NPO
- Systemic broad-spectrum antibiotics such as a fourth-generation fluoroquinolone
- Tetanus toxoid
- Antiemetics
- Pain medications

2.2 Prognosis

- Presenting visual acuity as most important factor to final outcome
- Use indirect opthalmoscope for light to determine visual acuity, especially if patient is no light perception

J.H. Tzu, MD
Department of Ophthalmology, Bascom Palmer Eye Institute, University of Miami,
900 NW 17th St., Miami, FL 33136, USA
e-mail: jtzu2@med.miami.edu

C.A. Medina et al. (eds.), *Manual of Retinal Diseases: A Guide to Diagnosis and Management*, DOI 10.1007/978-3-319-20460-4_2

- Presence of APD
- Primary enucleation rarely performed, only considered when eye is disorganized with significant extrusion of intraocular contents

2.3 Anesthesia

Local anesthesia (retro or peribulbar block with intravenous sedation) can be performed in smaller anterior open globes in adults. General anesthesia is preferred if extent of injury is significant or posterior and in children.

2.4 Principles of Repair

- Restore structural integrity of globe
- Watertight closure
- Reposit tissues or resect if needed
- Protect visual axis if possible
- Minimize iatrogenic damage

2.5 Location of Laceration

2.5.1 Cornea

- 10-0 nylon interrupted
- Deep stromal bites, equal length/depth each side
- Often need to replace sutures if they become loose as wound tightens
- Approximate original anatomy as much as possible
- Bury knots if possible
- Stellate lacerations, and use purse string suture, cyanoacrylate glue, or corneal patch graft if significant tissue loss
- Reposition uveal tissue if possible using cyclodialysis spatula or 27G cannula with viscoelastic, only excise if necrotic. Manipulation is easier after a few sutures are already placed. Assistant can reposition the iris, while surgeon places cornea sutures (Fig. 2.1)

2.5.2 Sclera

- Conjunctival peritomy for exposure
- 7-0 or 8-0 interrupted nonabsorbable sutures on spatulated needle

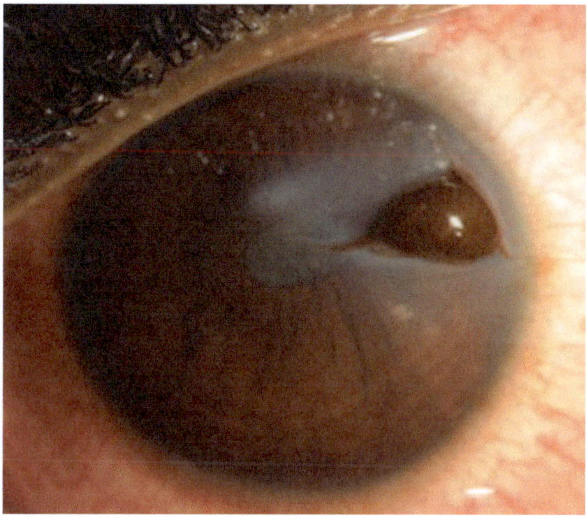

Fig. 2.1 Corneal laceration with iris prolapse

- If under muscle, a muscle hook can be used to expose the laceration, and if too much pressure, muscle can be taken down with a 6-0 Vicryl suture and resutured to insertion after laceration closed
- If significant loss of tissue, a scleral patch graft may be used
- Reposition any extruded uveal tissue. Excision can often cause significant bleeding
- Extruded vitreous should be cut with scissors or vitreous cutter
- Minimize excision of the retina or incarceration
- Often it is hard to identify retinal pathology because of media opacity during primary closure

2.5.3 Corneoscleral

- Limbal suture placed first as landmark
- Close limbal wounds with 9-0 nylon
- Then close corneal laceration after, followed by scleral portion

2.5.4 Other Considerations

- Generally defer AC washout, lensectomy, and/or vitrectomy as a secondary procedure
- There may be value in performing a scleral buckle in primary open globe repair

Small retrospective studies suggest benefit in lacerations extending >5 mm posterior to limbus in reducing vitreoretinal traction and subsequent detachment

- IOFB

  Should be removed at time of primary repair or within 24 h, risk of inflammatory complications, endophthalmitis if not quickly removed

- Use of prophylactic intravitreal antibiotics during repair

References/Suggested Reading

1. Miller DM, Eifrig CW, Banta JT. Open globe injuries: ruptures and lacerations. In: Banta JT, editor. Ocular trauma, 1st ed. London, New York, Oxford, St Louis, Sydney, Toronto: Elsevier; 2007, p. 163–79.
2. Mittra RA, Mieler WF. Controversies in the management of open globe injuries involving the posterior segment. Surv Ophthalmol. 1999;44(3):215–25.
3. Recchia FM, Sternberg P. Surgery for ocular trauma: principles and techniques of treatment. In: Ryan SJ, Wilkinson CP, Wiedemann P, editors. Retina, 5th ed. London, New York, Oxford, St Louis, Sydney, Toronto: Elsevier; 2013, p. 1852–75.
4. Scott IU, Mccabe CM, Flynn HW, Lemus DR, Schiffman JC, Reynolds DS, Pereira MB, Belfort A, Gayer S. Local anesthesia with intravenous sedation for surgical repair of selected open globe injuries. Am J Ophthalmol. 2002;134(5):707–11.

Chapter 3
Intraocular Foreign Body

Carlos A. Medina and Arun D. Singh

3.1 Definitions

- IOFB: Intraocular foreign body
- Penetration: There is no exit wound as the foreign body penetrates into the eye but not through and through
- Perforation: Perforating injuries have both entrance and exit wounds

3.2 Symptoms

- Similar to those of globe rupture
- Sometimes none except for a history of feeling something goes in the eye. More likely decreased vision, pain, epiphora or pseudo-epiphora (from aqueous), and foreign body sensation

3.3 Signs

- Similar to those of globe rupture
- Subconjunctival hemorrhage, hypotony, flat or shallow anterior chamber, hyphema, corectopia, lens disruption or cataract, vitreous hemorrhage, retinal tears, retinal hemorrhage, and entry wound

C.A. Medina, MD (✉)
Bascom Palmer Eye Institute, University of Miami,
900 NW 17th, St. Miami, FL 33136, USA
e-mail: camedina2020@gmail.com

A.D. Singh, MD
Department of Ophthalmic Oncology, Cole Eye Institute,
Cleveland Clinic, Cleveland, Ohio, USA

C.A. Medina et al. (eds.), *Manual of Retinal Diseases: A Guide to Diagnosis and Management*, DOI 10.1007/978-3-319-20460-4_3

3.4 Differential Diagnosis

- Penetrating/perforating globe injury with no IOFB
- Blunt trauma/ruptured globe

3.5 Etiology

Obtaining a full history is important for treatment and possible medicolegal implications. A detailed description of the injury may help ascertain the material and size of the IOFB (copper, iron, vegetable matter, etc.). Multiple foreign bodies may be present in certain events such as explosions and firearm injuries. Small high-velocity fragments of steel such as those encountered after hammering metal on metal or with high-speed machinery may be easily overlooked. The use of safety glasses should be documented.

3.6 Workup/Testing

A thorough examination of both eyes and adnexa is recommended. Slit-lamp examination may help identify an entry site. Corneal wounds are commonly Seidel negative and self-sealing. Transillumination of the iris may reveal iris stromal defect as the only sign of perforating injury. Presence of focal cataract should also raise suspicion of a perforating injury. A dilated fundus examination of both eyes should also be performed. Gonioscopy may be necessary in cases where angle involvement is suspected.

X-rays are usually sufficient to determine the presence of most radiopaque foreign bodies. A CT scan (without contrast) is better at determining the location as well as detecting less radiopaque foreign body such as glass (Fig. 3.1). Ultrasonography is helpful in detecting nonradiopaque IOFBs as well as their

Fig. 3.1 An 18-year-old male with glass fragment that entered the eye after the windshield shattered during a car accident. Visual acuity was CF at 1 foot. A 6 mm corneoscleral laceration was noted (**a**). Traumatic cataract and vitreous hemorrhage precluded detailed views of the fundus. CT scan showed foreign body on axial (**b**), coronal (**c**), and sagittal (**d**) cuts localizing the foreign body to the vitreous cavity. The patient underwent repair of the laceration, pars plana vitrectomy/lensectomy, with removal of 7 mm glass fragment from vitreous cavity through limbal wound grasped by Wilson forceps. Additionally, intravitreal antibiotics, endolaser, and silicon oil injection were also performed. Patient eventually recovered vision of 20/80 with attached retina (**e**) and normal macula (**f**, OCT) (Courtesy of Christopher R. Henry, MD (Miami, FL))

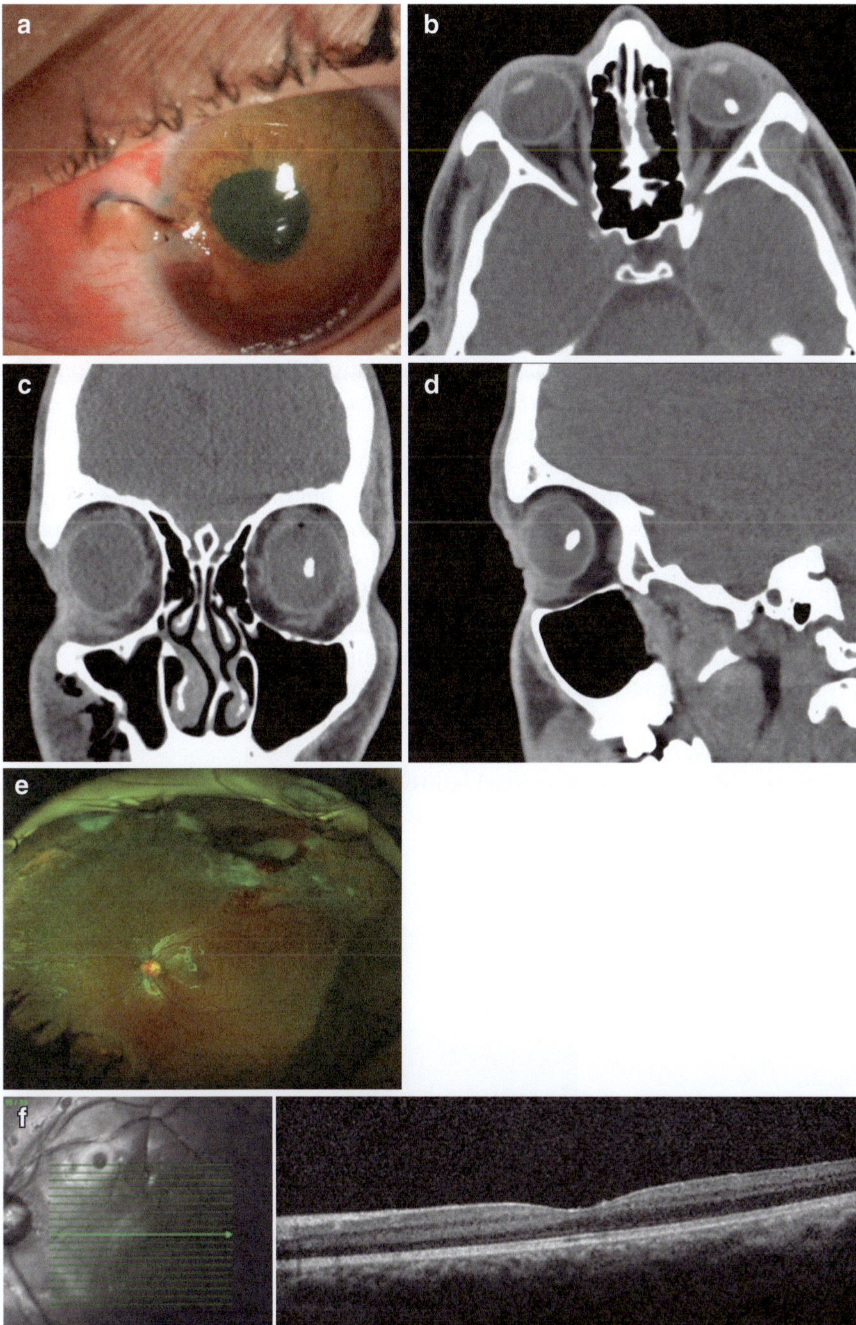
a
b
c
d
e
f

relationship to intraocular structures and the presence of an exit wound. Associated posterior segment alterations such as vitreous hemorrhage and retinal detachment are easily observed by ultrasonography (Fig. 3.2). Ultrasound biomicroscopy may be considered if the angle appears involved. MRI is contraindicated if a metallic foreign body is suspected.

3.7 Prognosis and Management

Prognosis largely depends upon the mechanism, location, and size of the injury as well as the material involved and the time to removal. Prior to surgical exploration, a fox shield, antiemetics, intravenous antibiotics, and update of tetanus coverage should be considered. Prompt surgical exploration, wound closure, removal of the IOFB (if possible), and antibiotic therapy should be initiated (Fig. 3.3).

Endophthalmitis occurs in 2–7 % of penetrating injuries. The incidence is higher in case with IOFB as well as those occurring in the rural setting, with dirty wounds, or where vegetable matter is involved. The risk of endophthalmitis may be reduced with prompt wound closure, removal of the IOFB, and use of prophylactic antibiotics (intravenous, subconjunctival, and intravitreal). *Bacillus cereus* (usually sensitive to intravitreal vancomycin or clindamycin) accounts for almost 25 % of posttraumatic endophthalmitis. It is notorious for its rapid and severe course that often leads to severe vision loss or loss of the eye. Intraoperative cultures should be taken if infection is suspected.

The reaction of the eye to retained IOFBs varies greatly depending on the material, sterility, and location. Materials such as stone, sand, glass, porcelain, and plastic are generally well tolerated. Other materials such as zinc, aluminum, copper, and

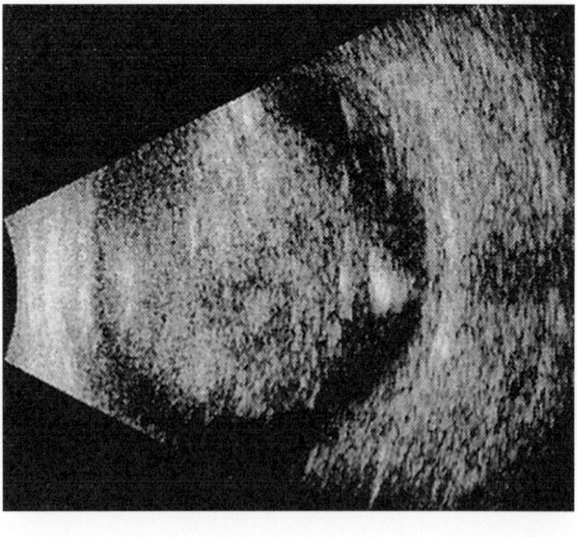

Fig. 3.2 A 60-year-old male with metallic foreign body sustained while moving an air conditioner. Visual acuity was NLP on presentation. B-scan ultrasonography detected a total retinal detachment and vitreous hemorrhage with metallic foreign body over the optic disk (Courtesy of Christopher R. Henry, MD (Miami, FL))

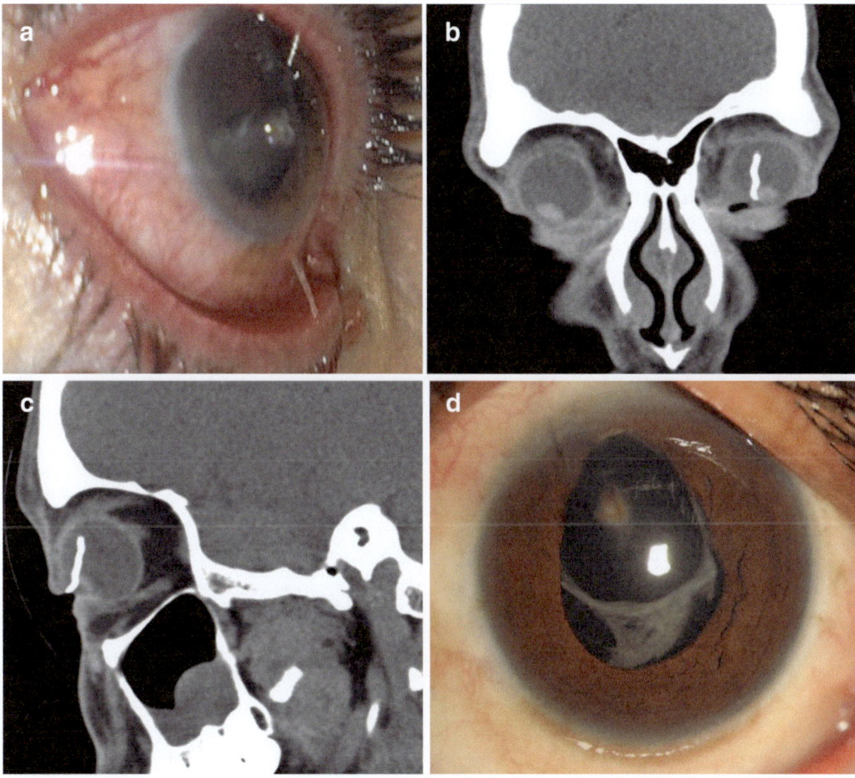

Fig. 3.3 A 32-year-old male with a nail injury that went through the cornea, iris, lens, and into vitreous cavity (**a**). CT scan showed foreign body on coronal (**b**) and sagittal (**c**) cuts localizing the nail (15 mm long) body to the vitreous cavity. Excellent outcome following removal of the foreign body through the anterior entry wound, wound closure, pars plana vitrectomy/lensectomy, and intravitreal antibiotics (**d**) (Courtesy of Christopher R. Henry, MD (Miami, FL))

iron appear to be more reactive and potentially toxic. Pure copper is especially toxic and prompt removal is usually recommended.

Iron or copper containing retained intraocular foreign body can cause delayed degenerative changes such as siderosis and chalcosis, respectively.

To reduce the risk of sympathetic ophthalmia, enucleation should be considered in a recently traumatized eye without hope for visual recovery (see Chap. 99).

3.8 Follow-Up

The patient should be followed closely (every 1–3 days) until the eye is deemed stable and the risk for infection reduces.

References and Suggested Reading

1. Essex RW, Yi Q, Charles PG, Allen PJ. Post-traumatic endophthalmitis. Ophthalmology. 2004;111(11):2015–22.
2. Jonas JB, Budde WM. Early versus late removal of retained intraocular foreign bodies. Retina. 1999;19(3):193–7.
3. Mieler WF, Mittra RA. The role and timing of pars plana vitrectomy in penetrating ocular trauma. Arch Ophthalmol. 1997;115(9):1191–2.
4. Reynolds DS, Flynn Jr HW. Endophthalmitis after penetrating ocular trauma. Curr Opin Ophthalmol. 1997;8(3):32–8.
5. Yeh S, Colyer MH, Weichel ED. Current trends in the management of intraocular foreign bodies. Curr Opin Ophthalmol. 2008;19(3):225–33.
6. Zhang Y, Zhang MN, Jiang CH, Yao Y, Zhang K. Endophthalmitis following open globe injury. Br J Ophthalmol. 2010;94(1):111–4.

Chapter 4
Commotio Retinae

Ashley M. Crane

4.1 Definitions

- Commotio retinae: Shearing of the photoreceptors giving the appearance of retinal opacification following blunt trauma. There is a notable absence of leakage (true edema) on fluorescein angiography.
- Berlin's edema: Often used interchangeably with commotion retinae, though more specifically refers to commotio retinae involving the macula.

4.2 Symptoms

Usually asymptomatic and can result in decreased vision if macula is involved.

4.3 Signs

Gray-white opacification of the retina following ocular blunt trauma (Fig. 4.1). When present at the posterior pole, it is referred to as Berlin's edema.

A.M. Crane, MD
Department of Ophthalmology, Bascom Palmer Eye Institute, University of Miami,
900 NW 17th, St. Miami, FL 33136, USA
e-mail: acrane@med.miami.edu

C.A. Medina et al. (eds.), *Manual of Retinal Diseases: A Guide to Diagnosis and Management*, DOI 10.1007/978-3-319-20460-4_4

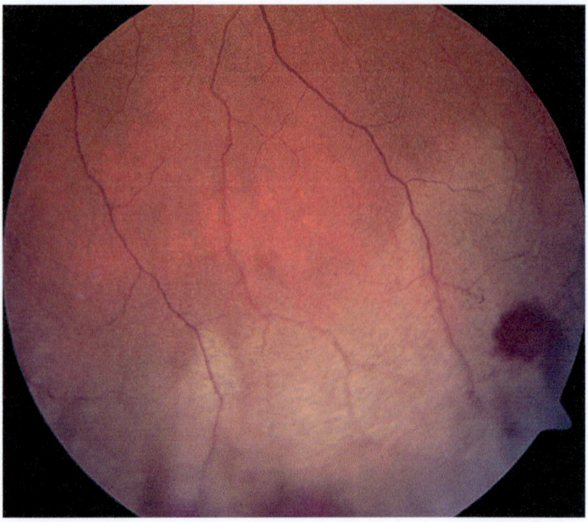

Fig. 4.1 Commotio retinae. Gray-white opacification of the retina following ocular blunt trauma

4.4 Epidemiology

Most commonly found in young men, following blunt trauma.

4.5 Predisposing Conditions

Blunt ocular trauma, often coexists with other sequelae of ocular trauma including orbital fractures, corneal injuries, hyphema/microhyphema, iritis, vitreous/retinal hemorrhages, and choroidal rupture.

4.6 Differential Diagnosis

Branch or central retinal artery occlusion, white without pressure, retinal detachment, myelinated nerve fiber layer, and Purtscher's retinopathy.

4.7 Etiology

Ocular blunt trauma results in photoreceptor and retinal pigment epithelium damage. The proposed etiologies include extracellular edema, disruption of photoreceptor outer segments, edema of Müller's cell processes, and retinal ganglion cell axons.

4.8 Workup/Testing

Clinical diagnosis with dilated fundus exam, including scleral depression except when contraindicated by coexisting injuries. Evaluate for other sequelae of blunt trauma. Optical coherence tomography may be used to evaluate retinal architecture when the macula is involved.

4.9 Prognosis and Management

Comprehensive clinical examination is essential as patients with commotio retinae often present with other coexisting pathology. Prognosis is generally good as the condition is self-limited. In the setting of Berlin's edema, it may be associated with traumatic maculopathy, and visual outcome can be limited by photoreceptor damage. Disruption of inner segment–outer segment junction and hyperreflectivity of overlying retina on optical coherence tomography are associated with worse visual outcomes. At this time, there is no effective treatment for traumatic maculopathy. Following blunt trauma, patients should be followed for development of peripheral retinal abnormalities such as retinal dialysis or breaks.

4.10 Follow-Up

Repeat dilated fundus exam approximately 2 weeks after injury. Best visual acuity may not be achieved for several months after initial injury.

References and Suggested Reading

1. Ahn SJ, et al. Optical coherence tomography morphologic grading of macular commotio retinae and its association with anatomic and visual outcomes. Am J Ophthalmol. 2013;156(5):994–1001.e1.
2. Blanch RJ, et al. Visual outcomes after blunt ocular trauma. Ophthalmology. 2013;120(8):1588–91.
3. Commotio retinae. In: Louis B. Cantor, Chrisopher J. Rapuano, George A. Cioffi (editors) Basic and clinical science course: retina and vitreous. San Francisco, CA: American Academy of Ophthalmology; 2014.
4. Mansour AM, Green WR, Hogge C. Histopathology of commotio retinae. Retina. 1992;12(1):24–8.
5. Souza-Santos F, et al. Spectral-domain optical coherence tomography in patients with commotio retinae. Retina. 2012;32(4):711–8.

Chapter 5
Traumatic Choroidal Rupture

Andrew J. McClellan

5.1 Definitions

- Choroidal rupture: A break involving the retinal pigmented epithelium (RPE), Bruch's membrane, and the choroid
- Sclopetaria: A break involving the retina and choroid but not sclera
- Open globe injury: Full-thickness wound of the eye wall
- Closed globe injury: Partial thickness wound of the eye wall
- CNV: Choroidal neovascular membrane

5.2 Symptoms

- History of eye trauma
- Decreased vision
- Metamorphopsia

5.3 Signs

Discontinuity of the red-orange color of the choroid, exposing the gray-white of the underlying sclera, with no overlying retinal break or tear.

A.J. McClellan, MD
Department of Ophthalmology, Bascom Palmer Eye Institute, University of Miami, 900 NW 17th St., Miami, FL 33136, USA
e-mail: andrew.mcclellan@med.miami.edu

C.A. Medina et al. (eds.), *Manual of Retinal Diseases: A Guide to Diagnosis and Management*, DOI 10.1007/978-3-319-20460-4_5

- Acute: commotio retinae, subretinal hemorrhage, rarely vitreous hemorrhage, or traumatic retinal breaks not overlying the area of rupture
  - *Direct* – located at the site of impact, which is often anterior. Rupture is aligned parallel to the ora serrata.
  - *Indirect* – located opposite the site of impact. Rupture is often curvilinear and concentric to the optic nerve to some degree.
- Chronic: choroidal neovascularization (CNV)

5.4 Epidemiology: Eye Injuries

- Age: 29 ± 26 years
- Gender: 4.6 male, 1 female
- Most often occur at home

5.5 Predisposing Conditions

- Blunt trauma to the eye.
- High-velocity projectile that passes in close proximity to the eye.

5.6 Differential Diagnosis

- Sclopetaria
- Globe rupture

5.7 Etiology

When the globe is distended from blunt trauma, the layers of the retinal pigment epithelium, Bruch's membrane, and choroid rupture as they are poorly distensible and weaker than adjacent layers of the eye. The overlying retina is protected by its elasticity and the underlying sclera is resistant to breakage due to high tensile strength. Ruptures are typically oriented latitudinally due to the expansion of the globe in this direction from blunt, traumatic compression in the anteroposterior plane (Fig. 5.1).

5.8 Workup/Testing

Choroidal rupture typically results from a large amount of blunt energy being imparted to the eye. A thorough ocular examination is imperative to rule out concurrent globe rupture. If suspicion is high, a CT scan of the orbits should be

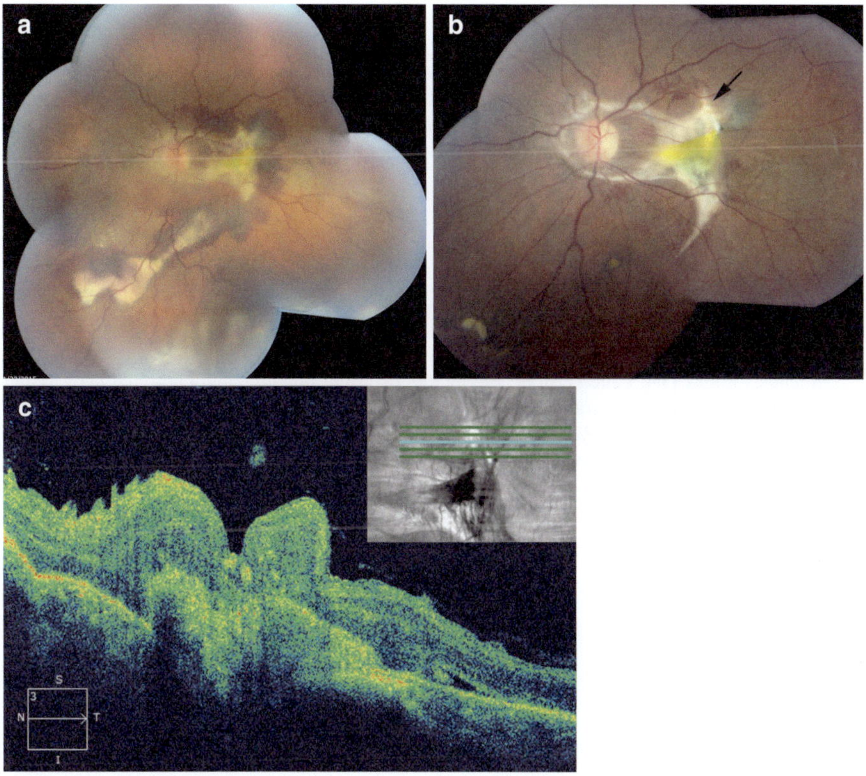

Fig. 5.1 Choroidal rupture. Following blunt trauma, there is widespread subretinal hemorrhage in the posterior pole (**a**). Several weeks later, hemorrhage is replaced by subretinal fibrosis with discontinuity of the red-orange color of the choroid, exposing the gray-white of the underlying sclera parallel to the disc margin (**b**, *arrow*). OCT confirms disruption of the RPE (**c**)

obtained. Likewise, blunt eye injuries can also cause orbital wall fractures. In the acute setting, cycloplegics and topical steroids should be considered for traumatic iritis.

5.9 Prognosis and Management

The prognosis of choroidal ruptures can be highly variable depending on the location. Posterior location of the rupture, multiple ruptures, and poor visual acuity at presentation have been shown to be associated with poor visual outcome. Older age and ruptures located within the posterior pole are more likely to develop CNV.

No treatment exists for choroidal rupture. However, sequelae, namely, CNV, should be treated accordingly with anti-VEGF agents, ablation, or photodynamic therapy.

5.10 Follow-Up

If concurrent iritis, commotio, or traumatic retinal breaks exist, patients may need more frequent follow-up to ensure resolution or stability of these issues. However, for isolated ruptures, patients should be followed on a monthly basis for some time to monitor for the development of CNV.

References and Suggested Reading

1. Ament C, Zacks DN, Lane A, et al. PRedictors of visual outcome and choroidal neovascular membrane formation after traumatic choroidal rupture. Arch Ophthalmol. 2006;124(7):957–66.
2. May DR, Kuhn FP, Morris RE, Witherspoon CD, Danis RP, Matthews GP, et al. The epidemiology of serious eye injuries from the United States Eye Injury Registry. Graefes Arch Clin Exp Ophthalmol. 2000;238(2):153–7.
3. Patel MM, Chee YE, Eliott D. Choroidal rupture: a review. Int Ophthalmol Clin. 2013; 53(4):69–78.

Chapter 6
Chorioretinitis Sclopetaria

Audrey C. Ko

6.1 Definitions

Chorioretinitis sclopetaria: A break involving the retina and choroid, but not sclera, usually following a high-velocity missile injury to the orbit.

6.2 Symptoms

Decreased or distorted vision after facial trauma involving a high-velocity projectile.

6.3 Signs

- Acute signs (Fig. 6.1)
  - Subretinal and intraretinal hemorrhage with overlying retinal breaks, typically involving the macula
  - Intact sclera
  - Vitreous hemorrhage
- Chronic signs (Fig. 6.2)
  - White fibrous scar with serrated edges
  - Retinal pigment epithelium changes
  - Fibrovascular proliferation and neovascularization

A.C. Ko, MD
Bascom Palmer Eye Institute, 900 NW 17th Street, Miami, FL 33136, USA
e-mail: ko.audrey@gmail.com

C.A. Medina et al. (eds.), *Manual of Retinal Diseases: A Guide to Diagnosis and Management*, DOI 10.1007/978-3-319-20460-4_6

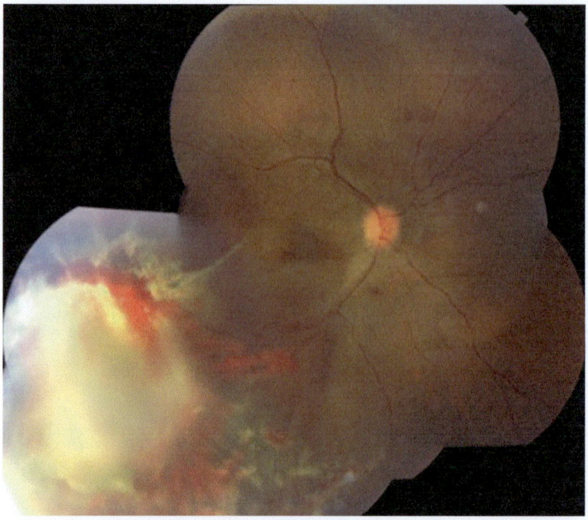

Fig. 6.1 Acute appearance of chorioretinitis sclopetaria, showing vitreous hemorrhage, retinal breaks with white fibrous scarring, and scattered subretinal and intraretinal hemorrhage (Photo credit: Eric Hansen, MD)

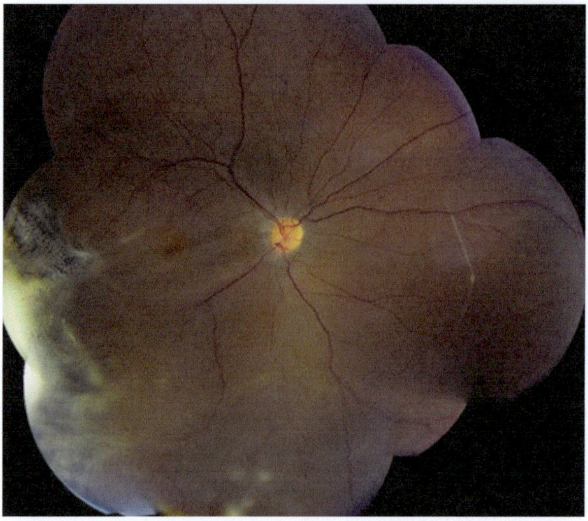

Fig. 6.2 Chronic appearance of chorioretinitis sclopetaria, showing white fibrous scar with serrated edges and retinal pigment epithelium changes (Photo credit: Eric Hansen, MD)

6.4 Epidemiology

Higher prevalence in young males.

6.5 Predisposing Conditions

Trauma involving a high-velocity projectile.

6.6 Differential Diagnosis

- Choroidal rupture
- Ruptured globe
- Commotio retinae

6.7 Etiology

A high-speed missile injury in which the shock waves generated by a projectile – passing adjacent to but without direct contact with the eye – cause a rupture of the choroid and retina while the sclera remains intact.

6.8 Workup/Testing

- Check for relative afferent pupillary defect to assess for corresponding optic nerve damage.
- If there is no posterior view, consider obtaining a B-scan ultrasound to evaluate the optic nerve and posterior pole and assess for the possibility of a ruptured globe.

6.9 Prognosis and Management

Patients are typically observed. Despite rupture of the retina and choroid, patients have low risk of retinal detachment due to marked scar formation. Patients with lesions involving the macula have a poor prognosis, as the vision typically does not improve.

6.10 Follow-Up

Follow-up examination is indicated to monitor for future development of neovascularization or retinal detachment. Consider obtaining optical coherence tomography (OCT) to assess for epiretinal membrane or intraretinal fluid suggestive of neovascularization. Consider obtaining fluorescein angiography (FA) if neovascularization is suspected.

References and Suggested Reading

1. Ahmadabadi MN, Karkhaneh R, Roohipoor R, Tabatabai A, Alimardani A. Clinical presentation and outcome of chorioretinitis sclopetaria: a case series study. Injury. 2010;41(1):82–5.
2. Dubovy SR, Guyton DL, Green WR. Clinicopathologic correlation of chorioretinitis sclopetaria. Retina. 1997;17(6):510–20.
3. Papakostas TD, Yonekawa Y, Skondra D, Vavvas DG. Traumatic chorioretinal rupture (sclopetaria). Int Ophthalmol Clin. 2013;53(4):119–25.
4. Rayess N, Rahimy E, Ho AC. Spectral-domain optical coherence tomography features of bilateral chorioretinitis sclopetaria. Ophthalmic Surg Lasers Imaging Retina. 2015;46(2):253–5.

Chapter 7
Valsalva Retinopathy

Ashley M. Crane

7.1 Definitions

Valsalva retinopathy: preretinal hemorrhage secondary to a sudden increase in intrathoracic pressure.

7.2 Symptoms

Asymptomatic or painless decreased vision.

7.3 Signs

Unilateral or bilateral sharply demarcated hemorrhage in the subhyaloid or sub-internal limiting membrane space (Fig. 7.1). The shape is usually approximately circular. The hemorrhage may contain an air-fluid level (boat shaped). It can result in vitreous hemorrhage if blood products escape the subhyaloid space.

A.M. Crane, MD
Department of Ophthalmology, Bascom Palmer Eye Institute, University of Miami,
900 NW 17th, St. Miami, FL 33136, USA
e-mail: acrane@med.miami.edu

C.A. Medina et al. (eds.), *Manual of Retinal Diseases: A Guide to Diagnosis and Management*, DOI 10.1007/978-3-319-20460-4_7

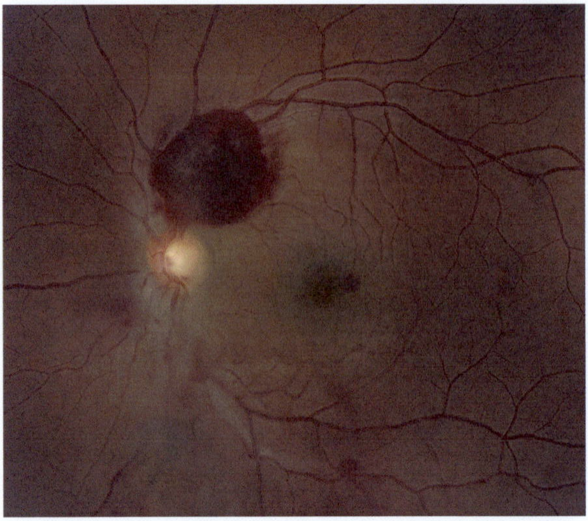

Fig. 7.1 Fundus photograph of Valsalva retinopathy with subhyaloid, intraretinal, and vitreous hemorrhage. (Courtesy of Nathan Blessing, MD)

7.4 Predisposing Conditions

History of Valsalva maneuver, especially during vigorous exercise, lifting/straining, coughing, vomiting, constipation, sexual intercourse, endoscopic gastrointestinal procedures, or labor/delivery. Impaired platelet function may also increase the risk for Valsalva retinopathy.

7.5 Differential Diagnosis: Table 7.1

- Ruptured retinal artery macroaneurysm
- Central retinal vein occlusion (CRVO)
- Branch retinal vein occlusion (BRVO)
- Hemorrhagic posterior vitreous detachment (PVD)
- Retinal tear
- Diabetic retinopathy
- Hematologic malignancy
- Terson syndrome

7.6 Etiology

Preretinal (subhyaloid or sub-internal limiting membrane) hemorrhage after forced exhalation against a closed glottis, causing a rise in intrathoracic or intra-abdominal pressure (Valsalva maneuver). During a Valsalva maneuver, high intraocular venous pressure is transmitted to perifoveal capillaries resulting in hemorrhage.

Table 7.1 Differential diagnosis of hemorrhage in multiple posterior layers

Valsalva retinopathy
Trauma
Retinal artery macroaneurysm
Terson syndrome
Wet Sickle Cell retinopathy

7.7 Workup/Testing

Careful history to evaluate for Valsalva maneuver. Clinical examination is usually sufficient for diagnosis. If diagnosis is in question, fundus fluorescein angiography can be performed to evaluate sources of leakage. Optical coherence tomography (OCT) can also be used to ascertain the level of hemorrhage.

7.8 Prognosis and Management

Prognosis is excellent for full recovery within weeks with observation alone. Nd:YAG laser membranotomy can be considered in some cases, especially in monocular patients or in those whose occupation requires prompt visual recovery. Vitrectomy is seldom required for persistent vitreous hemorrhage. Rarely, permanent visual loss can be caused by pigmentary maculopathies. Patients should be counseled about risk factors, as this condition can be recurrent.

7.9 Follow-Up

Observation every few weeks until clearance. If clearance does not occur after months, further intervention can be considered.

References and Suggested Reading

1. De Maeyer K, et al. Sub-inner limiting membrane haemorrhage: causes and treatment with vitrectomy. Br J Ophthalmol. 2007;91(7):869–72.
2. Duane TD. Valsalva hemorrhagic retinopathy. Trans Am Ophthalmol Soc. 1972;70:298–313.
3. Garcia Fernandez M, Navarro JC, Castano CG. Long-term evolution of Valsalva retinopathy: a case series. J Med Case Rep. 2012;6:346.
4. Pruett RC, Carvalho AC, Trempe CL. Microhemorrhagic maculopathy. Arch Ophthalmol. 1981;99(3):425–32.
5. Tassignon MJ, Stempels N, Van Mulders L. Retrohyaloid premacular hemorrhage treated by Q-switched Nd-YAG laser. A case report. Graefes Arch Clin Exp Ophthalmol. 1989;227(5):440–2.
6. Valsalva retinopathy. In: Louis B. Cantor, Christopher J. Rapuano, George A. Cioffi (editors). Basic and clinical science course: retina and vitreous. San Francisco, CA: American Academy of Ophthalmology; 2014.

Chapter 8
Solar Retinopathy

Sarah P. Read

8.1 Definitions

Solar retinopathy, Welder's maculopathy, foveomacular retinitis, eclipse retinopathy, and solar retinitis.

8.2 Symptoms

Headache, blurred vision, central scotoma, afterimage, and metamorphopsia. Vision can be decreased to 20/200. Symptoms can occur within hours of exposure.

8.3 Signs

Clinical signs can be subtle and often exam can appear normal immediately following injury. Acute findings can include yellow-white spot in the fovea with surrounding edema (Fig. 8.1). Within 24–48 hours, pigmentary changes around or near the fovea can appear.

S.P. Read, MD, PhD
Bascom Palmer Eye Institute, University of Miami,
900 NW 17th, St. Miami, FL 33136, USA
e-mail: read@med.miami.edu

C.A. Medina et al. (eds.), *Manual of Retinal Diseases: A Guide to Diagnosis and Management*, DOI 10.1007/978-3-319-20460-4_8

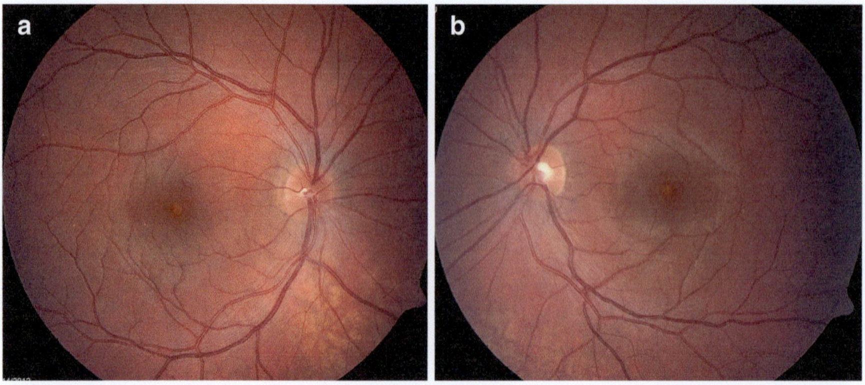

Fig. 8.1 Solar maculopathy: 19-year-old avid golfer. Bilateral solar maculopathy (visual acuity 20/25 OU) (**a** right eye, **b** left eye) (Courtesy of Anita Agarwal, MD, Nashville, TN)

8.4 Epidemiology

Younger patients with clearer lenses and patients taking drugs that photosensitize the eye, such as tetracyclines, are at a higher risk of solar retinopathy. Men have an increased incidence compared to women.

8.5 Predisposing Conditions

Ophthalmic instruments (endoillumination during vitrectomy or operating microscope light especially during cataract surgery), sun gazing (solar retinopathy), arc welding, industrial lasers. Solar retinopathy has been recorded in military personnel, sun gazers, sunbathers, and those under the influence of psychotropic substances.

8.6 Differential Diagnosis

Age-related macular degeneration, early macular or lamellar hole, macular dystrophy, and cystoid macular edema.

8.7 Etiology

Light-induced photochemical retinal damage and pathological specimen have shown localized necrosis of the retinal pigment epithelium and disruption of overlying photoreceptors.

8.8 Workup/Testing

OCT can show areas of hyper-reflectivity, disruption of the IS/OS junction, or foveal thinning with photoreceptor loss. After approximately 2 weeks, the damage may progress to lamellar hole or depression. Fluorescein angiography (FA) can show leakage in the early stages with later changes showing a window defect and staining but can also be normal.

8.9 Prognosis and Management

Observation. Vision may improve but depends on the extent of damage. Most patients with solar retinopathy have return of vision to 20/40 or better after 4–6 months. It can have permanent central/paracentral scotoma. Poor outcome is correlated with the degree of damage observed on optical coherence tomography (OCT). Prevention is important including public awareness surrounding sun gazing/eclipse watching, proper sunglasses/occupational protection, and using lower or oblique and decreasing exposure time of operating microscope illumination.

8.10 Follow-Up

Choroidal neovascular membrane is a rare potential complication and patients should be monitored, though no specific guidelines have been proposed.

References and Suggested Reading

1. Gass JDM. Stereoscopic atlas of macular diseases: diagnosis and treatment, vol. 4. St. Louis: Mosby; 1997. p. 760–3.
2. Green WR, Robertson DM. Pathologic findings of photic retinopathy in the human eye. Am J Ophthalomol. 1991;112:520.
3. Hatfield EM. Eye injuries and the solar eclipse. Sight Saving Rev. 1970;40:79.
4. Yannuzzi LA, Fisher YL, Krueger A, et al. Solar retinopathy: a photobiological and geophysical analysis. Trans Am Ophthalmol Soc. 1987;85:120.
5. Youssef PN, Sheibani N, Albert DM. Retinal light toxicity. Eye (Lond). 2011;25(1):1–14.

Chapter 9
Purtscher's Retinopathy

Sarah P. Read

9.1 Definitions

Purtscher's retinopathy: hemorrhagic and vasoocclusive vasculopathy first described in 1912 as a syndrome of sudden blindness associated with severe head trauma. It is most often seen after trauma but commonly associated with other causes. Also known as angiopathia retinae traumatica.

9.2 Symptoms

Severe vision loss occurring immediately or within 1–2 days following injury. Vision loss is more often bilateral but can be unilateral.

9.3 Signs

Findings are usually restricted to the posterior pole and include cotton wool spots, peripapillary retinal whitening, retinal hemorrhage, macular edema, dilated retinal vessels, and disk edema/pallor. Purtscher flecken are pathognomonic lesions described as polygonal cotton wool spots approximately a third disk diameter in size (Fig. 9.1). Chronic changes include optic atrophy and pigmentary retinal changes.

S.P. Read, MD, PhD
Bascom Palmer Eye Institute, University of Miami,
900 NW 17th, St. Miami, FL 33136, USA
e-mail: read@med.miami.edu

C.A. Medina et al. (eds.), *Manual of Retinal Diseases: A Guide to Diagnosis and Management*, DOI 10.1007/978-3-319-20460-4_9

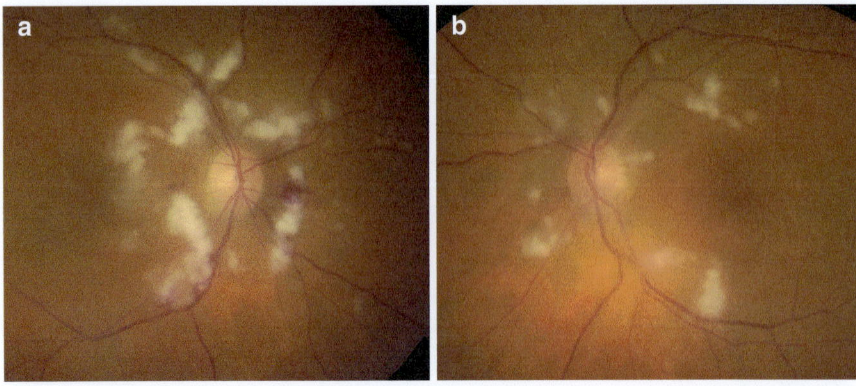

Fig. 9.1 Purtscher's retinopathy. Pathognomonic polygonal cotton wool spots approximately a third disk diameter in size restricted to posterior pole. Visual acuity: 20/25 OU) (**a** right eye, **b** left eye) (Courtesy of Anita Agarwal, MD, Nashville, TN)

9.4 Epidemiology

Rare disease seen most commonly in young men following trauma.

9.5 Predisposing Conditions

Retinal injury occurring following compression injury to the chest or head.

9.6 Differential Diagnosis

Hypertensive retinopathy, retinal vein occlusion, fat embolism from crush injuries or long-bone fractures, shaken baby syndrome, Terson's syndrome, pancreatitis (Purtscher-like retinopathy), connective tissue/vasculitis disease, commotio retinae, and HIV retinopathy.

9.7 Etiology

The exact pathophysiology of Purtscher's is not well understood. Injury may cause leukoembolization that leads intravascular platelet aggregation and consequently to vascular occlusion and retinal ischemia. Fat, air, or amniotic fluid can cause emboli that mimic the appearance of Purtscher's. Additionally, the concussive injury itself may cause damage to the retinal endothelium.

9.8 Workup/Testing

Fluorescein angiography (FA) can be useful to show the extent of retinal non-perfusion and ischemia (Fig. 9.2). In addition to non-perfusion, the FA can show leakage from injured vessels, perivascular staining, and retinal edema. Optical coherence tomography (OCT) may show inner retinal hyper-reflectivity consistent with nerve fiber layer infarction. Fundus autofluorescence (FAF) can show hypo-autofluorescence in areas of retinal ischemia with hyper-autofluorescence along the blood vessels correlating with stagnant blood. Given the history of trauma in these patients, it is important to refer for neurosurgical and/or general surgery evaluation. Additionally, it is important to rule out other systemic diseases that may mimic Purtscher's.

9.9 Prognosis and Management

Observation. Moderate spontaneous vision improvement is common. However, permanent vision loss can occur in proportion with duration of acute retinal injury with approximately half of patients reporting long-term central vision loss.

9.10 Follow-Up

Retinal atrophy can occur as a long-term complication that can be followed with retinal thinning on OCT.

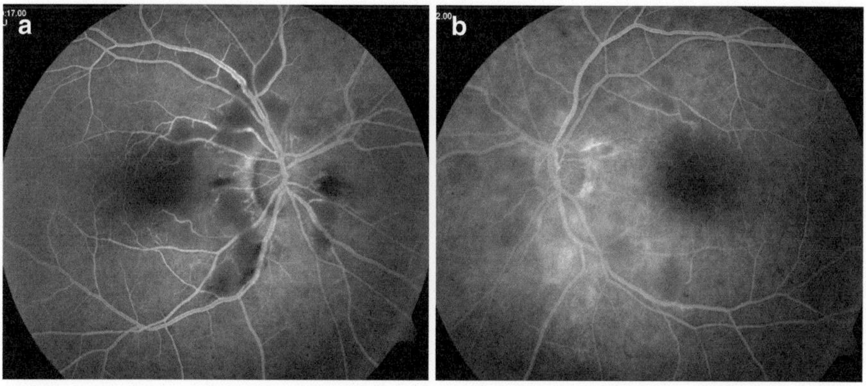

Fig. 9.2 Fluorescein angiogram showing retinal non-perfusion in early phase (**a** right eye) and late leakage from injured vessels and perivascular staining (**b** left eye) (Courtesy of Anita Agarwal, MD, Nashville, TN)

References and Suggested Reading

1. Agrawal A, McKibbin M. Purtscher's retinopathy: epidemiology, clinical features and outcome. Br J Ophthalmol. 2007;91(11):1456–9.
2. Behrens-Baumann W, Scheurer G, Schroer H. Pathogenesis of Purtscher's retinopathy. Graefes Arch Clin Exp Ophthalmol. 1992;230(3):286–91.
3. Miguel a IM, Henriques F, Azevedo LFR, Loureiro a JR, Maberley D a L. Systematic review of Purtscher's and Purtscher-like retinopathies. Eye (Lond). 2013;27(1):1–13.

Chapter 10
Traumatic Lens Dislocation

Andrew J. McClellan

10.1 Definitions

- Subluxation – incomplete or partial dislocation
- Luxation – complete dislocation

10.2 Symptoms

- Decreased visual acuity
- Photopsias

10.3 Signs

- Phacodonesis
- Iritis
- Vitreous prolapse

A.J. McClellan, MD
Bascom Palmer Eye Institute, University of Miami,
900 NW 17th, St. Miami, FL 33136, USA
e-mail: andrew.mcclellan@med.miami.edu

C.A. Medina et al. (eds.), *Manual of Retinal Diseases: A Guide to Diagnosis and Management*, DOI 10.1007/978-3-319-20460-4_10

10.4 Epidemiology: Eye Injuries

- Age: 29 ± 26 years
- Gender: 4.6 male, 1 female
- Most occur at home

10.5 Predisposing Conditions

- Trauma
- Homocystinuria
- Sulfite oxidase deficiency
- Marfan syndrome
- Weill-Marchesani syndrome
- Hyperlysinemia
- Ehlers-Danlos syndrome
- Crouzon disease
- Refsum syndrome
- Kniest syndrome
- Mandibulofacial dysostosis
- Sturge-Weber syndrome
- Conradi syndrome
- Pfaundler syndrome
- Pierre Robin syndrome
- Wildervanck syndrome
- Sprengel deformity

10.6 Inheritance

Autosomal or X-linked per associated syndrome.

10.7 Differential Diagnosis

See predisposing conditions.

10.8 Etiology

If partial or incomplete, zonular breakage will lead to lens subluxation. If complete, lens luxation will occur.

10.9 Workup/Testing

If lens dislocation is spontaneous or the inciting trauma is minimal, consider serum homocysteine level and evaluation for a genetic syndrome.

10.10 Prognosis and Management

Cycloplegia ± topical steroids are often needed for analgesia and to control inflammation. Phacomorphic glaucoma, corneal endothelial decompensation, capsular violation, or the need for posterior segment surgery may require early intervention. Otherwise, surgery should be deferred until intraocular inflammation is under control.

10.11 Follow-Up

Patients will likely require frequent follow-up initially, potentially daily, to assess control of inflammation and other sequelae from trauma. Once inflammation is controlled, patients can be followed less closely until the timing of pars plana lensectomy and vitrectomy is optimal.

References and Suggested Reading

1. Hoffman RS, Snyder ME, Devgan U, Allen QB, Yeoh R, Braga-Mele R. Management of the subluxated crystalline lens. J Cataract Refract Surg. 2013;39(12):1904–15.
2. May DR, Kuhn FP, Morris RE, Witherspoon CD, Danis RP, Matthews GP, et al. The epidemiology of serious eye injuries from the United States Eye Injury Registry. Graefes Arch Clin Exp Ophthalmol. 2000;238(2):153–7.

Section II
Pediatric Retinal Diseases

Ryan C. Young

Chapter 11
Approach to Leukocoria

Hershel Rajendrakumar Patel and Swetangi Bhaleeya

11.1 Definitions

Leukocoria (Greek "leucos" meaning white and "kore" meaning pupil), or white pupillary reflex, which can occur due to various ocular conditions.

11.2 Symptoms

- White pupillary reflex
- Strabismus
- Decreased vision

11.3 Signs

Leukocoria may not be evident in all aspects of gaze; thus, certain positions or conditions (e.g., dark environment/dilated pupil) allow for better visualization. The further peripheral a lesion is within the retina, the more important positioning and lighting become.

H.R. Patel, MS, MD (✉) S. Bhaleeya, MD
Department of Ophthalmology, USF Eye institute, University of South Florida, 13127 USF Magnolia Drive, Tampa, FL 33612, USA
e-mail: hershelrpatel@gmail.com; bhaleeya05@gmail.com

C.A. Medina et al. (eds.), *Manual of Retinal Diseases: A Guide to Diagnosis and Management*, DOI 10.1007/978-3-319-20460-4_11

11.4 Epidemiology

Greater than 50 % of leukocoria is secondary to retinoblastoma. Retinoblastoma represents 80 % of primary ocular tumors in children <15 years old and 17 % of neonatal cancers. The mean frequency of retinoblastoma is 1/20,000 live births with no strongly established increased risk related to sex/race/geographic location. A review of 2775 patients referred for management of retinoblastoma found 22 % were with simulating lesions. Persistent fetal vasculature (PFV), Coats's disease, and vitreous hemorrhage were most common in children <2 years old, while those >5 years most commonly had Coats's, toxocariasis, and familial exudative vitreoretinopathy (FEVR).

11.5 Inheritance

In the case of hereditary retinoblastoma, there is an autosomal dominant pattern of inheritance with a 90 % penetrance. These Individuals will be more likely to have an earlier and bilateral presentation. Coats's disease (primary retinal telangiectasia) is unilateral in 90 % of cases with the most common presenting patient being a young male between 5 and 10 years old. This congenital disease without a proven hereditary pattern presents with a triad of characteristics includes retinal telangiectasia, yellow exudate, and retinal detachment. PFV is also nonhereditary with a varied set of clinical manifestation including microphthalmia, failure of cleavage of the anterior segment, or uveal coloboma.

11.6 Differential Diagnosis

- Retinoblastoma
- Congenital cataract
- Persistent hyperplastic primary vitreous (PHPV)/persistent fetal vasculature (PFV)
- Coats's disease
- Retinal astrocytic hamartoma
- Coloboma of choroid or optic disk
- Toxocariasis
- Retinopathy of prematurity
- Organized vitreous hemorrhage
- Familial exudative vitreoretinopathy (FEVR)
- Incontinentia pigmenti
- Toxoplasmosis
- Norrie disease

11.7 Etiology

The etiologies of leukocoria are expansive and are listed above. Depending on the underlying cause of leukocoria, the treatment will differ. Most cases of retinoblastoma are believed to be associated with loss of the RB1 gene, an important regulator of the cell cycle. Knudson's two-hit hypothesis explains why the inherited form of retinoblastoma occurs at a younger age than the sporadic form, stating that those with the inherited form have the first of two hits required to cause cancer at birth. Other implicated genetic associations involve MYCN and a 13q deletion syndrome.

11.8 Workup/Testing

Immediate evaluation by an ophthalmologist with a comprehensive examination of the fundus is necessary in all cases of leukocoria. Examination of the dilated pupil under anesthesia should be considered. In the case where fundus examination does not allow definitive diagnosis, ultrasound or OCT can be used to evaluate the lesion. CT scan may be considered especially for determining if the lesion is calcified, though it should be noted that leukocoria is typically found in the pediatric population and x-ray exposure with serial examinations may be harmful. MRI can be used to detect associated intracranial tumors such as those associated with trilateral retinoblastoma and to distinguish between >2 mm solid tumors and Coats's disease or PFV, which has a characteristic of surrounding subretinal fluid. Coats's and PFV are the most common mimickers of retinoblastoma. In the case of ocular toxocariasis, serology, ultrasound, and neurodiagnostic imaging may be necessary. A full family history may provide insight with special attention paid to history of enucleation in first-degree relatives.

11.9 Prognosis and Management

Varies depending on the underlying etiology. Prompt referral and work-up are important especially in the case of retinoblastoma where delayed diagnosis can be more severely threatening to not only a child's vision but life.

11.10 Follow-Up

Close follow-up to monitor for amblyopia and progression of underlying pathology is recommended. Follow-up can be extended to every 6 months or 1 year after stability has been established over a minimum 12-month period.

References and Suggested Reading

1. Abdolvahabi A, Taylor BW, Holden RL, et al. Colorimetric and longitudinal analysis of leukocoria in recreational photographs of children with retinoblastoma. Bhattacharya S, ed. PLoS One. 2013;8(10):e76677.
2. Balmer A, Munier F. Differential diagnosis of leukocoria and strabismus, first presenting signs of retinoblastoma. Clin Ophthalmol (Auckland, NZ). 2007;1(4):431–9.
3. Balmer A, Munier F. Differential diagnosis of leukocoria and strabismus, first presenting signs of retinoblastoma. Clin Ophthalmol. 2007;1(4):431–9.
4. Canzano JC, Handa JT. Utility of pupillary dilation for detecting leukocoria in patients with retinoblastoma. Pediatrics. 1999;10(4):e44.
5. Ortiz MV, Dunkel IJ. Retinoblastoma. J Child Neurol. 2015;(2):253–64.
6. Rivas-Perea P, Baker E, Hamerly G, Shaw BF. Detection of leukocoria using a soft fusion of expert classifiers under non-clinical settings. BMC Ophthalmol. 2014;14:110.
7. Shields CL, Fulco EM, Arias JD, Alarcon C, Pellegrini M, Rishi P, Kaliki S, Bianciotto CG, Shields JA. Retinoblastoma frontiers with intravenous, intra-arterial, periocular, and intravitreal chemotherapy. Eye (Lond). 2013;27(2):253–64.
8. Tartarella MB, Britez-Colombi GF, Fortes Filho JB. Proposal of a novel classification of leukocorias. Clin Ophthalmol (Auckland, NZ). 2012;6:991–5.

Chapter 12
Retinopathy of Prematurity

Ryan C. Young and Brenda J. Fallas

12.1 Definitions

ROP: Retinopathy of prematurity is a disorder of the development of the retina in low birthweight premature infants.

12.2 Symptoms

Decreased vision, strabismus, nystagmus, and leukocoria.

12.3 Signs

The International Committee on Classification of Acute ROP defines the extent of ROP based on stage, location, and the presence of plus disease.

R.C. Young, MD (✉) • B.J. Fallas, CSA
Bascom Palmer Eye Institute, University of Miami,
900 NW 17th, St. Miami, FL 33136, USA
e-mail: youngrc@med.miami.edu

C.A. Medina et al. (eds.), *Manual of Retinal Diseases: A Guide to Diagnosis and Management*, DOI 10.1007/978-3-319-20460-4_12

12.3.1 Location (Fig. 12.1)

Zone I: posterior retina within a 60° circle centered on the optic nerve
Zone II: from the posterior circle (zone I) to the nasal ora serrate anteriorly
Zone III: remaining temporal peripheral retina

12.3.2 Stage (Fig. 12.2)

Stage 1: demarcation line between vascularized and nonvascularized retina
Stage 2: elevated avascular ridge with height, width, and volume
Stage 3: elevated ridge with fibrovascular proliferation
Stage 4: subtotal retinal detachment

4a: spares the fovea
4b: involves the fovea

Stage 5: total retinal detachment

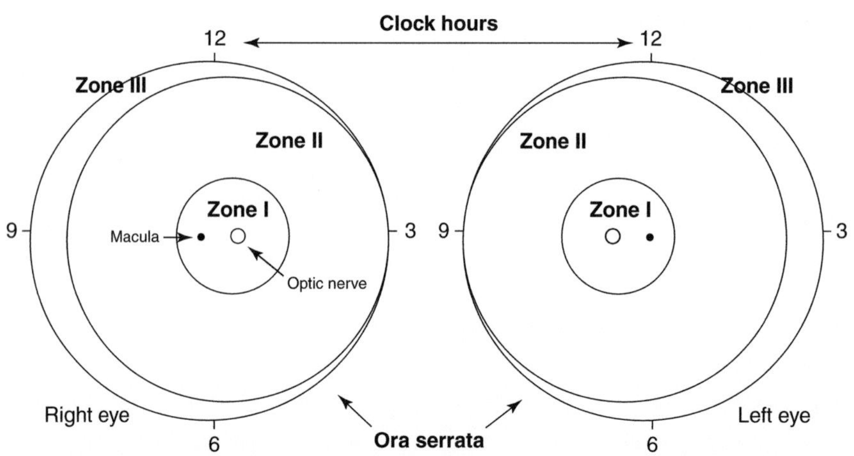

Fig. 12.1 Scheme of retina of the right and left eyes showing zone borders and clock hours used to describe the location and extent of ROP. Diagrammatic representation of the potential total area of the premature retina, with zone I (the most posterior) symmetrically surrounding the optic nerve head (the earliest to develop). A larger retinal area is present temporally (laterally) rather than nasally (medially) (zone III). Only zones I and II are present nasally. The retinal changes are usually recorded on a diagram such as this one (Reproduced with permission from: *American Academy of Pediatrics Section on Ophthalmology* 2013;131:189–195)

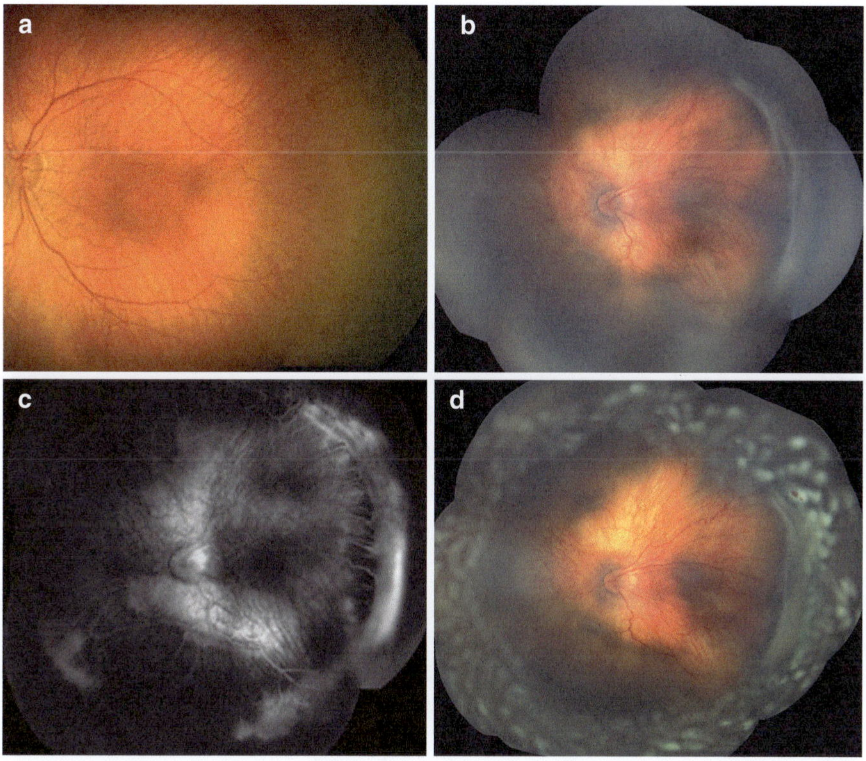

Fig. 12.2 Stages of ROP. Demarcation line between vascularized and nonvascularized retina (**a**, stage 1). Elevated avascular ridge with height, width, and volume (**b**, stage 2). Elevated ridge with fibrovascular proliferation (**c**, stage 3). Appearance after laser photocoagulation (**d**)

12.3.3 Plus Disease

Plus disease is characterized by the presence of retinal vascular dilation and tortuosity in the posterior pole.

12.4 Predisposing Conditions

The development and severity of ROP are most strongly correlated with low birthweight and low gestational age. Possible risk factors include supplemental oxygen, hypoxemia, hypercarbia, and concurrent systemic illness.

12.5 Differential Diagnosis

The differential diagnosis of ROP includes familial exudative vitreoretinopathy (FEVR), Coats's disease, persistent fetal vasculature/persistent hyperplastic primary vitreous (PHPV), retinoblastoma, Norrie's disease, and incontinentia pigmenti.

12.6 Etiology

ROP is a disorder of the development of the retina in low birthweight premature infants. Incomplete retinal vascularization and resulting ischemic retinopathy causes abnormal proliferation of developing blood vessels at the junction of vascular and avascular retina in these babies.

12.7 Workup and Testing

Evaluation of preterm infants at risk for ROP requires initial screening and follow-up dilated fundus examination with binocular indirect ophthalmoscopy and scleral depression. Fluorescein angiography, where available, is a useful tool that may help delineate the vasculature and extent and severity of the retinopathy.

12.8 Prognosis and Management

Spontaneous regression occurs in 85 %.

12.9 Follow-Up

Should be recommended by the examining ophthalmologist on the basis of retinal findings classified according to the international classification (Table 12.1). The detailed schedule can be followed according to the recommendations of the American Academy of Pediatrics as indicated in the Screening Examination of Premature Infants for Retinopathy of Prematurity available at www.pediatrics.org/cgi/doi/10.1542/peds.2012-2996 doi:10.1542/peds.2012-2996.

Table 12.1 Recommended follow-up intervals in the absence of plus disease

Stage	Zone I	Zone II	Zone II
Stage 3	Treatment	≤1 week	≤1 week
Stage 2	≤1 week	1–2 weeks	1–2 weeks
Stage 1	≤1 week	1–2 weeks	2–3 weeks
Immature vascularization but no ROP	1–2 weeks	2–3 weeks	2–3 weeks vs. discontinue exams
Regressing ROP	1–2 weeks	2 weeks	2–3 weeks

References and Further Reading

1. Dailey WA, Gryc W, Garg PG, Drenser KA. Frizzled-4 variations associated with retinopathy and intrauterine growth retardation: a potential marker for prematurity and retinopathy. Ophthalmology. 2015. pii: S0161-6420(15)00535-7.
2. Geloneck MM, Chuang AZ, Clark WL, Hunt MG, Norman AA, Packwood EA, Tawansy KA, Mintz-Hittner HA, BEAT-ROP Cooperative Group. Refractive outcomes following bevacizumab monotherapy compared with conventional laser treatment: a randomized clinical trial. JAMA Ophthalmol. 2014;132(11):1327–33.
3. Jayadev C, Vinekar A, Bauer N, Mangalesh S, Mahendradas P, Kemmanu V, Mallipatna A, Shetty B. Look what else we found – clinically significant abnormalities detected during routine ROP screening. Indian J Ophthalmol. 2015;63(5):373–7.
4. Lundgren P, Stoltz Sjöström E, Domellöf M, Smith L, Wu C, VanderVeen D, Hellström A, Löfqvist C. The specificity of the WINROP algorithm can be significantly increased by reassessment of the WINROP alarm. Neonatology. 2015;108(2):152–6.
5. Pertl L, Steinwender G, Mayer C, Hausberger S, Pöschl EM, Wackernagel W, Wedrich A, El-Shabrawi Y, Haas A. A systematic review and meta-analysis on the safety of vascular endothelial growth factor (VEGF) inhibitors for the treatment of retinopathy of prematurity. PLoS One. 2015;10(6):e0129383.
6. Vinekar A, Jayadev C, Mangalesh S, Shetty B, Vidyasagar D. Role of tele-medicine in retinopathy of prematurity screening in rural outreach centers in India – a report of 20,214 imaging sessions in the KIDROP program. Semin Fetal Neonatal Med. 2015;20:335–45.
7. Wang SK, Callaway NF, Wallenstein MB, Henderson MT, Leng T, Moshfeghi DM. SUNDROP: six years of screening for retinopathy of prematurity with telemedicine. Can J Ophthalmol. 2015;50(2):101–6.

Chapter 13
Familial Exudative Vitreoretinopathy

Ryan C. Young and Brenda J. Fallas

13.1 Definitions

Familial exudative vitreoretinopathy (FEVR) is a hereditary condition characterized by failure of vascular development of the temporal retina causing peripheral retinal ischemia, exudation, neovascularization, temporal dragging, and tractional retinal detachment.

13.2 Symptoms

Decreased vision
Leukocoria
Strabismus
Nystagmus

13.3 Signs

Failure of peripheral retinal vascular development results in retinal nonperfusion and ischemia. Clinical examination often reveals exudation with subretinal lipid deposition and exudative detachment, peripheral fibrovascular proliferation, straightening of retinal vessels with temporal macular dragging, and traction detachment in late stages of the disease (Fig. 13.1). Late-onset rhegmatogenous detachment may be seen. FEVR is often a bilateral disorder but may have an asymmetric presentation.

R.C. Young, MD (✉) • B.J. Fallas, CSA
Bascom Palmer Eye Institute, University of Miami,
900 NW 17th, St. Miami, FL 33136, USA
e-mail: youngrc@med.miami.edu

C.A. Medina et al. (eds.), *Manual of Retinal Diseases: A Guide to Diagnosis and Management*, DOI 10.1007/978-3-319-20460-4_13

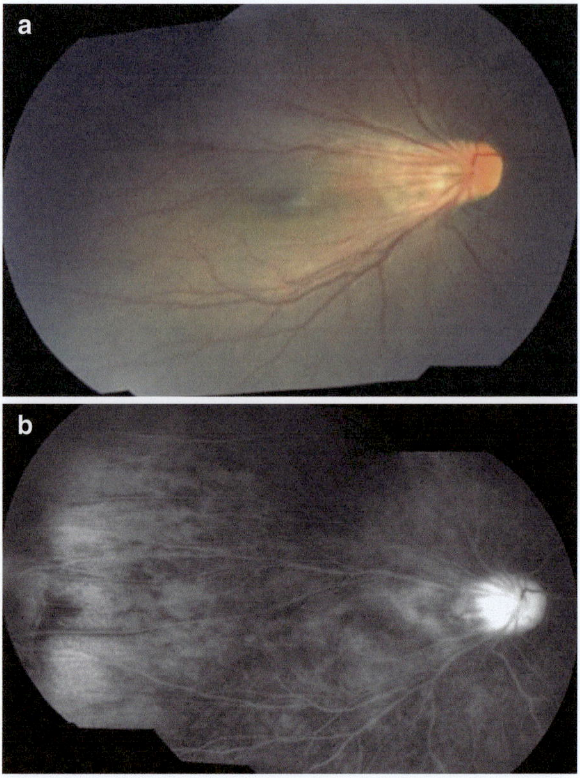

Fig. 13.1 FEVR. Fundus photo showing straightening of retinal vessels and macular dragging (**a**). Note retinal nonperfusion and leakage on fluorescein angiogram (**b**)

13.4 Predisposing Conditions

FEVR is a hereditary condition with autosomal dominant inheritance and variable penetrance. X-linked inheritance has been described and linked to the Norrie disease gene locus. In contrast to retinopathy of prematurity, affected individuals with FEVR are full term and of normal respiratory status.

13.5 Differential Diagnosis

The differential diagnosis includes retinopathy of prematurity, Coats' disease, Norrie disease, incontinentia pigmenti, Eales' disease, and sickle cell retinopathy.

13.6 Etiology

FEVR is a hereditary condition characterized by failure of vascular development of the temporal retina. Peripheral retinal ischemia, exudation, neovascularization, temporal dragging, and tractional retinal detachment occur as a result of arrested retinal vascular development. Presentation typically occurs in infancy and adolescence, though all age groups are affected.

13.7 Workup/Testing

Clinical examination is done with binocular indirect ophthalmoscopy with scleral depression. Fundus photography may be used to document baseline examination and disease progression. Fluorescein angiography is useful in assessing peripheral vasculature, including the extent and severity of disease, and in guiding therapy. Careful clinical examination of family members may help differentiate FEVR from retinopathy of prematurity. Though this is typically not necessary, fluorescein angiography of family members may identify peripheral vascular abnormalities, including peripheral ischemia and vascular straightening, and aid in the diagnosis of affected individuals. In cases of media opacity limiting visualization of the posterior pole, ultrasonography may be a useful adjunct.

13.8 Prognosis and Management

Observation is warranted for asymptomatic individuals without progression or late-stage complications, including tractional or rhegmatogenous retinal detachment. Peripheral retinal ablation with laser or cryotherapy is indicated in cases of fibrovascular proliferation secondary to peripheral nonperfusion. Scleral buckling or pars plana vitrectomy surgery is indicated for tractional or rhegmatogenous retinal detachment. Earlier age of presentation is associated with more severe disease course. The course of the disease and rate of progression is variable and generally slower in adults. Severe disease may result in total retinal detachment, neovascular glaucoma, and phthisis.

13.9 Follow-Up

Follow-up interval is dictated by the severity of the disease at presentation and subsequent clinical course.

References and Further Reading

1. Gilmour DF. Familial exudative vitreoretinopathy and related retinopathies. Eye (Lond). 2015;29(1):1–14.
2. Kang KB, Wessel MM, Tong J, D'Amico DJ, Chan RV. Ultra-widefield imaging for the management of pediatric retinal diseases. J Pediatr Ophthalmol Strabismus. 2013;50(5):282–8.

3. Kashani AH, Brown KT, Chang E, Drenser KA, Capone A, Trese MT. Diversity of retinal vascular anomalies in patients with familial exudative vitreoretinopathy. Ophthalmology. 2014;121(11):2220–7.
4. Kashani AH, Learned D, Nudleman E, Drenser KA, Capone A, Trese MT. High prevalence of peripheral retinal vascular anomalies in family members of patients with familial exudative vitreoretinopathy. Ophthalmology. 2014;121(1):262–8.
5. Ranchod TM, Ho LY, Drenser KA, Capone Jr A, Trese MT. Clinical presentation of familial exudative vitreoretinopathy. Ophthalmology. 2011;118(10):2070–5. doi:10.1016/j.ophtha.2011.06.020. Epub 2011 Aug 25. PubMed.
6. Shubert A, Tasman W. Familial exudative vitreoretinopathy: surgical intervention and visual acuity outcomes. Graefes Arch Clin Exp Ophthalmol. 1997;235(8):490–3.
7. Warden SM, Andreoli CM, Mukai S. The Wnt signaling pathway in familial exudative vitreoretinopathy and Norrie disease. Semin Ophthalmol. 2007;22(4):211–7.

Chapter 14
Persistent Fetal Vasculature

Norberto Mancera and Swetangi Bhaleeya

14.1 Definitions

Persistent hyperplastic primary vitreous (PHPV) or persistent fetal vasculature (PFV) is a rare developmental abnormality thought to be caused by failure of regression of the primary vitreous and or the fetal vessels. It is unilateral in 90 % of cases. PFV can be classified as anterior, posterior, and combined forms, according to the affected intraocular structures (Fig. 14.1).

14.2 Symptoms

- Leukocoria (white pupillary reflex)
- Decreased visual acuity (moderate to severe, including blindness)
- Strabismus

14.3 Signs

Anterior form (also known as persistent tunica vasculosa lentis):

- Retrolental opacity
- Leukocoria
- Elongated ciliary processes
- Shallow anterior chamber with secondary angle closure

N. Mancera, MD (✉) • S. Bhaleeya, MD
Department of Ophthalmology, University of South Florida,
12901 Bruce B Downs Blvd, Tampa, FL 33612, USA
e-mail: nmancera@health.usf.edu

C.A. Medina et al. (eds.), *Manual of Retinal Diseases: A Guide to Diagnosis and Management*, DOI 10.1007/978-3-319-20460-4_14

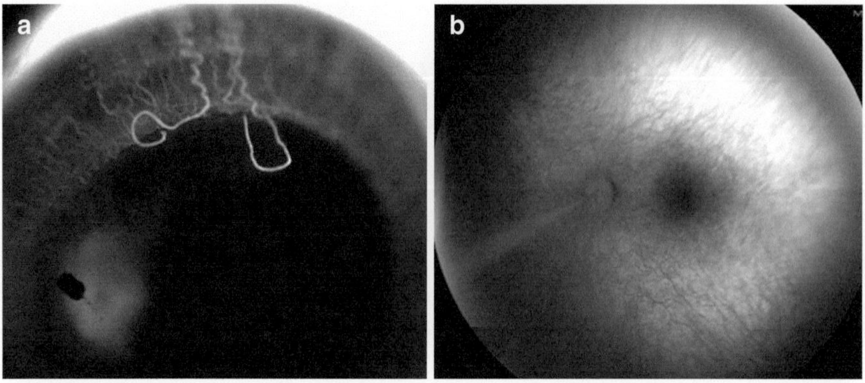

Fig. 14.1 PFV. Anterior segment FA showing prominent iris vessels that run across the pupil onto the anterior lens surface (**a**). Opaque membrane/prominent retinal fold attached to the disc (**b**)

- Cataract
- Amblyopia
- Glaucoma (due to incomplete anterior chamber angle development)
- Microphthalmia

Posterior form:

- Stalk of tissue emanating from the optic disc towards the retrolental region
- Retinal folds or dysplasia
- Retinal detachment
- Microphthalmia/phthisis
- Optic nerve abnormalities/hypoplasia

14.4 Predisposing Conditions

PFV is typically a sporadically occurring condition without associated systemic findings.

14.5 Differential Diagnosis

Retinoblastoma
Congenital cataract
Coat disease
Toxocariasis
Retinopathy of prematurity (ROP)
Familial exudative vitreoretinopathy (FEVR)
Norrie disease

14.6 Etiology

During embryogenesis the anterior portion of the eye receives nutrients from the hyaloid artery. As the fetus develops, this system is expected to regress. In the case of PFV, the primary vitreous and hyaloidal vessels do not regress during the second and third trimester.

Anterior PFV is most common and usually presents in one eye. As the name suggests, it affects the anterior segment with a retrolental mass and cataract. The lens may swell leading to a secondary angle-closure glaucoma. Posterior PFV is less common and involves the posterior segment with a white dense opaque membrane or a prominent retinal fold. Both optic disc and macular abnormalities can occur.

14.7 Workup/Testing

- Clinical exam (anterior segment changes on slit lamp biomicroscopy) and dilated fundus exam.
- Ultrasound and CT scan may be useful in differentiating PFV from retinoblastoma. In PFV the stalk reaching from the posterior pole to the lens can be seen. Calcifications are seen with retinoblastoma.
- Posterior forms of PFV should be differentiated from ROP, FEVR, Coats disease, and toxocariasis. Fluorescein angiography can be used to look for characteristic changes of each of the entities.

14.8 Prognosis and Management

Management of PFV can be medical, surgical, or close observation. Lensectomy and removal of the retrolental membrane may be indicated to prevent angle-closure glaucoma. Secondary complications such as amblyopia, glaucoma, and retinal detachment can be challenging to treat in these patients. Surgical interventions are done with the aim of preserving useful vision. In a study by Alexandrakis et al. approximately 50 % of patients undergoing surgery for PFV achieved useful vision. Visual acuity outcomes in patients with PFV are correlated with the nature and extent of ocular risk factors such as microphthalmia, retinal folds, and optic nerve abnormalities.

14.9 Follow-Up

It is important for patients with PFV to establish care with a vitreoretinal specialist and have prompt assessment. Early intervention to prevent secondary complications is essential to preserve as much functional visual acuity as possible.

References and Suggested Reading

1. Alexandrakis G, Scott IU, Flynn HW, et al. Visual acuity outcomes with and without surgery in patients with persistent fetal vasculature. Ophthalmology. 2000;107(6):1068–72.
2. Farber N, Shrier E. How to treat persistent fetal vasculature. Rev Ophthalmol. 2015. http://www.reviewofophthalmology.com/content/t/pediatrics/c/52898/.
3. Goldberg MF. Persistent Fetal Vasculature (PFV): an integrated interpretation of signs and symptoms associated with persistent hyperplastic primary vitreous (PHPV) LIV Edward Jackson Memorial Lecture. Am J Ophthalmol. 1997;124:587–626.
4. Shastry B. Persistent hyperplastic primary vitreous: congenital malformation of the eye. Clin Exp Ophthalmol. 2009;37:884–90.
5. Tartarella M, Takahagi R, Braga A, Filho J. Persistent fetal vasculature: ocular features, management of cataract and outcomes. Arq Bras Oftalmol. 2013;76:185–8.

Chapter 15
Shaken Baby Syndrome

Tayyeba K. Ali, Ryan C. Young, and Brenda J. Fallas

15.1 Definitions

Shaken baby syndrome (SBS) is a vitreo-chorioretinopathy secondary to nonaccidental trauma that occurs in children younger than 3–5 years old, and most frequently in infants less than 6–12 months old. SBS has been replaced with the term abusive head trauma (AHT) or inflicted childhood neurotrauma (ICN).

15.2 Symptoms

- Can range from an inconsolable, irritable child to a lethargic, unresponsive one
- Usually bilateral, though can be asymmetric
- Taking a good history from the care-giver is critical

15.3 Signs: (Fig. 15.1)

Ocular signs – present in 85–90 % of SBS

- Retinal hemorrhages in any or all layers of retina
- Cotton-wool spots
- Hemorrhagic schisis

T.K. Ali, MD (✉) • R.C. Young, MD • B.J. Fallas
Bascom Palmer Eye Institute, University of Miami,
900 NW 17th St., Miami, FL 33136, USA
e-mail: t.ali2@med.miami.edu

C.A. Medina et al. (eds.), *Manual of Retinal Diseases: A Guide to Diagnosis and Management*, DOI 10.1007/978-3-319-20460-4_15

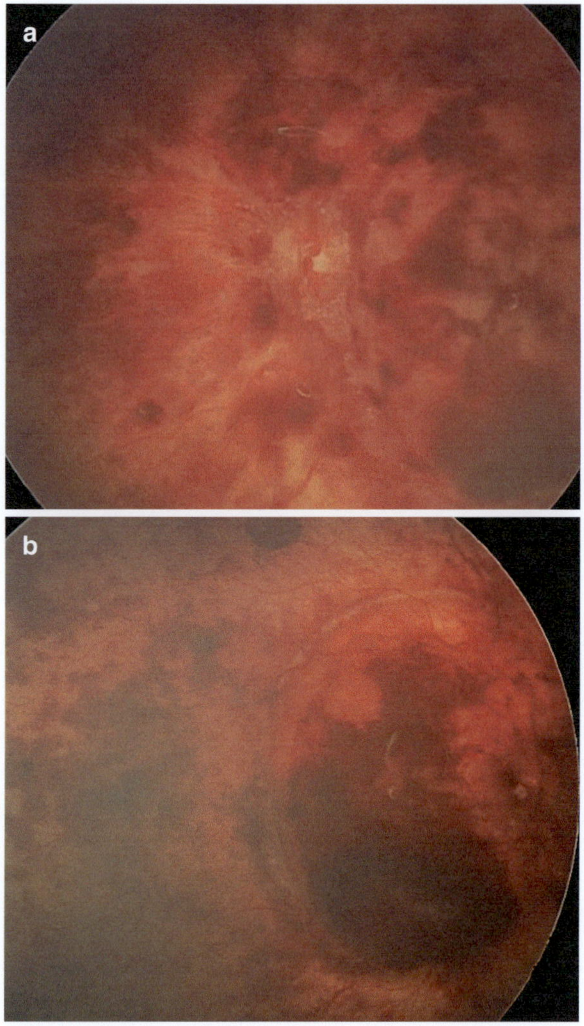

Fig. 15.1 Shaken baby syndrome. Note retinal hemorrhages in all layers (**a**) and schisis cavities (**b**). Courtesy of Ken Nischal, MD, Pittsburg, PA

- Vitreous hemorrhage
- Retinal and choroidal folds/rupture
- Optic nerve edema
- Macular edema

Systemic signs

- Bradycardia, apnea, hypothermia
- Failure to thrive
- Full or bulging fontanelles
- Spiral fractures of the long bones

- Systemic signs
- Subdural or subarachnoid hemorrhages
- Bruised skin

15.4 Epidemiology

- Occurs in younger infants and children
- Premature birth or congenital/hereditary birth issues put the baby at a higher risk
- No gender predilection

15.5 Differential Diagnosis

- Accidental trauma – although does not often present with retinal hemorrhaging or other classic SBS systemic findings
- Purtscher retinopathy – although it will not have extensive retinal hemorrhaging throughout all layers
- Central retinal vein occlusion (CRVO), which is exceedingly rare in children
- Coagulopathy
- Anemia
- Leukemia
- Increased intracranial pressure
- Retinopathy of prematurity

15.6 Etiology

- Acceleration-deceleration injury
- Severe whiplash injury

15.7 Workup/Testing

- A clinical diagnosis, as 85–90 % of patients with SBS will have ocular findings
- Neuroimaging such as CT or MRI, which may show intracranial bleeding, intracranial edema, ischemia, or contusion
- RetCam photos to document retinal pathology if present, as these cases often go to court
- Additional testing usually left to the discretion of the pediatric team

15.8 Prognosis and Management

- Almost 30 % of children, according to one study, died of injuries related to SBS.
- Vitrectomy can be considered for a nonclearing vitreous hemorrhage to prevent amblyopia.
- Most retinal hemorrhaging will clear in days to weeks.
- Schisis cavities can persist indefinitely.
- All physicians in the USA and Canada are required by law to report suspected child abuse to the appropriate governmental authority.

15.9 Follow Up

- Depends on the age and overall prognosis of the child.
- Infants and younger children will require more frequent (weeks) visits while older children may be able to extend their visits (several weeks to 1 month) between depending on the risk of amblyopia.

References and Suggested Reading

1. American Academy of Ophthalmology. Information statement. Abusive Head Trauma/Shaken Baby Syndrome. San Francisco: American Academy of ophthalmology; 2010. Available at: http://www.aao.org/clinical-statement/abusive-head-traumashaken-baby-syndrome--june-2010. Accessed 16 May 2015.
2. Basic and Clinical Science Course, Section 06: Pediatric Ophthalmology and Strabismus. American Academy of Ophthalmology, San Francisco, CA.
3. Matschke J, Mermann B, Sperhake J, et al. Shaken baby syndrome: a common variant of non-accidental head injury in infants. Dtsch Arztebl Int. 2009;106:211–7.
4. Tang J, Buzney SM, Lashkary K, et al. Shaken baby syndrome: a review and update on ophthalmologic manifestations. Int Opthalmol Clin. 2008;48:237–46.

Chapter 16
Coloboma

Hershel R. Patel and Swetangi Bhaleeya

16.1 Definitions

Coloboma is a developmental abnormality with defects of one or several ocular structures. Defects of the eyelids, cornea, iris, ciliary body, zonules, lens, retina, choroid, and/or optic nerve may be present and are caused by incomplete closure of the embryonic fissure.

16.2 Symptoms

Coloboma may be unilateral or bilateral, and the symptoms depend on which ocular structure is affected.

- Eyelid coloboma (eyelid abnormality or defect, symptoms occur secondary to exposure keratopathy)
- Iris coloboma ("keyhole, lightbulb, or inverted teardrop" appearance of the pupil)
- Lens coloboma (mostly asymptomatic, but decreased vision if there is associated lens opacity/cataract or lens subluxation with zonular involvement)
- Chorioretinal coloboma (usually asymptomatic; decreased vision or visual field defect noted in patient with optic nerve or macular involvement; symptoms due to secondary complications such as retinal tear or detachment)

H.R. Patel, MS, MD (✉) • S. Bhaleeya, MD
Department of Ophthalmology, USF Eye Institute, University of South Florida, 13127 USF Magnolia Drive, Tampa, FL 33612, USA
e-mail: hershelrpatel@gmail.com; bhaleeya05@gmail.com

C.A. Medina et al. (eds.), *Manual of Retinal Diseases: A Guide to Diagnosis and Management*, DOI 10.1007/978-3-319-20460-4_16

16.3 Signs

Eyelid coloboma is typically found in the upper lid and is often isolated. The exception is when it occurs in association with Goldenhar syndrome. In contrast, lower eyelid coloboma is often associated with Treacher Collins syndrome. Coloboma of the globe is typically located in the inferonasal quadrant of the affected structure, and there is a strong association with microphthalmia. Other associations include heterochromia, cataract, glaucoma, nystagmus, and posterior staphyloma (Fig. 16.1a). Lens coloboma is seen as flattening of the equator of the lens in an area of absence of zonular fibers. Posterior coloboma with retinal involvement appears as an area of whitening with pigment deposition where the defect meets normal retina (Fig. 16.1b). The sclera in this area may be covered by membrane which may be hypoplastic or gliotic retina. Eight to forty-three percent of posterior coloboma cases can eventually develop retinal detachment (both rhegmatogenous and non-rhegmatogenous).

16.4 Predisposing Conditions

Coloboma may be an isolated finding or associated with other systemic conditions:

- CHARGE syndrome
- Cat-eye syndrome
- Trisomy 13 (Patau syndrome)
- Trisomy 18 (Edwards syndrome)
- 13q deletion syndrome
- Basal cell nevus (carcinoma) syndrome

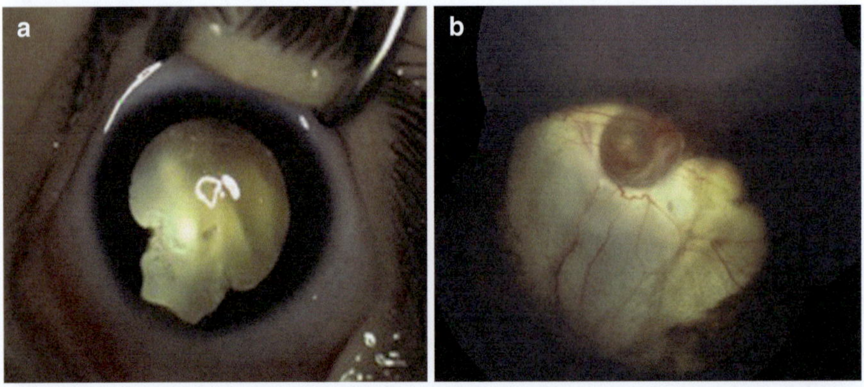

Fig. 16.1 Coloboma. External photograph showing inferonasal iris coloboma with secondary cataract (**a**). Posterior coloboma with retinal involvement appears as an area of whitening (**b**)

- Congenital contractural arachnodactyly
- Meckel-Gruber syndrome
- Sjogren-Larsson syndrome
- Humeroradial synostosis
- Oral-facial-digital syndrome (type VIII)
- Walker-Warburg syndrome
- Lenz microphthalmia syndrome
- Aicardi syndrome
- Catel-Manzke syndrome
- Wolf-Hirschhorn syndrome
- Linear sebaceous nevus syndrome
- Rubinstein-Taybi syndrome
- Kabuki syndrome

16.5 Differential Diagnosis

A coloboma can often be distinguished from other lesions by its typical appearance and location. Differential diagnosis can be considered according to the ocular structures involved (Table 16.1).

16.6 Epidemiology and Etiology

Ocular coloboma occurs due to failed closure of the embryonic fissure, and the prevalence is approximately 0.5 to 2.2 cases per 10,000 live births. It may be sporadic or inherited and is associated with systemic disorders in some cases. Typical colobomas which are anatomically in the inferonasal quadrant are believed to be secondary to failed closure of the embryonic fissure during the 5th week of gestation. Depending on the location/severity of failed closure, there may be a continuous uveal coloboma from posterior to anterior or "skip lesions" where some areas are spared. When an iris coloboma is in an area other than the inferonasal quadrant,

Table. 16.1 Differential diagnosis of Coloboma based on location

Eyelid	Iris	Retinochoroidal	Optic nerve
Eyelid trauma or laceration	Iris trauma	Trauma with choroidal rupture	Optic nerve pit
Entropion	Rieger syndrome	Chorioretinal scar	Morning glory disc
	Iris atrophy (ICE syndrome)		Congenital optic disc anomaly/ staphyloma
	Aniridia and heterochromia irides		Glaucomatous optic atrophy

the posterior uvea is not involved. The etiology in this case is believed to be secondary to fibrovascular remnants of the anterior hyaloid system and pupillary membrane.

16.7 Workup/Testing

Full ophthalmological exam should be conducted of all ocular structures. If there is concern for an associated syndrome, a tailored workup for the suspected disorder should be performed in conjunction with the primary physician.

16.8 Prognosis and Management

Treatment of patients with coloboma is typically conservative. Refractive error is corrected, with focus on optimizing visual acuity in the affected eye. Prevention of amblyopia is important in cases where there is asymmetry in visual potential.

Eyelid coloboma – lubrication for exposure keratopathy. Referral to oculoplastics for possible eyelid reconstruction.

Lens coloboma – correct refractive error. If significant cataract, consider lens extraction with intraocular lens placement. Surgery may be complicated by zonular abnormalities.

Chorioretinal coloboma – observation: monitor for retinal tear or detachment.

16.9 Follow-Up

Retinal detachment is a risk of posterior coloboma and must be monitored every 6–12 months via dilated fundoscopy. Genetic counseling to the patient and family members may be offered if indicated.

References and Suggested Reading

1. Kenneth W. Wright. Diseases of the cornea. anterior segment, and iris. In: Pediatric ophthalmology and strabismus, vol. 6. San Francisco: American Academy of Ophthalmology. p. 252, 356.
2. Warburg M. Classification of microphthalmos and coloboma. J Med Genet. 1993;30(8):664–9.
3. Stoll C, Alembik Y, Dott B, Roth MP. Epidemiology of congenital eye malformations in 131,760 consecutive births. Ophthalmic Paediatr Genet. 1992;13(3):179–86.

4. Schubert HD. Structural organization of choroidal colobomas of young and adult patients and mechanism of retinal detachment. Trans Am Ophthalmol Soc. 2005;103:457–72.
5. Facts About Uveal Coloboma (2012) Retrieved 12 July 2015, from https://nei.nih.gov/health/coloboma/coloboma.
6. Coloboma (2011) Retrieved 12 July 2015, from http://ghr.nlm.nih.gov/condition/coloboma.
7. Gregory-Evans CY, Williams MJ, Halford S, Gregory-Evans K. Ocular coloboma: a reassessment in the age of molecular neuroscience. J Med Genet. 2004;41(12):881–91. Review.

Chapter 17
Juvenile X-Linked Retinoschisis

Norberto Mancera and Swetangi Bhaleeya

17.1 Definitions

Juvenile X-linked retinoschisis is a hereditary disorder characterized by foveal schisis affecting males early in life. Schisis or splitting of the retina's neurosensory layers in the periphery can also be seen in some cases.

17.2 Symptoms

X-linked retinoschisis (XLRS) usually presents in males during school age, but can present as early as 3 months of age. Patients are often referred after they fail to pass school screening vision test. XLRS may be detected earlier in patients with known family history. Vision is only mildly reduced in younger patients but can gradually decrease to 20/200 or worse. Most patients are hyperopic. Peripheral visual field deficits can also occur secondary to a schisis cavity (present in up to 50 % of cases) or retinal detachment. With significant peripheral retinoschisis, vitreous hemorrhage can occur resulting in sudden loss of vision. There are no known systemic associations.

N. Mancera, MD (✉) • S. Bhaleeya, MD
Department of Ophthalmology, University of South Florida,
12901 Bruce B Downs Blvd, Tampa, FL 33612, USA
e-mail: nmancera@health.usf.edu

C.A. Medina et al. (eds.), *Manual of Retinal Diseases: A Guide to Diagnosis and Management*, DOI 10.1007/978-3-319-20460-4_17

17.3 Signs

- Stellate spokelike appearance of macula with microcysts (may be better visualized with red free)
- Retinal pigment epithelial changes in older patients
- Vitreous veils
- Vitreous hemorrhage
- Peripheral retinoschisis (usually inferotemporally) (Fig. 17.1)
- Vitreoretinal traction and retinal detachment
- Mizuo phenomenon or white flecks observed in some cases[1]
- Female carriers may only show white flecks or schisis in the periphery

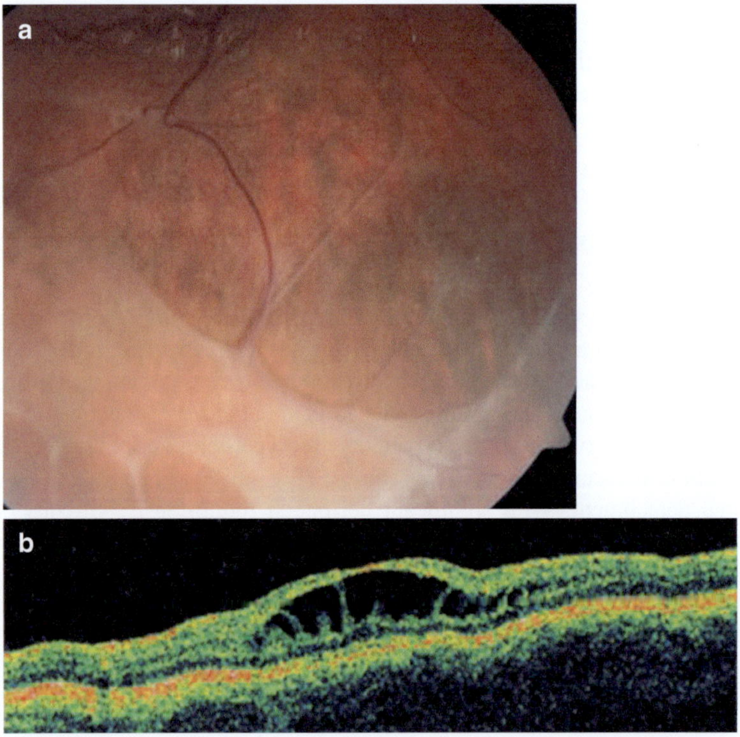

Fig. 17.1 Peripheral retinoschisis. Fundus photo showing peripheral schisis (**a**) visible on OCT (**b**) (Courtesy of Sami Uwaydat, MD, and Scott Lowery, MD, Little Rock, Arkansas)

[1] Mizuo-Nakamura phenomenon is a change in the color of the fundus from red in the dark-adapted state to golden immediately or shortly after exposure to light. The color of the fundus reflex can be either homogeneous or streaky.

17.4 Predisposing Conditions

Inherited disorder occurring in males with complete penetrance and variable expressivity. Females are carriers.

17.5 Differential Diagnosis

- Goldmann-Favre syndrome
- Retinitis pigmentosa
- Familial exudative vitreoretinopathy
- Stargardt's disease
- Macular dystrophy or macular degeneration

17.6 Etiology

Inherited disorder secondary to mutations in the RS1 gene located on Xp22.2-p22.1. It encodes for protein retinoschisin, which is expressed in photoreceptor and bipolar cells. Function of retinoschisin is not fully understood, but it appears to function as a cell adhesion protein to maintain the cellular organization of the retina and the structural integrity of the photoreceptor-bipolar synapse. The prevalence of this condition can range from 1 in 5,000 to 1 in 25,000, with several reports indicating the highest prevalence in Finland.

17.7 Workup/Testing

- Optical coherence tomography (OCT) can show cystic spaces in various retinal layers, including nerve fiber layer, inner nuclear, and outer plexiform layers.
- Fluorescein angiography does not show leakage of fluorescein in the macula but can be used to distinguish foveal schisis from cystoid macular edema.
- Electroretinogram (ERG) shows selective reduction of the amplitude of the dark-adapted b-wave with relative preservation of the a-wave amplitude (ERG responses can be variable and are not always diagnostic).

17.8 Prognosis and Management

- No current medical treatment for XLRS. Use of dorzolamide and oral acetazolamide may be useful in decreasing cystic spaces and foveal thickness in some cases.
- Research is ongoing for gene therapy as an option in the future.

- Laser photocoagulation of peripheral schisis can be performed but is not commonly recommended due to the possibility of causing a retinal detachment.
- Surgical management may be necessary for vitreous hemorrhage and retinal detachments.
- With large schisis cavities in the periphery, there is risk of vitreous hemorrhage with minor trauma. Eye protection should be recommended when playing sports and or avoidance of high-contact sports.
- Low vision aids.
- Genetic counseling should be offered. Genetic testing is not necessary as the diagnosis is clinical and will not change management.

17.9 Follow-Up

- During the first decade of life, routine dilated fundus exams are recommended to monitor for any complications such as vitreous hemorrhage or retinal detachment and correct any associated refractive errors to prevent amblyopia or strabismus.
- Referral to a vitreoretinal specialist for complicated cases and vitreous hemorrhage or detachment.

References and Suggested Reading

1. George ND, Yates JR, Moore AT. X linked retinoschisis. Br J Ophthalmol. 1995;79(7):697–702.
2. Molday R, Kellner U, Weber B. X-linked juvenile retinoschisis: Clinical diagnosis, genetic analysis, and molecular mechanisms. Prog Retinal Eye Res. 2012;31:195–212.
3. Mooy CM, Van Den Born LI, Baarsma S, Paridaens DA, Kraaijenbrink T, Bergen A, Weber BH. Hereditary X-linked juvenile retinoschisis: a review of the role of Muller cells. Arch Ophthalmol. 2002;120:979–84.
4. Tantri A, Vrabec TR, Cu-Unjieng A, Frost A, Annesley Jr WH, Donoso LA. X-linked retinoschisis: a clinical and molecular genetic review. Surv Ophthalmol. 2004;49:214–30.

Chapter 18
Toxocariasis

Tayyeba K. Ali and Ryan C. Young

18.1 Definitions

Ocular toxocariasis is a unilateral infectious uveitis secondary to tissue invasion by roundworm *Toxocara canis* or *Toxocara cati*, which leads to a severe inflammatory reaction and significant chorioretinitis in children.

18.2 Symptoms

- Decreased vision
- Floaters
- Pain/photophobia
- Scotomas
- Leukocoria
- Strabismus
- Usually unilateral

T.K. Ali, MD (✉) • R.C. Young, MD
Bascom Palmer Eye Institute, University of Miami,
900 NW 17th St., Miami, FL 33136, USA
e-mail: t.ali2@med.miami.edu

C.A. Medina et al. (eds.), *Manual of Retinal Diseases: A Guide to Diagnosis and Management*, DOI 10.1007/978-3-319-20460-4_18

18.3 Signs

- The anterior segment is typically quiet, though it can present with non-granulomatous inflammation and posterior synechiae.
- Severe vitritis is often present.
- Funduscopic examination reveals one of three syndromes: (1) leukocoria mimicking endophthalmitis, (2) macular granuloma, and (3) peripheral granuloma (Fig. 18.1).
- Rarely, it can present as a unilateral pars planitis with significant exudation.
- Although toxocariasis is secondary to ingestion of a roundworm larva, ocular toxocariasis rarely has concurrent systemic manifestations or presents with visceral larva migrans (VLM).

18.4 Epidemiology

- Occurs in children and young adults.
- No gender predilection.
- Caucasians and Hispanics most often affected.
- 2 % of children worldwide infected with toxocariasis.
- Some studies suggest 1 % prevalence of toxocara chorioretinitis.
- Caused by nematode *Toxocara canis* or *Toxocara cati.*

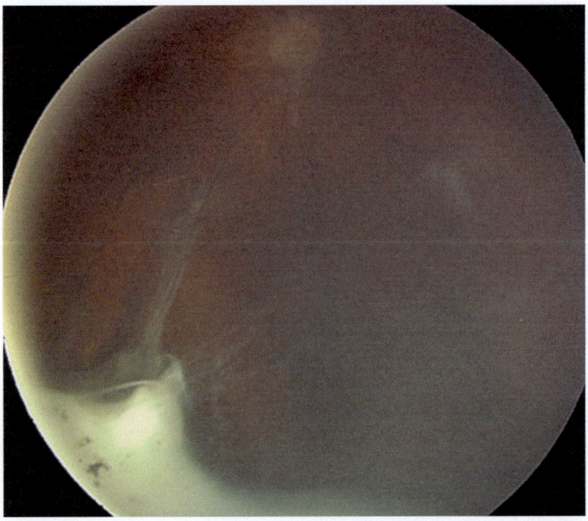

Fig. 18.1 Toxocara granuloma. Peripheral granuloma with characteristic vitreous traction (Courtesy Jonathan Sears, MD, Cole Eye Institute, Cleveland Clinic, Cleveland, OH. Reproduced with permission from Kim JW, Singh AD. Chapter 2: Differential diagnosis of leukocoria. In: Singh AD, Murphree AL, Damato BE, editors. Clinical ophthalmic oncology retinoblastoma. 2nd ed. Springer; 2015. p. 13–28)

18.5 Predisposing Conditions

- Ingestion of contaminated food
- Fecal-oral route

18.6 Differential Diagnosis

- Retinoblastoma (will often show calcium on CT, have limited inflammation, and present at a younger age)
- Infectious endophthalmitis
- Toxoplasmosis
- Pars planitis
- Retinopathy of prematurity
- Persistent fetal vasculature
- Coat disease
- Familial exudative vitreoretinopathy (FEVR)

18.7 Etiology

- Complete ocular immunology unknown.
- Children ingest Toxocara eggs that mature in the gut, leading to a strong immunological response and production of IgM, IgG, and IgE.
- Hematogenous spread leads to chorioretinal invasion.
- Th-2 medicated response leads to eosinophilic granuloma along with a B-lymphocyte response and antibody-dependent cytotoxicity.

18.8 Workup/Testing

- A clinical diagnosis.
- Serum ELISA.
- Vitreous biopsy showing Toxocara antibodies may be useful, though rarely necessary.
- Laboratory testing for syphilis, with syphilis IgG and rapid plasma regain (RPR); TB, with either PPD or TB-specific interferon-gamma release assay (e.g., QuantiFERON-TB Gold®) as well as chest X-ray; and toxoplasmosis, with serum IgM and IgG levels should be performed to rule out other infectious etiologies.

- *Color fundus photography*: useful in documenting lesions and in monitoring for progression of disease.
- *Optical coherence tomography (OCT):* may show cystoid macular edema (CME).
- *Echography (B* scan): to rule out retinal detachment (RD) (or the presence of calcium if trying to rule out retinoblastoma).

18.9 Prognosis and Management

- Systemic anti-helminthic medication rarely useful.
- Aggressive periocular and systemic steroids often necessary to control the inflammatory response.
- Vitreoretinal surgery may be required to manage tractional retinal detachment.
- Laser photocoagulation has been used if larvae are visible and motile, though this may exacerbate the inflammatory response.

18.10 Follow-Up

Patient should be seen frequently during the acute phase until inflammatory response has subsided. Depending on the age of the patient, and if she is out of the amblyopic age group, she may be followed every 4–6 months to monitor for any retinal sequelae, such as CME, glaucoma, or tractional RD.

References and Suggested Reading

1. Ahn SJ, Ryoo NK, Woo SJ. Ocular toxocariasis: clinical features, diagnosis, treatment, and prevention. Asia Pac Allergy. 2014;4(3):134–41.
2. Ahn SJ, Woo SJ, Jin Y, Chang YS, Kim TW, Ahn J, Heo JW, Yu HG, Chung H, Park KH, Hong ST. Clinical features and course of ocular toxocariasis in adults. PLoS Negl Trop Dis. 2014;8(6):e2938.
3. Cella W, Ferreira E, Torigoe AM, Macchiaverni-Filho N, Balarin V. Ultrasound biomicroscopy findings in peripheral vitreoretinal toxocariasis. Eur J Ophthalmol. 2004;14(2):132–6.
4. Giuliari GP, Ramirez G, Cortez RT. Surgical treatment of ocular toxocariasis: anatomic and functional results in 45 patients. Eur J Ophthalmol. 2011;21(4):490–4.
5. Stewart JM, Cubillan LD, Cunningham Jr ET. Prevalence, clinical features, and causes of vision loss among patients with ocular toxocariasis. Retina. 2005;25(8):1005–13.
6. Woodhall D, Starr MC, Montgomery SP, Jones JL, Lum F, Read RW, Moorthy RS. Ocular toxocariasis: epidemiologic, anatomic, and therapeutic variations based on a survey of ophthalmic subspecialists. Ophthalmology. 2012;119(6):1211–7.

Section III
Retinal Dystrophies

Veeral S. Shah

Chapter 19
Retinitis Pigmentosa

Salman A. Rahman and Veeral S. Shah

19.1 Definitions

Retinitis pigmentosa (RP) is a progressive retinal degenerative disorder with varying patterns of inheritance.

19.2 Symptoms

- *Early*: Nyctalopia and loss of peripheral vision
- *Late*: Decrease in central vision and photophobia

19.3 Signs

- *Early*: Vessel attenuation, vitreous cell, abnormal testing (ERG), and pigmentary deposits resembling bone spicules (perivascular) in the periphery (early-mid stage) (Fig. 19.1).
- *Late*: Waxy optic nerve pallor, RPE atrophy, posterior subcapsular cataract, cystoid macular edema, abnormal testing (ERG absent), and pigment deposition involving the macula.

S.A. Rahman, MD • V.S. Shah, MD, PhD (✉)
Department of Ophthalmology, Baylor College of Medicine,
Texas Children's Hospital, Houston, TX, USA
e-mail: vsshah@texaschildrens.org

C.A. Medina et al. (eds.), *Manual of Retinal Diseases: A Guide to Diagnosis and Management*, DOI 10.1007/978-3-319-20460-4_19

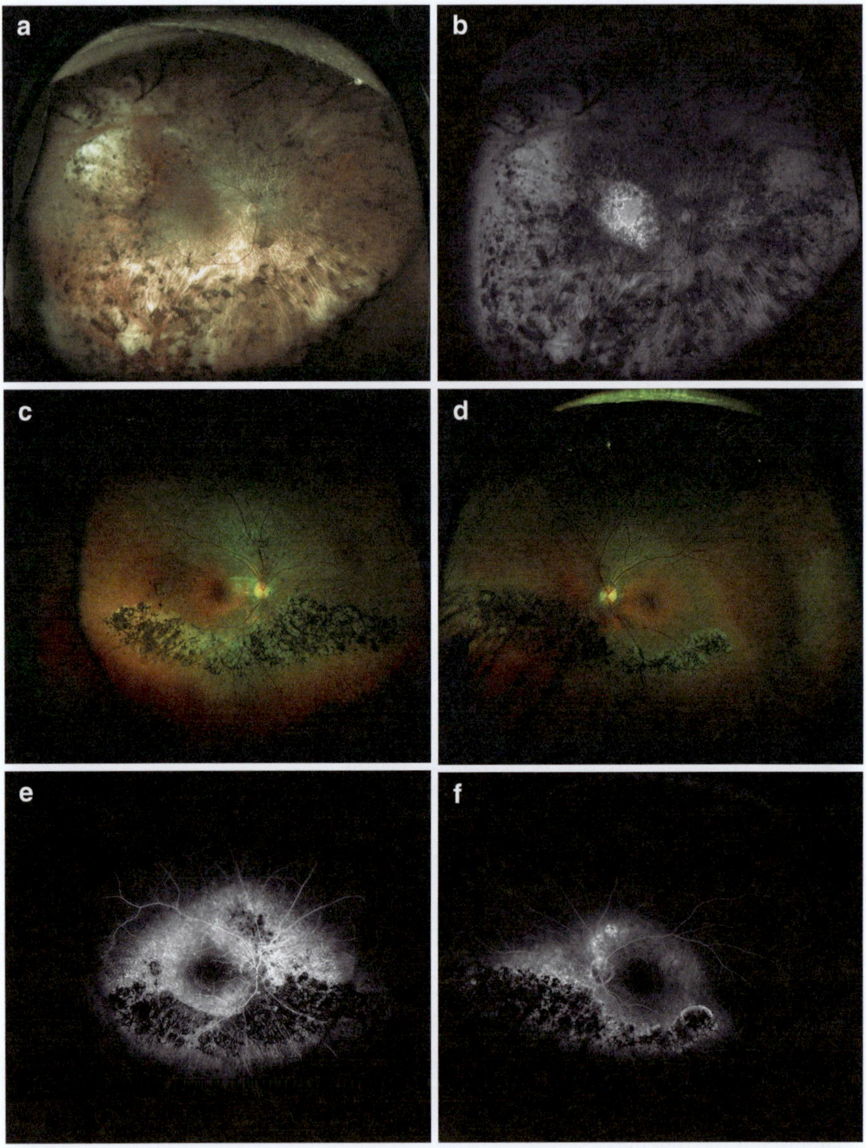

Fig. 19.1 Advance stages of retinitis pigmentosa; the right eye demonstrating RPE atrophy, pigmentary deposits, and waxy optic nerve (**a**). Fundus autofluorescence shows a parafoveal ring of hyperfluorescence with edge corresponding to loss of peripheral retina (**b**). Fundus photo and fluorescein angiogram demonstrate sectoral RP with focal RPE hypertrophy atrophic area extending towards the macular and vascular attenuation (**c**, **e** Right eye, **d**, **f** Left eye) (Courtesy of Hassan Rahman, MD, and Emmanuel Chang, MD, Houston, TX)

19.4 Epidemiology

Prevalence of 1 in 4000 to 1 in 5000 with over 1 million cases worldwide. Age of onset varies from early childhood to middle ages.

19.5 Inheritance

Non-syndromic: Over 50 genes and loci associated with non-syndromic RP (– 65 % of all RP).

- *Autosomal recessive*: 15–20 % of all RP with over 30 genes and loci associated with this form. RPE65 is involved in 2 % recessive RP and 16 % of Leber's congenital amaurosis (human gene replacement trials involving RPE65 underway).
- *Autosomal dominant*: Mildest form characterized by onset in adulthood (20–25 % of all RP). Mutations in RHO associated with 30 % of AD. Mutant form of rhodopsin is toxic to rods by interfering with metabolism. Over 20 different genes associated with autosomal dominant form.
- *X-linked*: Rarest form of non-syndromic RP with early-onset and severe vision loss (8–15 % of all RP). Female carriers may have fundus pigmentary changes. Associated with myopia. Mutations in RPGR associated with 55–70 % of X-linked and 25 % of sporadic.
- *Digenic*: Heterozygous mutation in ROM1 in combination with a heterozygous mutation in RDS causes RP. Children of affected patients have a 1/4 risk of developing RP.
- *Sporadic.*

Syndromic: 25 % of all RP with over 30 different syndromes identified.

- *Usher syndrome*: Typically, autosomal recessive and mutations in USH2A in 30–50 % of cases (also in 16–20 % AR, non-syndromic RP). At least 11 other genes related to Usher syndrome.
- *Bardet-Biedl syndrome*: Autosomal recessive, 17 genes related to this systemic disease.

19.6 Associated Diseases

- *Usher syndrome*: The most frequent systemic disease with RP (10–20 % of all RP). Prevalence of 1 in 12,000 to 1 in 30,000. Characterized by sensorineural hearing loss. Three different forms: type 1 with profound deafness and ataxia, type 2 with moderate deafness and no ataxia, and type 3 with hearing loss that presents in childhood and progressively worsens.

- *Bardet-Biedl syndrome*: Prevalence is 1 in 150,000. Characterized by obesity, mental retardation, polydactyly, hypogenitalism, mild psychomotor delay, and renal abnormalities. 5 % of all RP.
- *Refsum's disease*: Deficiency of phytanoyl-CoA hydroxylase deficiency. Associated with elevated phytanic acid, deafness, ataxia, anosmia, liver disease, polyneuropathy, and cardiac abnormalities. Treat by restricted intake of milk products, green leafy vegetables, and animal fats (low phytanic acid diet).
- *Abetalipoproteinemia (Bassen-Kornzweig syndrome)*: Deficiency in apolipoprotein B leads to inability to absorb lipids and a deficiency in fat-soluble vitamins (A, D, E, and K). Findings include progressive ataxia, steatorrhea, and growth retardation. Diagnosis is based on lack of apolipoprotein B. Treat with vitamin A, E, and K supplements.
- *Cockayne syndrome*: Associated with dwarfism, mental retardation, deafness, and premature aging.
- *Neuronal ceroid lipofuscinosis (Batten disease)*: Findings include seizures, ataxia, and dementia.
- *Zellweger*: Associated with hepatosplenomegaly, hypotonia, and renal abnormalities.
- *Alstom*: Hearing loss, obesity, renal abnormalities, and hypogenitalism.

19.7 Differential Diagnosis

- *Leber's congenital amaurosis*: Severe visual impairment in infancy or early childhood. Frequently defined as an early form of RP.
- *Congenital stationary night blindness*: Relatively normal visual field and vision, nonprogressive.
- *Vitamin A deficiency*: Associated with keratitis or history of poor nutrition and malabsorption.
- *Congenital infections TORCH*: Pigmentary retinopathy from rubella or syphilis.
- *Kearns-Sayre syndrome*: Mitochondrial disorder associated with salt-and-pepper fundus, chronic progressive external ophthalmoplegia, ptosis, and cardiac conduction defects.
- *Cone-rod dystrophy*: Presenting symptom is decreased central acuity. ERG with a diminished waver form. Late stages of RP and CRD can appear very similar with flat ERGs. Differentiate by history of initial symptoms.
- *Secondary RP*: trauma, previous vascular occlusion, prior retinal detachment, uveitis, infection, metallic intraocular foreign body, or drug toxicity (chloroquine, phenothiazines).
- *Choroideremia*: X-linked disease caused by mutation in the CMH gene. Scalloped RPE atrophy early. Presence of RPE and choriocapillaris only in the macula in late stage.
- *Gyrate atrophy*: Autosomal recessive due to a deficiency in ornithine aminotransferase. Scalloped areas of absent RPE and choriocapillaris.

- *Workup/testing*: Obtain a detailed family history. Dilated fundus exam with above findings. Reduction of a- and b-wave amplitudes on ERG. Both rod and cone-isolated signals are reduced, but scotopic loss predominates. ERG is unrecordable in late stage. Visual field with ring scotoma that progresses to a central island. OCT may aid in diagnosing cystoid macular edema and reveal structural abnormalities in the photoreceptor layer. Unilateral RP is very almost nonexistent (single case confirmed genetically in publication), and acquired etiology should be ruled out. Non-syndromic RP can present in localized forms, which include sectoral RP (only 1–2 quadrants involved bilaterally), central RP (macula involvement early with visual field loss centrally that progresses peripherally), and pericentral RP (ring scotoma around central vision).

19.8 Prognosis and Management

Most patients are legally blind by 40s–50s due to severely constricted visual fields. Tinted glasses may aid with photophobia. Vitamin A therapy (15,000 IU daily) may reduce the rate in loss of ERG amplitude, but liver function should be monitored. Do not prescribe in women planning for pregnancy. Remove cataracts and treat cystoid macular edema with oral or topical carbonic anhydrase inhibitors. Experimental treatments currently being investigated include gene therapy, use of neuroprotective growth factors, tissue transplantation, and retinal prosthesis, promising genetic research involving the replacement of RPE65 gene (associated with autosomal recessive RP and Leber's congenital amaurosis).

- Family counseling and genetic testing. Low vision aids as need.
- Diet low in phytanic acid if Refsum disease. Supplementation with vitamin A, E, and K for abetalipoproteinemia.
- Refer to cardiology if suspicion for Kearns-Sayre syndrome.

19.9 Follow-Up

Annually.

References and Suggested Reading

1. Daiger SP, Bowne SJ, Sullivan LS. Perspective on genes and mutations causing retinitis pigmentosa. Arch Ophthalmol. 2007;125:151–8.
2. Daiger SP, Sullivan LS, Bowne SJ. Genes and mutations causing retinitis pigmentosa. Clin Genet. 2013;84(2):132–41.

3. Ferrari S, Di Ioro E, Barbaro V, Ponzin D, Sorrentino FS, Parmeggiani F. Retinitis pigmentosa: genes and disease mechanisms. Curr Genom. 2011;12(4):238–49.
4. Hamel C. Retinitis pigmentosa. Orphanet J Rare Dis. 2006;1:40.
5. Hartong DT, Berson EL, Dryja T. Retinitis pigmentosa. Lancet. 2006;368:1795–809.
6. Rivolta C, Sharon D, DeAngelis MM, Dryja TP. Retinitis pigmentosa and allied diseases: numerous diseases, genes, and inheritance patterns. Hum Mol Genet. 2002;11(10):1219–27.

Chapter 20
Cone-Rod Dystrophies

Salman A. Rahman and Veeral S. Shah

20.1 Definitions

Cone-rod dystrophy (CRD) is a progressive degenerative disorder predominantly of retinal cones with varying patterns of inheritance.

20.2 Symptoms

Early: Decreased vision, dyschromatopsia, photophobia, and central scotoma
Late: Nyctalopia and progressive loss of peripheral vision

20.3 Signs

- *Early:* Normal-appearing fundus or fine, pigmentary changes (possibly resembling a bull's-eye maculopathy), and abnormal testing (OCT, FAF, ERG) (Fig. 20.1).
- *Late:* Vessel attenuation, waxy pallor of the optic nerve head, pigmentary changes resembling bone spicules in periphery and macula, RPE atrophy, and abnormal testing (ERG) (Fig. 20.2). Rod photoreceptor involvement will frequently occur late in cone dystrophy.

S.A. Rahman, MD • V.S. Shah, MD, PhD (✉)
Department of Ophthalmology, Baylor College of Medicine,
Texas Children's Hospital, Houston, TX, USA
e-mail: vsshah@texaschildrens.org

C.A. Medina et al. (eds.), *Manual of Retinal Diseases: A Guide to Diagnosis and Management*, DOI 10.1007/978-3-319-20460-4_20

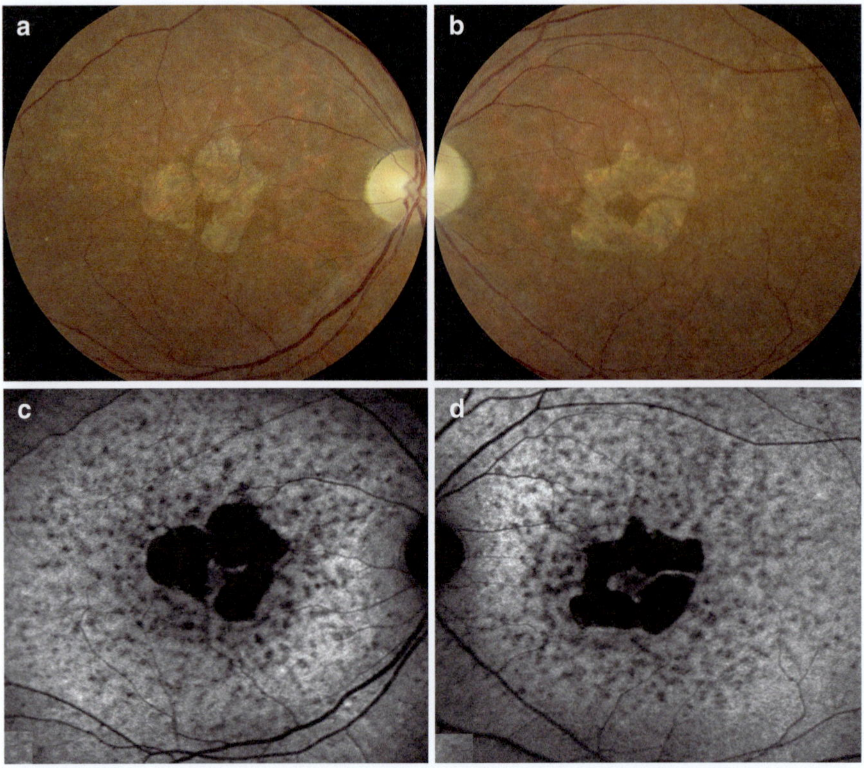

Fig. 20.1 Fundus photos of advanced "bull's-eye" maculopathy with discrete parafoveal RPE atrophy (**a**, right eye; **b**, left eye). Fundus autofluorescence shows a parafoveal ring of increased autofluorescence and central foveolar atrophy (**c**, right eye; **d**, left eye) (Courtesy of Hassan Rahman, MD, Houston, TX)

20.4 Epidemiology

Prevalence 1 in 40,000. One study found the mean age of onset as 12 years and mean age of legal blindness at 35 years. Cone dystrophy has been described in the literature and possibly represents a disease in the spectrum of cone rod dystrophy rather than an isolated disease process.

20.5 Inheritance

- Autosomal dominant, autosomal recessive, or X-linked depending on mutation.
  - Autosomal dominant: GUCY2D (also associated with Leber's congenital amaurosis) and CRX.

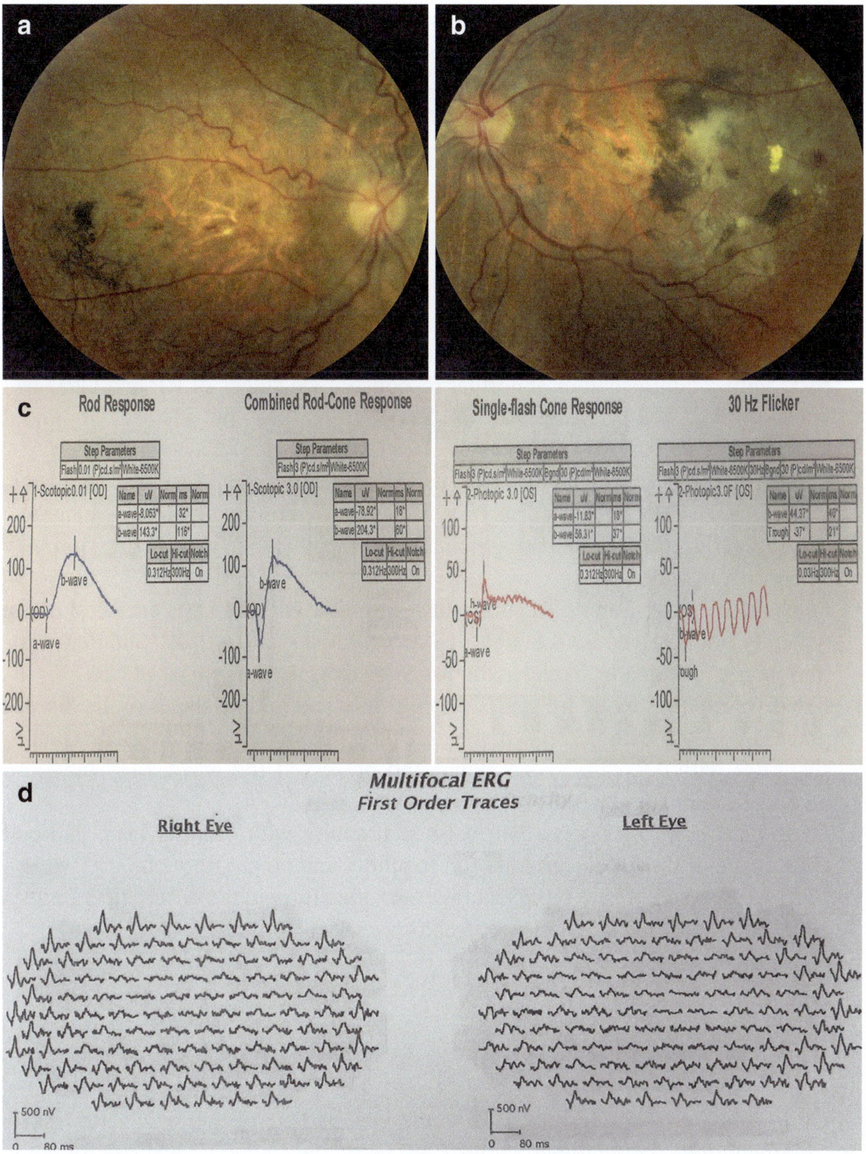

Fig. 20.2 Fundus photos of cone dystrophy (**a**, right eye; **b**, left eye), with a representative ERG demonstrating marked reduced and delay cone response with relatively normal rod response (**c**). Multifocal ERG demonstrated reduced waveform centrally (**d**) (Courtesy of Emmanuel Chang, MD, and Byron Lam, MD, Houston, TX)

- Autosomal recessive: ABCA4 (associated with Stargardt disease) causes 30–60 % of autosomal recessive disease.
- X-linked: RPGR (associated with X-linked RP). Also associated with both Bardet-Biedl syndrome and spinocerebellar atrophy type 7.

- Additional information available at the RetNet website.

20.6 Differential Diagnosis

- *Retinitis pigmentosa:* Initial symptom is nyctalopia with normal central vision. ERG with a diminished or abnormal response. Late stages of RP and CRD can appear very similar with flat ERGs. Differentiate by history of initial symptoms.
- *Leber's congenital amaurosis:* Can have reduced function of cones and rods. Poor visual acuity identified at or within a few months of birth, nystagmus, severely reduced ERG, and a pigmentary retinopathy. Delay in progression may be consistent with CRD.
- *Stargardt disease:* Early CRD may share a similar appearance. Peripheral retina typically not involved with Stargardt. Also, whitish-yellow flecks and dark choroid on FA, which are characteristic for Stargardt, are not typical of CRD.
- *Cone dystrophies:* Rods are spared during early and middle stages of the disease process. Present with decreased visual acuity, photophobia, and dyschromatopsia. ERG with decreased cone signal and preserved rod wave. May have rod involvement in later stages.
- *Congenital color blindness:* Normal visual acuity with onset at birth. Normal appearance of the fundus, normal rod function, and no progression.
- *Bull's-eye maculopathy:* If present on exam, then refer to the differential diagnosis of bull's-eye maculopathy in the chloroquine toxicity section.

20.7 Workup/Testing

Obtain a detailed family history. Due to the genetic heterogeneity, genetic testing not routinely done, but commercial tests are being developed to evaluate for some of the more frequently involved genes. Perform a complete ophthalmic exam including evaluation of color vision and dilated fundus examination. Consider obtaining fundus autofluorescence, (FAF) electroretinogram (ERG), and optical coherence tomography (OCT). These may show the following characteristic findings:

- FAF – may help identify RPE disturbances
- ERG – predominantly decreased photopic responses (flicker response, single-flash photopic response) early with development of abnormal rod signals. Severely reduced or flat ERG in late stage
- OCT – abnormalities of outer retinal layers

20.8 Prognosis and Management

Visual prognosis is poor with mean age of legal blindness at 35 years old. Tinted spectacles and miotic drops may help minimize photophobia. Genetic counseling and low vision aids should be prescribed as needed. Consider repeating ERG 1–2 years after initial diagnosis is made.

20.9 Follow-Up

Annually.

References and Suggested Reading

1. Hamel CP. Cone rod dystrophies. Orphanet J Rare Dis. 2007;2:7.
2. Michaelides M, Hardcastle AJ, Hunt DM, Moore AT. Progressive cone and cone-rod dystrophies: phenotypes and underlying molecular genetic basis. Surv Ophthalmol. 2006;51(3):232–58.
3. Thiadens AAHJ, Phan TML, Zekveld-Vroon RC, Leroy BP, Van den Born LI, et al. Clinical course, genetic etiology, and visual outcome in cone and cone-rod dystrophy. Ophthalmology. 2012;119(4):819–26.

Chapter 21
Stargardt Disease

Salman A. Rahman and Veeral S. Shah

21.1 Definition

Stargardt disease is the most common juvenile-onset macular dystrophy.

21.2 Symptoms

- Decreased vision (slow, progressive, bilateral vision loss).
- Acquired dyschromatopsia.

21.3 Signs

- *Early:* Vision decreases prior to visible macular changes. Bilateral, variable pigmentary changes in the macula (including bull's-eye maculopathy or beaten bronze metal appearance), yellow-white flecks at the level of the RPE in the posterior pole and mid-periphery (classically in a pisciform shape) with a distribution that typically expands radially from the fovea (Fig. 21.1).
- *Late:* Atrophy of RPE and choriocapillaris, abnormal testing (ERG, EOG), resorbed flecks, "dark or silent" choroid.

S.A. Rahman, MD • V.S. Shah, MD, PhD (✉)
Department of Ophthalmology, Baylor College of Medicine,
Texas Children's Hospital, Houston, TX, USA
e-mail: vsshah@texaschildrens.org

C.A. Medina et al. (eds.), *Manual of Retinal Diseases: A Guide to Diagnosis and Management*, DOI 10.1007/978-3-319-20460-4_21

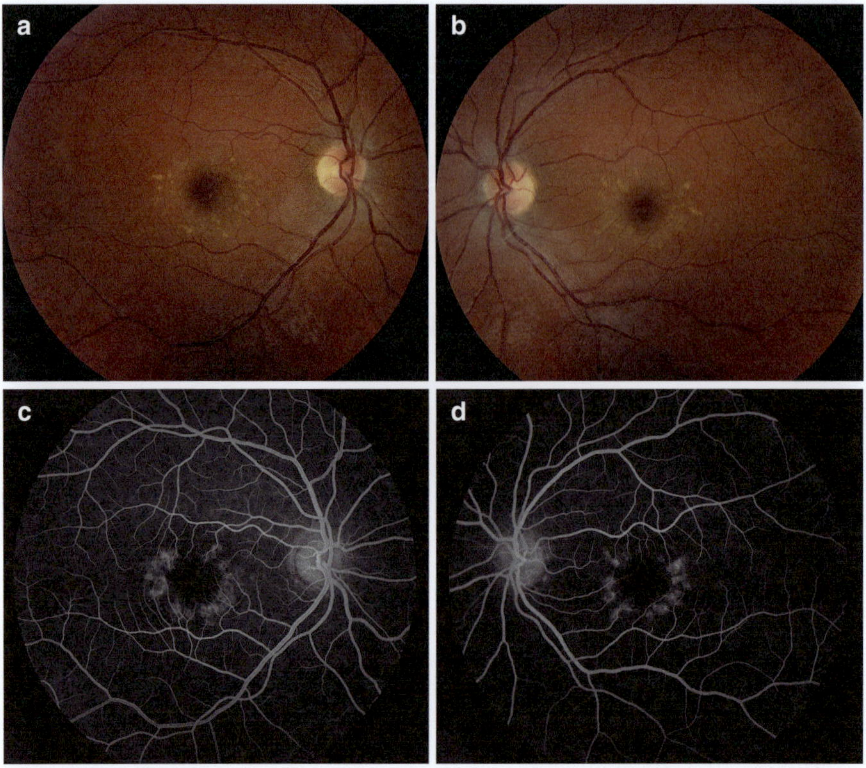

Fig. 21.1 Fundus photo of Stargardt's disease demonstrates a number of yellow, discrete "pisciform" fleck at the level of the RPE and clustered in posterior pole (**a**, right eye; **b**, left eye). Mid-phase fluorescein angiogram shows parafoveal pisciform flecks with features of "dark" choroid (**c**, right eye; **d**, left eye)

21.4 Epidemiology

It is the most common juvenile-onset macular dystrophy (age of onset between 10 and 20 years) with prevalence of 1 in 8,000 to 1 in 10,000 in the United States.

21.5 Inheritance

Primarily autosomal recessive caused by a mutation in the ABCA4 gene (95 % of cases) that codes for an ATP-binding cassette transmembrane protein in the photoreceptor discs. Five percent of cases are caused by mutations in EVOL4, PRPH2, or BEST1 genes.

21.6 Differential Diagnosis

- *Age-related macular degeneration* – Age of onset will differ; drusen are hyperfluorescent on FA.
- *Cone-rod dystrophy* – Early cone-rod dystrophy may share a similar appearance. Peripheral retina typically not involved with Stargardt. Also, whitish-yellow flecks and dark choroid on FA, which are characteristic for Stargardt, are not typical of cone-rod dystrophy.
- *Fundus albipunctatus* – Normal visual acuity. Diffuse, small, white lesions in mid-peripheral fundus that spare the fovea. Do not develop atrophy of RPE or choriocapillaris or pigmentary changes.
- *Retinitis punctata albescens* – Variant of RP with nyctalopia and progressively worsening vision and visual field. Similar fundus appearance to fundus albipunctatus.
- *Chloroquine/hydroxychloroquine* – History of use with increased macular pigmentation and bull's-eye maculopathy.

21.7 Etiology

Abnormal deposition of lipofuscin in RPE due to accumulation of all-trans-retinal leading to RPE degeneration and subsequent photoreceptor degeneration. First described by Karl Stargardt in 1909.

Fundus flavimaculatus was initially described in 1963 by Franceschetti to describe ill-defined yellow-white flecks in the deep retinal layers of the posterior pole. Stargardt disease and fundus flavimaculatus later found to be the same disease. Fundus flavimaculatus diagnosis may be reserved for cases with diffusely scattered flecks.

21.8 Workup/Testing

Obtain a detailed family history and consider genetic testing with genotyping microarray to identify mutations in ABCA4. A complete ophthalmic examination including dilated fundus exam should be performed. Consider fundus autofluorescence (FAF), fluorescein angiography (FA), optical coherence tomography (OCT), electroretinogram (ERG), electrooculogram (EOG), and formal perimetry. These may show the following characteristic findings:

- FAF – Hyperautofluorescence due to lipofuscin accumulation.
- FA – Characteristic dark choroid due to blockage of fluorescence by lipofuscin in the RPE, can be present in 50–80 % of patients.

- OCT – Absence of the photoreceptor outer segments and IS/OS junction at the fovea.
- ERG – Abnormally late (scotopic and photopic ERG may be decreased; pattern ERG can be abnormal) in the disease.
- EOG – Subnormal ratios for light peak to dark trough.
- Perimetry – Central field loss that can involve the periphery with disease progression.

21.9 Prognosis and Management

Visual acuity ranges from 20/20 to 20/400. Moderate visual acuity may be retained in one eye. Patients that present later (>20 years old) with visual acuity of 20/40 or better tend to maintain visual acuity >20/200 longer than patients who present <20 years old. Absence of foveal atrophy is associated with good vision.

Genetic counseling and low vision aids should be prescribed as needed.

Experimental gene replacement studies are underway.

21.10 Follow-Up

Annually.

References and Suggested Reading

1. Abdollahi SH, Hirose T. Stargardt-Fundus flavimaculatus: recent advancements and treatment. Semin Ophthalmol. 2013;28(5–6):372–6.
2. Koenekoop RK, Lopez I, den Hollander AI, Allikmets R, Cremers FPM. Genetic testing for retinal dystrophies and dysfunctions: benefits, dilemmas, and solutions. Clin Exp Ophthalmol. 2007;35:473–85.
3. Lois N, Holder GE, Bunce C, Fitzke FW, Bird AC. Phenotypic subtypes of Stargardt macular dystrophy-fundus flavimaculatus. Arch Ophthalmol. 2001;119:359–69.
4. Rotenstreich Y, Fishman GA, Anderson RJ. Visual acuity loss and clinical observations in a large series of patients with Stargardt disease. Ophthalmology. 2003;110(6):1151–8.
5. Walia S, Fishman GA. Natural history of phenotypic changes in Stargardt macular dystrophy. Ophthalmic Genet. 2009;30:63–8.

Chapter 22
Best's Disease

Salman A. Rahman and Veeral S. Shah

22.1 Definitions

Best's vitelliform macular dystrophy (BVMD) due to to abnormal processing of photoreceptor outer segments and lipofuscin accumulation in RPE cells.

22.2 Symptoms

Decreased visual acuity, metamorphopsia, or asymptomatic.

22.3 Signs (6 Stages): (Fig. 22.1)

- *Early:*
  - *Stage 1* – Previtelliform: Initial stage with a normal fovea or mild RPE changes (abnormal testing) (EOG with reduced ratio of light peak to dark trough [Arden ratio], normal ERG),
  - *Stage 2* – Vitelliform elevated subretinal yellowish macular lesion composed of lipofuscin at the fovea
  - *Stage 3* – Pseudohypopyon layering of lipofuscin within a serous subretinal cavity yellowish lesion breaks up
  - *Stage 4* – "Scrambled egg" or "vitelliruptive" deposition
    Typically a single lesion is observed; multifocal lesions are rare.

S.A. Rahman, MD • V.S. Shah, MD, PhD (✉)
Department of Ophthalmology, Baylor College of Medicine,
Texas Children's Hospital, Houston, TX, USA
e-mail: vsshah@texaschildrens.org

C.A. Medina et al. (eds.), *Manual of Retinal Diseases: A Guide to Diagnosis and Management*, DOI 10.1007/978-3-319-20460-4_22

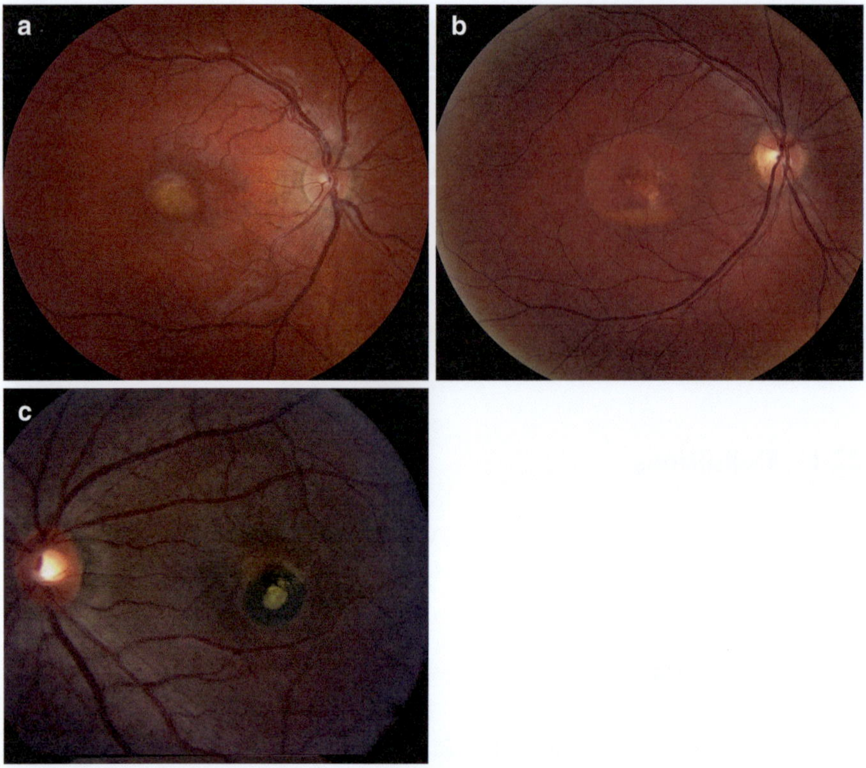

Fig. 22.1 Fundus photo of Best disease vitelliform stage, characterized with an "egg yolk" deposition at the level RPE (**a**). In the pseudohypopyon stage of Best disease, there is a subretinal layering of the yellowish lipofuscin (**b**). Progression to the vitelliruptive stage leads in the breakdown of deposition with a "scrambled egg" appearance and RPE atrophy (**c**) (Courtesy of Hassan Rahman, MD, and Emmanuel Chang, MD, Houston, TX)

- *Late:*
  - *Stage 5* – Chorioretinal atrophy.
  - *Stage 6* – 2–9 % develop choroidal neovascular membrane with scarring.

22.4 Epidemiology

Onset in childhood, but may not present until later in life.

22.5 Inheritance

Autosomal dominant – BEST1 gene (chromosome 11q12, previously called VMD2) that encodes bestrophin-1, which forms a Ca2+ activated Cl– channel. Bestrophin-1 is found on the basolateral plasma membrane and intracellularly in RPE cells. Variable penetrance and expressivity.

22.6 Differential Diagnosis

- *Age-related macular degeneration* – Older age of onset and AMD will not evolve through the stages characteristic of Best disease. More likely to have multifocal findings (scattered drusen) than with Best.
- *Adult-onset vitelliform dystrophy* – Type of pattern dystrophy characterized by onset at a later age (mean fifth decade) with slower disease progression. Patients are asymptomatic or complain of mild blurriness and metamorphopsia. Typically isolated, but has been linked to mutations in BEST1 and peripherin/RDS. Visual acuity usually good but can decline with RPE atrophy or CNV formation (up to 15 %). Fundus exam reveals bilateral, solitary, subfoveal, round yellow lesion sometimes with a central pigmented spot (1/3-1/2 DD in size) that do not break up. Normal or slightly subnormal EOG. FA shows central area of hypofluorescence surrounded by a small ring of hyperfluorescence. FAF shows variable hyperautofluorescence. OCT with a hyperreflective lesion causing an exudative detachment of the neurosensory retina. Treat CNV if present.
- *Basal laminar (cuticular) drusen* – Variable-sized drusen surround this area of confluent drusen that may have a vitelliform appearance.

22.7 Etiology

Disruption of fluid transport in RPE cells due to dysfunction of bestrophin-1 leading to abnormal processing of photoreceptor outer segments and lipofuscin accumulation in RPE cells. The major fluorescent component of lipofuscin is A2E (N-retinylidene-N-retinylethanolamine), which is a retinal metabolite.

22.8 Workup/Testing

Obtain a detailed family history and consider examining family members. A complete ophthalmic examination including dilated fundus exam should be performed. Consider fundus autofluorescence (FAF), fluorescein angiography (FA), optical coherence tomography (OCT), electroretinogram (ERG), electrooculogram (EOG), and formal perimetry (Fig. 22.2). These may show the following characteristic findings:

- FA – Blockage from vitelliform material and hyperfluorescence in areas of RPE atrophy.
- FAF – Hyperautofluorescence due to lipofuscin and hypoautofluorescence in areas of RPE atrophy.
- OCT – reveals a subretinal lesion causing a central macular detachment of the neurosensory retina in the vitelliform, scrambled egg, and pseudohypopyon stages. Scars and CNVM will appear hyperreflective, and the transparent fluid during the pseudohypopyon stage is hyporeflective on OCT.
- ERG – Abnormally late (scotopic and photopic ERG may be decreased; pattern ERG can be abnormal) in the disease.
- EOG with reduced Arden ratio (ratio of light peak to dark trough).

22.9 Prognosis and Management

Visual acuity mildly decreased during early stages. Moderate-severe decrease in vision during the later stages if scarring or CNV forms (20/100–20/200). Can treat CNV with intravitreal anti-vascular endothelial growth factor agents, laser photocoagulation (outside fovea), or PDT (no clinical trials for anti-VEGF medications and CNV in Best disease). Genetic counseling.

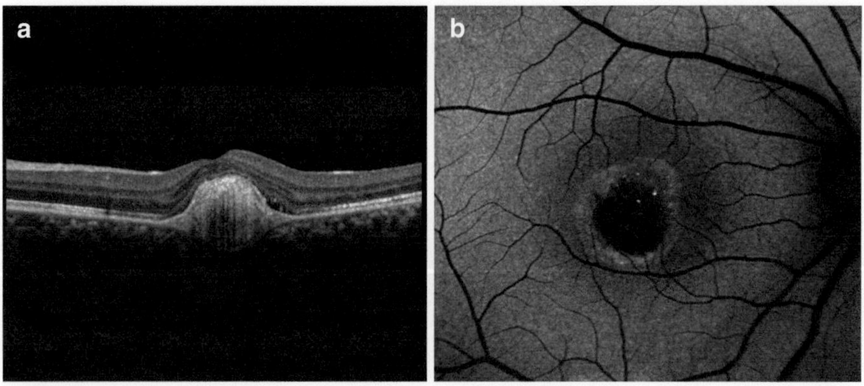

Fig. 22.2 Cross-sectional OCT of Best disease in the vitelliform stage demonstrates large hyperreflective proteinaceous deposition (**a**). (**b**) At late stage of Best disease, fundus autofluorescence shows a parafoveal ring of increased autofluorescence and central foveolar atrophy (**b**) (Courtesy of Emmanuel Chang, MD, Houston, TX)

22.10 Follow-Up

Annually.

References and Suggested Reading

1. Boon CJF, Klevering BJ, Leroy BP, Hoyng CB, Keunen JEE, den Hollander AI. The spectrum of ocular phenotypes caused by mutations in the BEST1 gene. Prog Retin Eye Res. 2009;28:187–205.
2. Hartzell HC, Qu Z, Yu K, Xiao Q, Chien L. Molecular physiology of bestrophins: multifunctional membrane proteins linked to best disease and other retinopathies. Physiol Rev. 2008;88:639–72.
3. Marmorstein AD, Marmorstein LY, Rayborn M, Wang X, Hollyfield JG, Petrukhin K. Bestrophin, the product of the best vitelliform dystrophy gene (vmd2), localizes to the basolateral plasma membrane of the retinal pigment epithelium. Proc Natl Acad Sci U S A. 2000;97(23):12758–63.
4. Xiao Q, Hartzell HC, Yu K. Bestrophins and retinopathies. Pflugers Arch. 2010;460(2): 559–69.

Chapter 23
Pattern Dystrophy

Veeral S. Shah

23.1 Definitions

Synonymous names: Pattern dystrophy or pattern-like dystrophy; butterfly dystrophy; acquired vitelliform deposit.

23.2 Symptoms

Spectrum from asymptomatic, mild metamorphopsia, or gradual but limited central vision loss.

23.3 Signs

- Visual acuity testing typically is normal until the fifth or sixth decade, where they may become symptomatic with mild metamorphopsia or mild progressive central vision loss. Peripheral vision is spared and demonstrated on Amsler grid and visual field testing.
- Multiple clinical subtypes; characteristically, there can be yellow, orange, or brown sub-RPE deposition in various patterns.
  - *Butterfly dystrophy.* It is the most common and is a bilateral, tri-radial, or peculiar "butterfly" pattern of yellow pigment deposition at the level of the

V.S. Shah,MD, PhD
Department of Ophthalmology, Baylor College of Medicine,
Texas Children's Hospital, Houston, TX, USA
e-mail: vsshah@texaschildrens.org

C.A. Medina et al. (eds.), *Manual of Retinal Diseases: A Guide to Diagnosis and Management*, DOI 10.1007/978-3-319-20460-4_23

RPE in the central macula. Both fluorescein angiogram and OCT demonstrate loss of RPE and photoreceptor layers adjacent to the pigmentary deposition.
- *Adult-onset foveomacular vitelliform dystrophy.* Circular, yellowish vitelliform deposition in the central macula which is a result of accumulation of lipofuscin pigments and an infiltration of pigment engulfing macrophages leading to local RPE and photoreceptor loss in the central macula.
- *Reticular dystrophy of RPE.* Characteristic yellowish-gray deposition in a fishnet or lattice-like network located in the central macula and extending in the periphery.
- *Multifocal pattern dystrophy syndrome simulating fundus flavimaculatus.* Yellow depositions found at the level of the RPE that resemble fleck typical of Stargardt's disease. Fluorescein angiogram is helpful with the absence of dark choroid, which is a sign of Stargardt's disease.
- *Fundus pulverulentus.* Large radial, coarse pigmentary changes that have a "punctiform" or mottled appearance in the central macula RPE. Fluorescein angiogram demonstrates large areas of hypofluorescence due to pigmentary deposition at the level of the RPE.

• Pedigree studies have demonstrated that there is variable expression and penetrance of pattern dystrophy, such that individuals may have different patterns in a given family and have different patterns in the fellow eye and temporally patterns can change to another clinical subtype.

23.4 Epidemiology

Onset typically begins in middle ages or even later in life.

23.5 Inheritance

Pattern dystrophy represents heterogeneous group of related conditions that are inherited in an autosomal dominant manner. Ten percent of these patients have a mutation in the PRPH2 (peripherin/RDS) on the short arm of chromosome 6. Mutations in PRPH2 have multiple phenotypes and penetrance that are linked to other retinal degenerative disease, thus not exclusive to pattern dystrophies. Pattern dystrophy has also been linked to the VDM2 gene.

23.6 Differential Diagnosis

• Stargardt's disease – fundus flavimaculatus
• Early Best vitelliform disease
• Dominant drusen (malattia leventinese)
• Age-related macular degeneration

23.7 Etiology

Pattern dystrophies are caused by various mutations in the human retinal degeneration slow (RDS)/peripherin gene chromosome 6P21.2. RDS/peripherin gene encodes for a photoreceptor glycoprotein that is involved in the development and maintenance of the photoreceptor outer segment layer. It is hypothesized that mutations in this gene disrupt the integrity of the photoreceptor membrane in the macula resulting in the collection of extracellular material derived from the photoreceptor outer segment and the RPE. Accumulation of this deposit progressively results in RPE hypertrophy and then subsequent atrophy and attenuation.

23.8 Workup/Testing

Given the autosomal dominant inheritance pattern, it is important to obtain a detailed family history and consider examining family members. Confrontational and formalized visual field testing is typically normal with minimal depression in sensitivity of the macular region. Consider fundus autofluorescence (FAF), fluorescein angiography (FA), optical coherence tomography (OCT), electroretinogram (ERG), electrooculogram (EOG), and formal perimetry. These may show the following characteristic findings:

- FAF – Hyperautofluorescence due to lipofuscin and hypoautofluorescence in areas of RPE atrophy and closely follows the multiple clinical subtype patterns (Fig. 23.1).
- FA – Pattern dystrophy demonstrates hypofluorescence with blockage from extracellular deposition and hyperfluorescence in areas of RPE atrophy.
- OCT – Can show hyperreflectivity between the RPE, Bruch's complex, and the IS/OSS junction for receptors.
- ERG/EOG – Full-field flash ERG is normal, and EOGs may be normal to mildly subnormal (with a light to dark ratio of greater than 150 %).

23.9 Prognosis and Management

Visual prognosis of pattern dystrophy is quite good even in the setting of significant morphological changes in the central macula. The likelihood of retaining central vision in at least one eye is excellent. Genetic counseling can be obtained to identify genetic mutations, but no effective treatment is available at this time. There is a lifetime risk of 18 % of developing secondary choroidal neovascularization; secondary choroidal neovascularization can be managed and treated with anti-VEGF therapy.

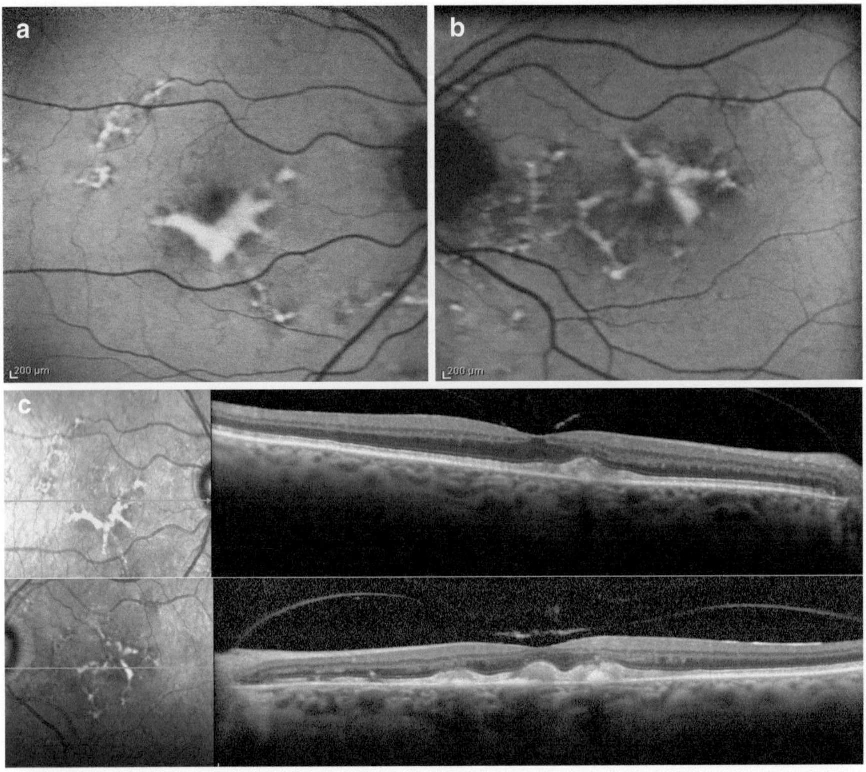

Fig. 23.1 Autofluorescence imaging of pattern dystrophy shows areas of discrete hyperautofluorescence and hypoautofluorescence (**a**, right eye; **b**, left eye). Cross-sectional OCT imaging shows hyperreflective proteinaceous material between the RPE, Bruch's complex, and the IS/OS junction (**c**, *upper panel*, right eye; *lower panel*, left eye)

23.10 Follow-Up

Annual follow-up.

References and Suggested Reading

1. Ayazi S, Fagan R. Pattern dystrophy of pigment epithelium. Retina. 1981;1:287–9.
2. Boon CJ, den Hollnader AI, Hoyng CB. The spectrum of retinal dystrophies caused by mutations in the peripherin/RDS gene. Prog Retin Eye Res. 2008;27:213–35.
3. Boon CJ, van Schooneveld MJ, den Hollander AI, et al. Mutations in the peripherin/RDS gene are an important cause of multifocal pattern dystrophy simulating STGD1/fundus flavimaculatus. Br J Ophthalmol. 2007;91:1504–11.
4. Chen MS, Chang CC, Tsai TH, et al. Reticular dystrophy of the retinal pigment epithelium. J Formos Med Assoc. 2007;106:490–4.

5. Deutman AF, Blommestein JD, Henkes HE, et al. Butterfly-shaped pigment dystrophy of the fovea. Arch Ophthalmol. 1970;83:558–69.
6. Gaffe GJ, Schatz H. Histopathologic features of adult-onset foveomacular pigment epithelial dystrophy. Arch Ophthalmol. 1988;106:958–60.
7. Kohl S, Christ-Adler M, Apfelstedt-Sylla E, et al. RDS/peripherin gene mutations are frequent causes of central retinal dystrophies. J Med Genet. 1997;34:620–6.
8. Parodi MB. Choroidal neovascularization in fundus pulverulentus. Acta Ophthalmol Scan. 2002;80:559–60.
9. Wells J, Wroblewski J, Keen J, et al. Mutations in the human retinal degeneration slow (RDS) gene can cause either retinitis pigmentosa or macular dystrophy. Nat Genet. 1993;3:213–8.
10. Yang Z, Li Y, Jiang L, Karan G, et al. A novel RDS/peripherin gene mutation associated with diverse macular phenotypes. Ophthalmic Genet. 2004;25:133–45.
11. Zhang K, Garibaldi DC, Li Y, et al. Butterfly-shaped pattern dystrophy: a genetic, clinical, and histopathological report. Ophthalmic Mol Genet. 2002;120:485–90.

Chapter 24
Congenital Stationary Night Blindness

Veeral S. Shah

24.1 Definition

Congenital stationary night blindness (CSNB); Hemeralopia-myopia disease.

Congenital stationary night blindness (CNSB) is a clinically and genetic diverse group of nonprogressive retinal disorders that is characterized by stable poor vision in low light (night blindness). CNSB can be classified either functionally by electrophysiology or fundus phenotypes. ERG can distinguish a "complete" form or CNSB type 1 with absent rod function, from an "incomplete" form or CNSB type 2 with reduced rod and cone function. Phenotypically, CNSB can have a normal appearing fundus or an abnormal fundus (includes Oguchi's disease and fundus albipunctatus) (Fig. 24.1).

24.2 Symptoms

Nonprogressive decreased vision and nyctalopia

24.3 Signs

- Visual acuity can range from normal to subnormal vision with impaired night vision. CSNB patients can also have high myopia, strabismus, and nystagmus. Dilated fundus exam can be normal or abnormal.

V.S. Shah, MD, PhD
Department of Ophthalmology, Baylor College of Medicine,
Texas Children's Hospital, Houston, TX, USA
e-mail: vsshah@texaschildrens.org

C.A. Medina et al. (eds.), *Manual of Retinal Diseases: A Guide to Diagnosis and Management*, DOI 10.1007/978-3-319-20460-4_24

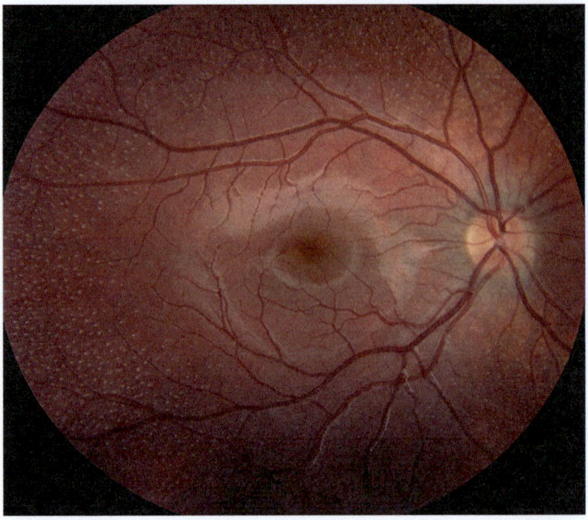

Fig. 24.1 CSNB. Diffuse, small, white lesions in mid-peripheral fundus that spare the macula diagnostic of fundus albipunctatus

- *Abnormal fundus exam.*
  - *Fundus albipunctatus* is a retinal disorder with normal visual acuity and fundus with diffuse, small, white lesions in the mid-peripheral fundus that spare the macula. This disorder does not develop atrophy of RPE/choriocapillaris or pigmentary changes.
  - *Oguchi's disease* is a retinal disorder where the fundus has a metallic silver sheen with accentuated retinal vessels. With prolonged dark adaptation, this sheen disappears, and the fundus appears normal which is referred to as the *Mizuo-Nakamura phenomenon.*

24.4 Epidemiology

Rare, prevalence is unknown.

24.5 Inheritance/Etiology

CSNB has multiple modes of inheritance including autosomal dominant, autosomal recessive, and X-linked (Table 24.1). The X-linked form is the most common and can be distinguished from the autosomal form by the association of myopia.

- *Fundus albipunctatus* is an autosomal recessive condition with a mutation in RDH5 gene on chromosome 12q13-q14. The RDH5 gene encodes for 11-cis-retinol dehydrogenase enzyme, and mutation in this gene is believed to affect the rate of photoreceptor recovery

Table 24.1 List of genes associated with CSNB and their pattern of inheritance

Genes	Location	Inheritance
GNAT1	3p22	Autosomal dominant CSNB
RHO	3q21-24	Autosomal dominant CSNB
PDE6B	4p16.3	Autosomal dominant CSNB
NYX	Xp11.4	X-linked CSNB
CACNA1F	Xp11.23	X-linked CSNB
GRM6	5q35	Autosomal recessive CSNB
TRPM1	15q13.3	Autosomal recessive CSNB
CABP4	11q13.1	Autosomal recessive CSNB
SLC24A1	15q22.31	Autosomal recessive CSNB
GPR179	17q12	Autosomal recessive CSNB
LRIT3	4q25	Autosomal recessive CSNB

– *Oguchi's disease* is an autosomal recessive disorder with a mutation in either SAG or ROK, which encodes the gene product arrestin and rhodopsin kinase, respectively. The photoreceptor pigments are normal; however, defects in these genes presumably affect phototransduction in the retina resulting in abnormal ERGs.

24.6 Differential Diagnosis

- *Cone-rod dystrophy*: Early cone-rod dystrophy may share a similar appearance but has a progressive clinical course.
- *Retinitis punctata albescens*: Variant of RP with nyctalopia and progressively worsening vision and visual field. Similar fundus appearance to fundus albipunctatus.

24.7 Workup/Testing

Obtain a detailed family history and complete ophthalmic exam including visual field, color vision, and dilated fundus exam. Fundus albipunctatus can present normal visual acuity, no visual field defect, normal caliber of retinal vessels, and normal perfusion of optic disc.

Dark adaptometry is a test to examine vision in the dark in which a patient acclimates in a dark room and then is exposed to different intensities of dim light and alerts examiner when they can see the light. The results are graphed and are compared to a normal dark adaptation curve. Dark adaptometry in both rod and cones is delayed from reaching threshold.

Consider fundus autofluorescence (FAF), fluorescein angiography (FA), optical coherence tomography (OCT), electroretinogram (ERG), electrooculogram (EOG), and formal perimetry. These may show the following characteristic findings:

- FAF – can have hyperautofluorescence due to lipofuscin accumulation.
- OCT – can reveal a smaller or absence of the photoreceptor outer segments and IS/OS junction at the fovea.
- ERG – abnormal with reduced b-wave and a-wave in both scotopic and photopic conditions. In some conditions like Oguchi's disease and fundus albipunctatus, dark-adapted ERGs normalize.

24.8 Prognosis and Management

Visual acuity ranges from normal to 20/200, with severe vision loss associated to high myopia. Unlike retinitis pigmentosa, the visual function is stable throughout life. Low vision aids as needed. Genetic testing and counseling is recommended. At this time, there is no available treatment.

24.9 Follow-Up

Annually

References and Suggested Reading

1. Berger W, Kloeckener-Gruissem B, Neidhardt J. The molecular basis of human retinal and vitreoretinal diseases. Prog Retin Eye Res. 2010;29(5):335–75.
2. Boycott K, Pearce W, Musarella M, Weleber R, Maybaum T, Birch D, Miyake Y, Young R, Bech-Hansen N. Evidence for genetic heterogeneity in X-linked congenital stationary night blindness. Am J Hum Genet. 1998;62(4):865–75.
3. Khouri G, Mets MB, Smith VC, Wendell M, Pass AS. X-linked congenital stationary night blindness: review and report of a family with hyperopia. Arch Ophthalmol. 1988;106: 1417–22.
4. Miyake Y, Yagasaki K, Horiguchi M, Kawase Y, Kanda T. Congenital stationary night blindness with negative electroretinogram: a new classification. Arch Ophthalmol. 1986;104: 1013–20.
5. Peachey NS, Ray TA, Florijn R, Rowe LB, Sjoerdsma T, Contreras-Alcantara S, Baba K, Tosini G, Pozdeyev N, Iuvone PM, Bojang Jr P, Pearring JN, Simonsz HJ, van Genderen M, Birch DG, Traboulsi EI, Dorfman A, Lopez I, Ren H, Goldberg AF, Nishina PM, Lachapelle P, McCall MA, Koenekoop RK, Bergen AA, Kamermans M, Gregg RG. GPR179 is required for depolarizing bipolar cell function and is mutated in autosomal-recessive complete congenital stationary night blindness. Am J Hum Genet. 2012;90(2):331–9.
6. Pusch CM, Zeitz C, Brandau O, Pesch K, Achatz H, Feil S, Scharfe C, Maurer J, Jacobi F, Pinckers A, Andreasson S, Hardcastle A, Wissinger B, Berger W, Meindl A. The complete form of X-linked congenital stationary night blindness is caused by mutations in a gene encoding a leucine-rich repeat protein. Nat Genet. 2000;26(3):324–7.

Chapter 25
Choroideremia

Veeral S. Shah

25.1 Definitions

Choroideremia is hereditary progressive retinal degeneration that specifically affects the choriocapillaris, retinal pigment epithelium-photoreceptor complex, and the retina.

25.2 Symptoms

Nyctalopia (night blindness) or dark adaptation in males between the ages 5 and 10 with a slow and progressive peripheral visual field loss.

25.3 Signs

- *Early*: mid-peripheral rods are severely affected and exhibit a "salt and pepper" RPE mottling extending from the equator to the posterior pole. Female carriers tend to a nonprogressive "salt and pepper" RPE mottling, with normal choroidal vasculature.
- *Late*: progressive atrophy resulting to RPE dropouts that aggregate and collectively progress centrally to the posterior pole.

V.S. Shah, MD, PhD
Department of Ophthalmology, Baylor College of Medicine,
Texas Children's Hospital, Houston, TX, USA
e-mail: vsshah@texaschildrens.org

C.A. Medina et al. (eds.), *Manual of Retinal Diseases: A Guide to Diagnosis and Management*, DOI 10.1007/978-3-319-20460-4_25

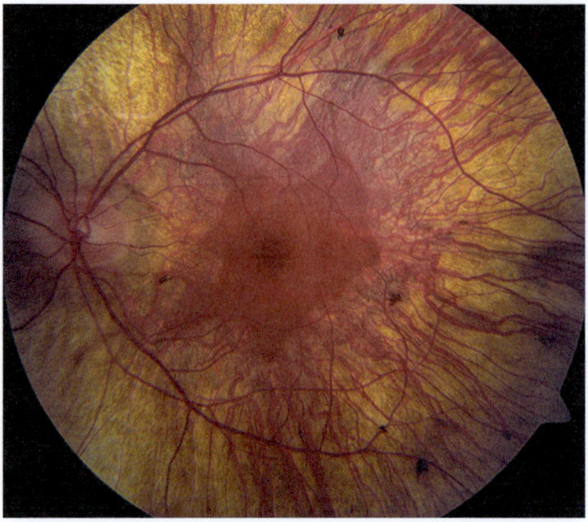

Fig. 25.1 Choroideremia. Typical fundus features at terminal stage. Note atrophy of choroidal vessels revealing yellow-white reflex of the underlying sclera that spares the macula (Fig. 25.1) (Courtesy of Elias Traboulsi, MD, Cleveland, OH)

- *Terminal stage*: the atrophy reveals the choroidal vessels and the yellow-white reflex of the underlying sclera but spares the macula and scattered areas of intact choroid (Fig. 25.1).

25.4 Epidemiology

The onset of symptoms typically occurs in the first and second decade of life, most commonly affecting males between the ages of 5 and 10.

25.5 Inheritance

Choroideremia is an X-linked recessive retinal degeneration that affects the RPE, retina, and choroid. Thus, males are affected and females are carriers. Choroideremia is caused by various mutations in the CHM gene found on Xq21.2 and encodes Rab escort protein-1 (REP-1).

25.6 Differential Diagnosis

- *Gyrate atrophy*: may share a similar appearance at final stages of choroideremia, but the mode of inheritance can be a distinguishing factor.

- *Retinitis pigmentosa*: have bone spicule degeneration and attenuated retinal vessels, neither typical of choroideremia.
- *Salt and pepper retinopathy*: history TORCH or metabolic disease.

25.7 Etiology

Mutations in the *CHM* gene lead to a functional loss or knockdown of REP-1 protein, thus preventing its primary role of as chaperone protein. REP-1 escorts Rab protein to reach and bind to plasma membrane of organelles and to allow normal intracellular exchange. Disruption of this intracellular function leads to early cell death.

25.8 Workup/Testing

Obtain a detailed family history with an X-linked recessive mode of inheritance; consider examining family members, given the potential of female carriers to demonstrate partial phenotype. Consider fundus autofluorescence (FAF), fluorescein angiography (FA), optical coherence tomography (OCT), electroretinogram (ERG), electrooculogram (EOG), and formal perimetry. These may show the following characteristic findings:

- FA – early stages would demonstrate normal choroid with scatter areas of choriocapillaris loss; however, in the late stage it would show global loss of the choriocapillaris.
- OCT – absence of the photoreceptor outer segments and IS/OS junction with peripheral to central progression.
- ERG – normal to subnormal in the early stages of the disease; however, at later stages there is clearly an extinction of the scotopic ERG and severely reduced amplitude of the photopic response.
- Perimetry – serial visual field testing would demonstrate a progressive peripheral constriction in both eyes.

25.9 Prognosis and Management

Vision loss is slow and progressive. While peripheral vision may start in the first decade of life, central vision is not affected until the third to fourth decade with profound central vision loss not occurring until the fifth to seventh decade. Genetic counseling is necessary to describe X-linked recessive inheritance and educate female carriers about the risk of transmitting the mutation to future. Female carriers typically have normal vision throughout their life. Choroidal neovascularization is extremely rare but can occur. Presently, there is no treatment for choroideremia.

25.10 Follow-Up

Six months to annually.

References and Suggested Reading

1. Cheung MC, Nune GC, Wang M, McTaggart KE, MacDonald IM, Duncan JL. Detection of localized retinal dysfunction in a choroideremia carrier. Am J Ophthalmol. 2004;137(1): 189–91.
2. Forsius HR, Eriksson AW, Karna J. Choroideremia. In: Eriksson AW, Forsius HR, Nevanlinna HR, Workman PL, Norio RK, editors. Population structure and genetic disorders. New York: Academic; 1980. p. 592–5.
3. Karna J. Acta Ophthalmol Suppl. 1986;176:1–68.
4. Mura M, Sereda C, Jablonski MM, MacDonald IM, Iannaccone A. Clinical and functional findings in choroideremia due to complete deletion of the CHM gene. Arch Ophthalmol. 2007;125:1107–13.
5. Ohba N, Isashiki Y. Clinical and genetic features of choroideremia. Jpn J Ophthal. 2000;44:317 only.
6. Siu VM, Gonder JR, Jung JH, Sergovich FR, Flintoff WF. Choroideremia associated with an X-autosomal translocation. Hum Genet. 1990;84:459–64.

Chapter 26
Gyrate Atrophy

Veeral S. Shah

26.1 Definitions

Hyperornithinemia with gyrate atrophy of choroid and retina (HOGA) or Ornithine aminotransferase deficiency (OAT) or Gyrate atrophy is auto-recessive chorioretinal dystrophy that leads to progressive myopia and retina/choroidal degeneration.

26.2 Symptoms

Nyctalopia or night blindness, myopic astigmatism, and peripheral vision loss during childhood.

26.3 Signs

- *Early*: Bilateral, variable but sharply demarcated circular areas of peripheral chorioretinal atrophy. Typically these areas of chorioretinal atrophy have hyper-pigmented margins that are found in the mid-peripheral retina.
- *Late*: These discrete areas of chorioretinal atrophy progressively enlarge into "scalloped" edges of geographic atrophy expanding both anteriorly and posteriorly to encroach the macula. At later stages, there is widespread choroidal atrophy extending from the periphery to posterior pole, with islands of preserved retina,

V.S. Shah, MD, PhD
Department of Ophthalmology, Baylor College of Medicine,
Texas Children's Hospital, Houston, TX, USA
e-mail: vsshah@texaschildrens.org

C.A. Medina et al. (eds.), *Manual of Retinal Diseases: A Guide to Diagnosis and Management*, DOI 10.1007/978-3-319-20460-4_26

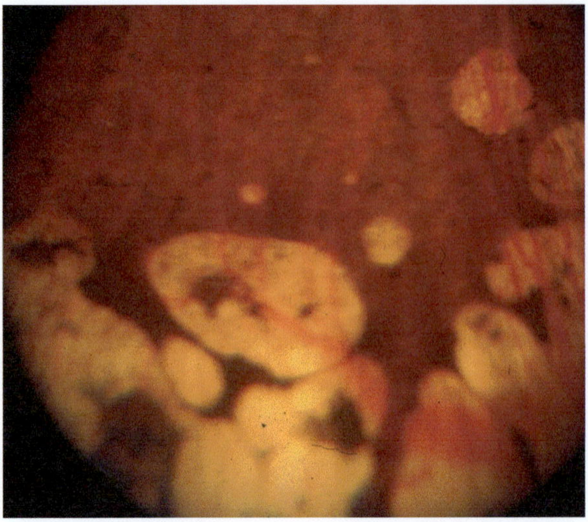

Fig. 26.1 Gyrate atrophy. Late-stage fundus changes showing peripheral discrete areas of chorioretinal atrophy with scalloped edges (Courtesy of Elias Traboulsi, MD, Cleveland, OH)

typically sparing the macula to some degree (Fig. 26.1). Macular involvement can be progressive atrophic changes or from the development of macular edema.

- *Associated clinical findings*: While majority of patients with gyrate atrophy have no systemic disease with the exception of the vision loss, there are several associated clinical findings of this inherited disorder. Newborn with gyrate atrophy can develop hyperammonemia and present with vomiting, failure to thrive, seizures, comatose, and lethargy. Patients are commonly myopic and develop posterior subcapsular cataracts in the second decade. Systemically, they develop tubular aggregates in type II skeletal muscle that lead to muscle weakness with subclinical changes noted on imaging. Within the central nervous system, these patients may acquire white matter lesions and premature atrophic changes within the brain that can lead to seizures and/or abnormal EEGs. Intelligence is not affected in this disorder.

26.4 Epidemiology

The symptoms nyctalopia and progressive myopic astigmatism typically occur in the first decade of life.

26.5 Inheritance/Etiology

Gyrate atrophy is autosomal recessive chorioretinal dystrophy that results in a progressive degeneration of the retina and choroid. Mutation in the gene for ornithine-delta-aminotransferase (OAT) enzyme on chromosome 10q26 leads to an absence or deficiency of this enzyme and leads into elevated plasma levels of ornithine of 10–20 times the normal level. The OAT is found in the mitochondria matrix and plays an important role protein metabolism by breaking down the ornithine into pyrroline-5-carboxylate (P5C), which eventually converted into glutamate and proline. How this directly leads to retina and choroid degeneration is unclear, but there is evidence that suggests that a lack of P5C may be responsible for this degeneration.

26.6 Differential Diagnosis

- *Choroideremia*: In late stage of both gyrate atrophy and choroideremia, the fundus may look quite similar; however, distinction can be made with investigation into the genetic pedigree and examination of the female carrier in choroideremia.
- *Retinitis pigmentosa*: May look similar in later stages, but RPE commonly has bone spicule degeneration and attenuated retinal vessels, neither typical of gyrate atrophy.

26.7 Workup/Testing

Obtain a detailed family history for mode of inheritance and complete ophthalmic exam including evaluation of cataract and refraction. Dilated fundus exam with characteristic findings of chorioretinal atrophy mentioned above. Based on clinical suspicion, evaluation of amino acid plasma levels for elevated ornithine level. Genetic testing and OAT enzyme immunoassay are available to aid in diagnosis.

- FA – hyperfluorescence in areas of chorioretinal atrophy and leakage at the margins of healthy and degenerative tissue.
- ERG – early stages, scotopic, and photopic ERG would be reduced and eventually become absence with progression of the disease.
- Perimetry – serial visual field testing demonstrates progressive peripheral constriction of the visual field in both eyes.

26.8 Prognosis and Management

The mainstay of treatment of gyrate atrophy is to normalize the plasma ornithine levels. Pyridoxine or vitamin 6 supplementation has shown to decrease plasma ornithine in the subtype of gyrate atrophy responsive. Alternatively, arginine (precursor of ornithine)-restricted diet has demonstrated delayed progression in chorioretinal atrophy and visual field losses. The visual prognosis of gyrate atrophy follows the pattern of peripheral constriction progressing into posterior pole, with majority having central vision loss ranging between the fourth and seventh decade. Genetic counseling can be obtained to identify genetic mutations, but no effective treatment is available at this time. Secondary choroidal neovascularization can be managed and treated with anti-VEGF therapy.

26.9 Follow-Up

Three to twelve months follow-up depending on normalization of ornithine levels and monitoring for cataracts.

References and Suggested Reading

1. Cleary MA, Dorland L, de Koning TJ, Poll-The BT, Duran M, Mandell R, Shih VE, Berger R, Olpin SE, Besley GT. Ornithine aminotransferase deficiency: diagnostic difficulties in neonatal presentation. J Inherit Metab Dis. 2005;28(5):673–9.
2. Fleury M, Barbier R, Ziegler F, Mohr M, Caron O, Dollfus H, Tranchant C, Warter JM. Myopathy with tubular aggregates and gyrate atrophy of the choroid and retina due to hyperornithinaemia. J Neurol Neurosurg Psychiatry. 2007;78(6):656–7. Epub 2006 Nov 6.
3. Kaiser-Kupfer MI, Caruso RC, Valle D, Reed GF. Use of an arginine-restricted diet to slow progression of visual loss in patients with gyrate atrophy. Arch Ophthalmol. 2004; 122(7):982–4.
4. Peltola KE, Jääskeläinen S, Heinonen OJ, Falck B, Näntö-Salonen K, Heinänen K, Simell O. Peripheral nervous system in gyrate atrophy of the choroid and retina with hyperornithinemia. Neurology. 2002;59(5):735–40.
5. Santinelli R, Costagliola C, Tolone C, D'Aloia A, D'Avanzo A, Prisco F, Perrone L, del Giudice EM. Low-protein diet and progression of retinal degeneration in gyrate atrophy of the choroid and retina: a twenty-six-year follow-up. J Inherit Metab Dis. 2004;27(2):187–96.
6. Valtonen M, Nanto-Salonen K, Jaaskelainen S, Heinanen K, Alanen A, Heinonen OJ, Lundbom N, Erkintalo M, Simell O. Central nervous system involvement in gyrate atrophy of the choroid and retina with hyperornithinaemia. J Inherit Metab Dis. 1999;22:855–66.

Chapter 27
Leber Congenital Amaurosis

Veeral S. Shah

27.1 Definitions

Leber congenital amaurosis (LCA) or congenital retinal blindness (CRB) is a group of early-onset retinal dystrophies characterized by severe vision loss, nystagmus, and retinal dysfunction demonstrated with severely abnormal ERG.

27.2 Symptoms

Vision loss from birth, mild to moderate photophobia

27.3 Signs

- *Severe vision impairment*: Nonresponsive to minimal sensitivity for visual stimuli (no blinking with light nor fixation or following eye movements).
- *Abnormal eye movements*: Manifestation of involuntary eye movements or nystagmus which is typically horizontal and present at birth. LCA patients may also have absent or sluggish pupillary reaction to light.

V.S. Shah, MD, PhD
Department of Ophthalmology, Baylor College of Medicine,
Texas Children's Hospital, Houston, TX, USA
e-mail: vsshah@texaschildrens.org

C.A. Medina et al. (eds.), *Manual of Retinal Diseases: A Guide to Diagnosis and Management*, DOI 10.1007/978-3-319-20460-4_27

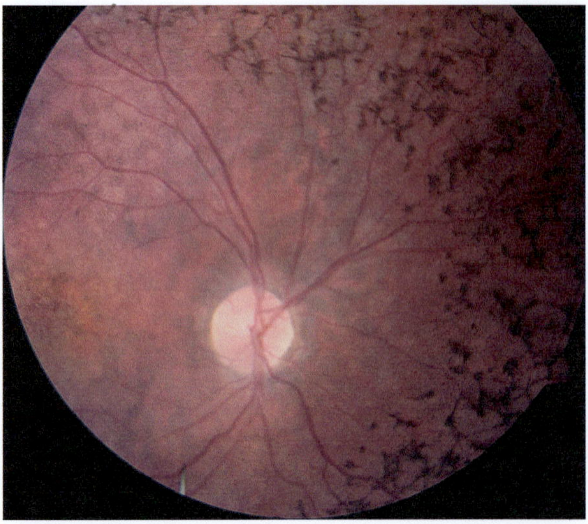

Fig. 27.1 LCA. Typical ophthalmoscopic features including pigment epithelial atrophy/hyperplasia and optic nerve atrophy (Courtesy of Elias Traboulsi, MD, Cleveland, OH)

- A unique feature of LCA is the *Franceschetti's or oculo-digital sign,* which refers to self-stimulatory behavior of eye poking, pressure, or rubbing to incite mechanical retinal stimulation.
- *Dilated fundus exam*: Can range from normal appearing at birth but can have:
  - Progressive retinal and pigment epithelial atrophy
  - Pigment epithelial hyperplasia
  - Scattered white dots or flecks
  - Retinal vascular sheathing and optic nerve atrophy (Fig. 27.1)
- Retinoscopy or refraction; a vast number of LCA children have high hyperopia. LCA children can develop associated cataracts and keratoconus in the first and second dacade of life.
- *Associated clinical findings*: There are several systemic clinical findings associated with LCA which include mental retardation, skeletal abnormalities, renal disease, and multiple neurological abnormalities.

27.4 Epidemiology

Signs and symptoms are from birth or have early onset during the newborn period. LCA has an incidence of 2–3 per 100,000 newborns.

27.5 Inheritance/Etiology

The primary mode of inheritance is autosomal recessive, and many genes have been identified that present with clinical findings consistent with LCA diagnosis. A list of genes that account for roughly 70 % of LCA diagnosis are listed in Table 27.1.

Table 27.1 Genes associated with Leber congenital amaurosis

Genes	Location
GUCY2D	17p13.1
RPE65	1p31
CRX	19q13.3
AIPL	17p13.1
CRB1	1p31-q32.1
RPGRIP1	14q11.2
MERTK	2q14.1
RDH12	14q24.1
IMPDH1	7q31.3-32
TULP1	6p21
CEP290	12q21-q22
LCA5	6q11-q16
SPATA7	14q24
OTX2	14q21-22
IQCB1	3q21.1
PDE6G	17q25
KCNJ13	2q37.1
RD3	1q32
NMNAT1	1p36
DTHD1	4p14

This panel of genes accounts for roughly 70 % of LCA cases

There are only few gene mutations that cause LCA in an autosomal dominant manner. In 20–30 % of LCA, the genetic cause is unknown.

27.6 Differential Diagnosis

- Early-onset retinal dystrophy associated with renal disease (Senior-Loken syndrome), cerebellar vermis hypoplasia + neonatal respiratory distress (Joubert syndrome), or diabetes mellitus/sensorineural hearing loss (Alstrom syndrome)
- Albinism
- Congenital stationary blindness
- Blue cone monochromatism
- Achromatopsia
- Neuronal ceroid lipofuscinosis

27.7 Workup/Testing

Obtain a detailed family history for mode of inheritance and complete ophthalmic exam including evaluation of anterior segment (cataract and keratoconus) and refraction (hyperopia). Dilated fundus exam may be normal or with characteristic findings of progressive pigmentary atrophy and degeneration as mentioned above.

- ERG – would be profoundly abnormal or extinguished.

27.8 Prognosis and Management

Early profound vision loss affects development in terms of cognitive and motor skills. Little to no vision from the onset and typically by the third or fourth decade completes blindness in both eyes. There is no treatment for this disorder at this time, but genetic therapy trials are ongoing.

27.9 Follow-Up

Six to twelve months follow-up to optimize vision.

References and Suggested Reading

1. Khan AO, Al-Mesfer S, Al-Turkmani S, Bergmann C, Bolz HJ. Genetic analysis of strictly defined Leber congenital amaurosis with (and without) neurodevelopmental delay. Br J Ophthalmol. 2014;98:1724–8.
2. Maguire AM, Simonelli F, Pierce EA, Pugh EN, Mingozzi F, Bennicelli J, Banfi S, Marshall KA, Testa F, Surace EM, Rossi S, Lyubarsky A, Arruda VR, Konkle B, Stone E, Sun J, Jacobs J, Dell'Osso L, Hertle R, Ma JX, Redmond TM, Zhu X, Hauck B, Zelenaia O, Shindler KS, Maguire MG, Wright JF, Volpe NJ. McDonnell safety and efficacy of gene transfer for Leber's congenital amaurosis. N Engl J Med. 2008;358:2240–8.
3. Weleber RG, Francis PJ, Trzupek KM, et al. Leber Congenital Amaurosis. 2004 Jul 7 [Updated 2013 May 2]. In: Pagon RA, Adam MP, Ardinger HH, et al., editors. GeneReviews® [Internet]. Seattle (WA): University of Washington, Seattle; 1993–2016. Available from: http://www.ncbi.nlm.nih.gov/books/NBK1298/
4. Schroeder R, Mets MB, Maumenee IH. Leber's congenital amaurosis: retrospective review of 43 cases and a new fundus finding in two cases. Arch Ophthalmol. 1987;105:356–9.
5. Zernant J, Kulm M, Dharmaraj S, den Hollander AI, Perrault I, Preising MN, Lorenz B, Kaplan J, Cremers FPM, Maumenee I, Koenekoop RK, Allikmets R. Genotyping microarray (disease chip) for Leber congenital amaurosis: detection of modifier alleles. Invest Ophthalmol Vis Sci. 2005;46:3052–9.

Chapter 28
Paraneoplastic Retinopathy

Veeral S. Shah

28.1 Definitions

Paraneoplastic retinopathy is a syndrome where one's immune system response to a tumor leads to generation of antibodies to the tumor antigen that cross-reacts with retinal proteins. These autoantibodies to the retina lead to rod and cone photoreceptor dysfunction. There are several classifications of paraneoplastic retinopathies; we discuss the three most common types carcinoma-associated retinopathy (CAR), melanoma-associated retinopathy (MAR), and bilateral diffuse uveal melanocytic proliferation (BDUMP).

28.2 Symptoms

Initial symptoms are a painless dimming or blurring of vision in both eyes. Mild decreased vision, peripheral visual field loss, and nyctalopia are commonly encountered. Many patients describe a range for episodic positive visual disturbances including visual distortions, shimmering or flashing lights, or peculiar images. Photophobia and intense visual glare have also been reported. These symptoms are typically bilateral but asymmetric and gradually worsen in the course of several weeks to months.

V.S. Shah, MD, PhD
Department of Ophthalmology, Baylor College of Medicine,
Texas Children's Hospital, Houston, TX, USA
e-mail: vsshah@texaschildrens.org

C.A. Medina et al. (eds.), *Manual of Retinal Diseases: A Guide to Diagnosis and Management*, DOI 10.1007/978-3-319-20460-4_28

28.3 Signs

In early stage of paraneoplastic syndrome, symptomatic patient may have normal visual function and funduscopic exam. Invariably, these patients develop decreased central visual acuity with sparing of color vision, and visual field defects can range and include central, ring/paracentral, and peripheral scotomas. Disruption in cone function would demonstrate decreased central visual acuity, central scotoma, decreased color vision, and increased photosensitivity. Alternatively, rod dysfunction can manifest as ring or peripheral scotoma and nyctalopia.

- *MAR and CAR*, fundus exam can demonstrate optic disc pallor, retinal vessel attenuation, and retinal pigmentary changes (Fig. 28.1).
- *BDUMP* is characterized with diffuse uveal thickening that presents as orange or greenish pigmentary choroidal mass. These orange or pigment changes can appear as polygonal lesion known as "giraffe sign" (Fig. 28.2).

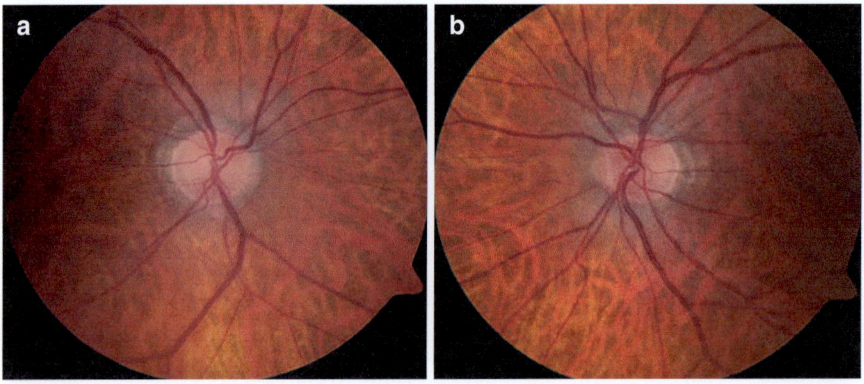

Fig. 28.1 A 61-year-old white male presented to the neuro-ophthalmology service in consultation for bilateral progressive decrease in vision that started approximately 1 year prior to presentation. He saw an ophthalmologist 1 month prior to his presentation who noted mild sheathing of his retinal vessels without anterior uveitis or vitritis. Past medical history was significant for asthma, and the patient had previous hernia repair and sinus surgery. He denied diabetes, known malignancies, or autoimmune diseases. On ophthalmic examination, his best-corrected visual acuity was 20/80 OD and 20/40 OS. IOP was 19 OU and pupils were equal and reactive without an afferent pupillary defect. His extraocular movements were full OU, and a Goldmann visual field showed peripheral constriction with the I-4 targets OU. Dilated fundus exam showed mildly attenuated retinal arterioles but was otherwise unremarkable (**a** *right eye*; **b** *left eye*). There was no sheathing noted on fundus examination. Multifocal ERG revealed severe attenuation of a- and b-waves centrally OU. Serum anti-retinal antibody tests showed the presence of anti-α enolase antibodies with staining of the inner nuclear layer on immunohistochemistry. The patient was diagnosed with probable cancer-associated retinopathy. Further workup revealed the presence of a peripheral lung nodule whose biopsy showed the presence of signet ring cell carcinoma (Courtesy of Martin Heur MD and Gregory S. Kosmorsky, MD, Cleveland, OH. Reproduced with permission from Courtney et al. [5])

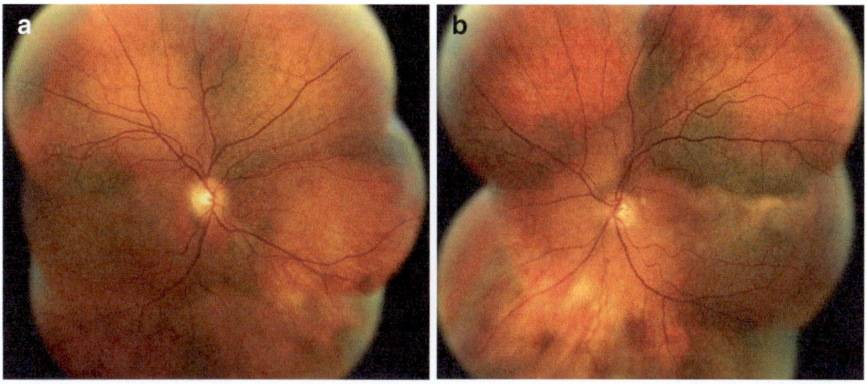

Fig. 28.2 A 56-year-old woman presented with progressive deteriorating vision in both eyes for the last 6 months. The onset of visual symptoms coincided with the diagnosis of large cell carcinoma of the lung. She was not known to have metastasis and was receiving chemotherapy. The corrected visual acuity was 20/40 in the right eye and 20/60 in the left eye. Anterior segment examination was unremarkable. On ophthalmoscopic examination, the choroid was diffusely thickened in both eyes (**a** *right eye*; **b** *left eye*). The choroid was also markedly hypermelanotic with scattered areas of orange pigmentation. The choroidal thickening was confirmed by B-scan ultrasonography. The patient had recently noticed new onset-pigmented lesions on her forearms and thighs for the last few months. Patients' visual status worsened for the next 6 months when she died from metastatic disease (Reproduced with permission from Singh et al. [6])

28.4 Epidemiology

There is no sex or age predilection. The incidence of the paraneoplastic is associated with known or occult malignancy. The most common associated malignancies include small cell lung cancer; breast cancer; and endocrine, gynecologic, and visceral tumors. CAR and BDUMP have been found in other malignancies such as colon cancer, kidney cancer, pancreatic cancer, prostate cancer, lymphoma, basal cell cancer, and skin squamous cancer. Typically, majority of MAR patient have the diagnosis of melanoma and subsequently develop visual symptoms up to and greater than ten years after the diagnosis and suggestive of possible metastatic progression.

28.5 Etiology

The underlying mechanism of paraneoplastic retinopathies is the presence of tumor cells that triggers the immune system to generate antibodies that cross-react with retinal proteins. In these retinopathies there can be many single or multiple autoantibodies, and not all the autoantibodies are known. The following are identified retinal antigens found in CAR and BDUMP: recoverin, a-enolase, carbonic anhydrase, transducin B, and arrestin. In particular, the recoverin is most common and is a calcium-binding protein found in rods and cone. Alternatively, MAR does not commonly have autoantibodies that react to recoverin but instead have antibodies to bipolar cells in the outer plexiform area and has distinct ERG pattern.

28.6 Differential Diagnosis

The following are several retinal disorders that can be ruled out with medical, family, and medication history; complete ophthalmic exam; and ancillary testing like fluorescein angiogram, OCT, and ERG:

- Retinitis pigmentosa
- Cone dystrophy
- Stargardt's disease
- Toxic nutritional retinopathy
- Acute zonal outer occult retinopathy (AZOOR)
- Hereditary optic neuropathy
- Artery and vein occlusion

28.7 Workup/Testing

Obtain complete medical, family history, and social with particular detail to cancer history. Complete ophthalmic exam including visual field testing, color vision, and dark adaptometry:

- Dark adaptometry – prolonged dark adaptation.
- ERG – significantly reduced a-wave and b-wave amplitudes.

28.8 Prognosis and Management

Systemic steroids and immunosuppressive therapy (including plasma exchange and IVIG) can lead to improved vision in many paraneoplastic retinopathy patients. Early diagnosis and intervention may lead to improve visual outcomes.

28.9 Follow-Up

Follow closely during interval tumor management. Once tumor is remitted and symptoms stabilize, follow-up can be extended.

References and Suggested Reading

1. Hecklenlively JR, Ferreyra HA. Autoimmune retinopathy: a review and summary. Semin Immunopathol. 2008;30:127–34.
2. Keltner JL, Roth AM, Chang S. Photoreceptor degeneration – a possible autoimmune disease. Arch Ophthalmol. 1983;101:564–9.
3. Ferreyra HA, Jayasundera T, Kahn NW, et al. Management of autoimmune retinopathies with immunosuppression. Arch Ophthalmol. 2009;127(4):390–7.
4. Chan JW. Paraneoplastic retinopathies and optic neuropathies. Surv Ophthalmol. 2003;48(1):12–38.
5. Courtney RJ, Singh RP, Aronow MB, Singh AD. Ocular paraneoplastic diseases. In: Singh AD, Damato BE, editors. Retinal tumors. Clinical ophthalmic oncology. Heidelberg: Springer; 2015. p. 133–52.
6. Singh AD, Rundle PA, Slater DN, et al. Uveal and cutaneous involvement in paraneoplastic melanocytic proliferation. Arch Ophthalmol. 2003;121(11):1637–40.

Section IV
Disorders of the Vitreous and Vitreo-Retinal Interface

Carlos A. Medina

Chapter 29
Posterior Vitreous Detachment

Xiongfei Liu and Carlos A. Medina

29.1 Definition

Posterior vitreous detachment (PVD) is a separation between the internal limiting membrane (ILM) of the retina and the posterior vitreous cortex. It is usually spontaneous and age related but may also be associated with trauma.

29.2 Symptoms

Early stages are asymptomatic and occult in most eyes until separation from the glial disc margin (area of Martegiani) occurs (Table 29.1). This is accompanied by the appearance of a Weiss ring on fundoscopic examination and symptoms such as floaters, photopsia under dim light, and blurred vision.

29.3 Signs

Weiss ring: complete or incomplete circular vitreous density over the optic disc (Fig. 29.1). Detached posterior hyaloid membrane.

Retinal break, retinal detachment, vitreous opacities, vitreous hemorrhage, and retinal or optic disc hemorrhage may be observed.

X. Liu, MD • C.A. Medina, MD (✉)
Department of Ophthalmology, Bascom Palmer Eye Institute,
University of Miami, 900 NW 17th Street, Miami, FL 33136, USA
e-mail: camedina2020@gmail.com

C.A. Medina et al. (eds.), *Manual of Retinal Diseases: A Guide to Diagnosis and Management*, DOI 10.1007/978-3-319-20460-4_29

Table 29.1 Stages of posterior vitreous detachment

Stage 1	Perifoveal PVD with residual vitreofoveal adhesion
Stage 2	Complete separation of vitreous from the macula
Stage 3	Extensive PVD with only vitreous adhesion to the disc
Stage 4	Complete vitreous detachment from retina

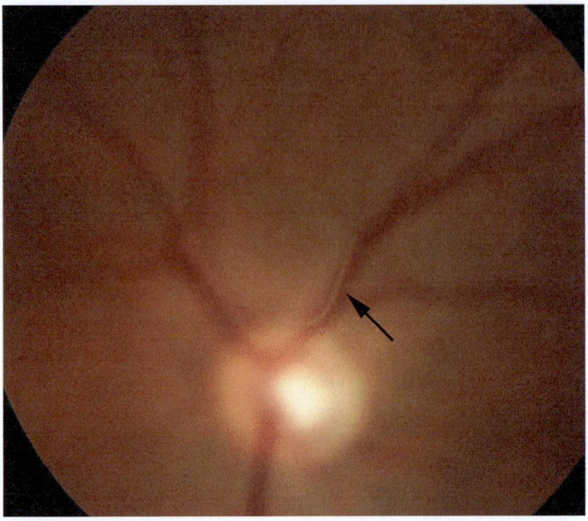

Fig. 29.1 Weiss ring corresponds to the site of previous vitreous attachment to the optic disc. It is characterized by vitreous density over the optic disc (*arrow*)

Vitreous pigment cells (Schaffer sign or "tobacco dust") may also be observed. This is associated with retina tear in 92 % of patients with acute PVD. Vitreous hemorrhage may arise from rupture of retinal vessels that cross retinal tears or from avulsion of superficial or peripheral retinal vessels.

29.4 Epidemiology

A PVD usually occurs between the ages of 45 and 65 in the general population. The incidence correlates with aging as 53 % of adults develop PVD by age 50 and 65 % by age 65. The prevalence increases with the axial length of the eye and age of the patient. There is a female predilection as well.

29.5 Predisposing Conditions

Those with health conditions such as diabetes mellitus, myopia, Marfan syndrome, and retinal vascular diseases are at increased risk for developing PVD. Furthermore, history of ocular trauma, previous cataract surgery, aphakia, uveitis, and vitreous hemorrhage elevate the risk as well. Postmenopausal women are at increased risk secondary to declining estrogen levels.

29.6 Differential Diagnosis

Since patients with symptomatic PVD often present with floaters and photopsia, the differential diagnosis for floaters and photopsia includes retinal tear/detachment, vitreous hemorrhage, vitritis, rapid eye movement, oculodigital stimulation, and migraine.

29.7 Etiology

Two concurrent processes are at work. First, there is a progressive age-related degeneration of the adhesion between the posterior vitreous cortex and the ILM. Second, aging of the human vitreous leads to gel liquefaction (syneresis) and fluid-filled pockets. As these pockets enlarge, the posterior wall becomes thin, eventually leading to microbreaks in the perifoveal region. Combined with gradual dissolution of the adhesion, liquid vitreous enters the retrohyaloid space leading to posterior vitreous detachment. Further rotational eye movements contribute to subsequent dissection of the remaining adhesion between the vitreous cortex and the ILM, leading to progressive PVD. The vitreous gel is attached most firmly at the vitreous base, a circumferential zone straddling the ora serrata extending approximately 2 mm anterior and 4 mm posterior to the ora serrata. Vitreous collagen fibers are also firmly attached at the margin of the optic disc, the macula, along major vessels, around areas of lattice degeneration, and chorioretinal scars.

29.8 Workup/Testing

- Ocular Examination
  - Anterior vitreous for pigmented cells or hemorrhage.
  - Dilated fundus exam with indirect ophthalmoscopy and scleral depression or 3-mirror contact lens examination to rule out retinal break and detachment.
- SD-OCT may help establish a diagnosis when a frank PVD is not visualized on examination.
- Ultrasonography is recommended if there is poor view to the fundus secondary to media opacity.
- When a retinal tear is suspected based on presence of Shaffer sign, hemorrhage, or significant symptoms but cannot be identified on clinical exam, repeat examination or ultrasonography within 1–2 weeks of the initial examination is recommended.

29.9 Prognosis and Management

The prognosis tends to be good, with no management needed unless there is suspicion for retinal tear/detachment. Furthermore, PVD symptoms tend to diminish over the span of several months. If floaters are still symptomatic after such period, some vitreoretinal surgeons may perform a pars plana vitrectomy. Patients should be instructed on the warning signs of retinal detachment: increase in floaters and photopsia, blurring vision, or persistent curtain in field of vision.

29.10 Follow-Up

Approximately 15 % of all patients with acute symptomatic PVD have a retina tear and 3.7 % of patients with initial uncomplicated PVD can develop subsequent retinal tears at 6 weeks follow-up. For those with symptomatic PVD without retinal tear, follow-up should be scheduled at 1–8 weeks and then 6–12 months depending on risk factors and clinical findings. Since vitreous hemorrhages and vitreous pigment increase the likelihood of retinal tear, the follow-up interval can be shortened based on the presence of these signs. For those without a retinal break but clinical exam is positive for mild vitreous hemorrhages or peripheral punctate retinal hemorrhages, follow-up should be scheduled at 1 week, 2–4 weeks, 3 months, and then 6 months afterward. Similarly, for patients without a retinal break but with significant vitreous hemorrhages or anterior vitreous pigment cells, ocular examination should be repeated within 1 week and consideration should be given to repeat B scan ultrasonography to visualize the dynamic movement of the vitreous body and any persistent vitreoretinal adhesions.

Reference and Suggested Reading

1. American Academy of Ophthalmology Retina/Vitreous Panel. Preferred Practice Pattern® Guidelines. Posterior Vitreous Detachment, Retinal Breaks, and Lattice Degeneration. San Francisco: American Academy of Ophthalmology; 2014. Available at: www.aao.org/ppp.
2. Gerstenblith A, Rabinowitz M. Posterior vitreous detachment. In: The wills eye manual: office and emergency room diagnosis and treatment of eye disease. 6th ed. Philadelphia: LWW; 2012. p. 293–4.
3. Hikichi T, Yoshida A. Time course of development of posterior vitreous detachment in the fellow eye after development in the first eye. Ophthalmology. 2004;111(9):1705–7.
4. Hollands H, Johnson D, Brox A, Almeida D, Simel D, Sharma S. Acute-onset floaters and flashes: is this patient at risk for retinal detachment? JAMA. 2009;302(20):2243–9.
5. Johnson M. Posterior vitreous detachment: evolution and complications of its early stages. Am J Ophthalmol. 2010;149(3):371–82.
6. Kaiser P, Friedman N, Pineda R. Posterior vitreous detachment. In: The Massachusetts Eye and Ear Infirmary Illustrated Manual of Ophthalmology. 4th ed. Philadelphia: Saunders; 2014. p. 322–3.

7. Larsson L, Osterlin S. Posterior vitreous detachment. A combined clinical and physiochemical study. Graefes Arch Clin Exp Ophthalmol. 1985;223(2):92–5.
8. Sarrafizadeh R, Hassan R, Ruby A, et al. Incidence of retinal detachment and visual outcome in eyes presenting with posterior vitreous separation and dense fundus-obscuring vitreous hemorrhage. Ophthalmology. 2001;108(12):2273–8.
9. Tanner V, Harle D, Tan J, Foote B, Williamson T, Chignell A. Acute posterior vitreous detachment: the predictive value of vitreous pigment and symptomatology. Br J Ophthalmol. 2000;84:1264–8.
10. van Overdam K, Bettink-Remeijer M, Klaver C, Mulder P, Moll A, van Meurs J. Symptoms and findings predictive for the development of new retinal breaks. Arch Ophthalmol. 2005;123(4):479–84.

Chapter 30
Vitreous Hemorrhage

Angelica Ortiz and Carlos A. Medina

30.1 Definition

Vitreous hemorrhage is the presence of extravasated blood within the space outlined by the internal limiting membrane of the retina posteriorly and laterally, the nonpigmented epithelium of the ciliary body laterally, and the lens zonular fibers and posterior lens capsule anteriorly. Hemorrhage into Berger's space, the canal of Petit, and Cloquet's canal is also considered vitreous hemorrhage. Although visually compromising, vitreous hemorrhage actually serves as a symptom of an underlying disease process.

30.2 Symptoms

Patients may present clinically with a complaint of haze, floaters, photophobia, and/or the perception of shadows and cobwebs. Visual acuity in eyes with vitreous hemorrhage and retained macular function is determined by the location and density of hemorrhage. If the patient reports that the loss of vision was preceded by sudden onset of floaters and flashing lights, then one should consider possibility of posterior vitreous detachment and look for an associated retinal break.

A. Ortiz, MD • C.A. Medina, MD (✉)
Department of Ophthalmology, Bascom Palmer Eye Institute,
University of Miami, 900 NW 17th St., Miami, FL 33136, USA
e-mail: camedina2020@gmail.com

C.A. Medina et al. (eds.), *Manual of Retinal Diseases: A Guide to Diagnosis and Management*, DOI 10.1007/978-3-319-20460-4_30

30.3 Signs

Red blood cells in the anterior vitreous.

Hemorrhage within Berger's space or canal of Petit can lead to formation of a crescent-shaped pool of blood, with the hyaloideocapsular ligament forming a border.

Afferent pupillary defect (APD) may be present.

Some patients may have retinal break, posterior vitreous detachment, or iris neovascularization depending on the etiology of the vitreous hemorrhage.

30.4 Epidemiology

There are approximately 7 cases of spontaneous vitreous hemorrhage per 100,000 population each year. Among patients younger than 40 years of age, trauma is the most common cause of vitreous hemorrhage, with a mean patient age of 28 years and a higher incidence in males. Among black patients with spontaneous vitreous hemorrhage and sickle cell retinopathy, the mean age is 39 years.

30.5 Predisposing Conditions

Patients with diabetes mellitus, sickle cell disease, and inflammatory diseases that produce an occlusive vasculitis are predisposed to vitreous hemorrhage as a result of ischemic damage, which leads to retinal neovascularization. Patients with systemic hypertension, recent stroke, history of leukemia, age-related macular degeneration, and high myopia are also at higher risk for vitreous hemorrhage.

30.6 Differential Diagnosis

Conditions in which vitreous opacities are present include amyloidosis of the vitreous, asteroid hyalosis, uveitis (vitritis), and ocular or systemic lymphoma. To distinguish other opacities from vitreous blood, one can examine the anterior vitreous with the slit-lamp biomicroscope. Vitreous blood has characteristic small cells with reddish pigmentation. In older vitreous hemorrhages, the cells appear grayish white in color because of loss of hemoglobin.

30.7 Etiology

The most common causes of spontaneous vitreous hemorrhage are proliferative diabetic retinopathy (32 %), retinal tear (30 %), proliferative retinopathy after retinal vein occlusion (11 %), and posterior vitreous detachment without retinal tear (8 %). Proliferative diabetic retinopathy accounts for 64 and 89 % of vitreous hemorrhages in patients with noninsulin-dependent diabetes mellitus and insulin-dependent diabetes mellitus, respectively. Proliferative diabetic retinopathy is also the most common cause of bilateral intraocular hemorrhage. Spontaneous posterior vitreous detachment with a retinal tear is more common in high myopia. In patients with systemic hypertension, retinal vein occlusion or a macroaneurysm should be considered as possible causes of vitreous hemorrhage. Vitreous bleeding is found in approximately 20 % of patients with subarachnoid hemorrhages (Terson's syndrome). In black patients, the principal cause of spontaneous nondiabetic vitreous hemorrhage is proliferative sickle retinopathy. Congenital retinoschisis is a cause of vitreous hemorrhage in young males, and there is often a positive family history. Hyperviscosity syndromes, as seen in leukemia, may rupture retinal vessels, causing a vitreous hemorrhage.

30.8 Workup/Testing

- Ocular Examination
  - A low intraocular pressure (IOP) may indicate a retinal detachment, while a high IOP may suggest ghost cell or neovascular glaucoma.
  - Examination for APD should be performed.
  - Slit-lamp examination can be done to evaluate for iris neovascularization.
  - Fundus examination is usually performed with indirect ophthalmoscopy.
  - The anterior vitreous should be examined for RBCs. Pigmented cells may indicate a retinal tear or detachment (tobacco dust or Shafer's sign).
  - In a mild hemorrhage, the retinal vessels can be seen, while in a moderate hemorrhage, only the optic nerve can be identified. In a severe hemorrhage, no retinal details can be visualized.
  - B-scan ultrasonography is the standard method for evaluation of vitreoretinal diseases with vitreous hemorrhage.
  - The density of the hemorrhage can be ascertained, which may allow one to estimate the rate of spontaneous clearing.
  - In mild vitreous hemorrhages, fluorescein angiography or angioscopy may make it possible to find abnormalities in the retinal vasculature.
- Systemic testing
  - In a patient with possible ocular ischemic syndrome, a noninvasive carotid Doppler study should be ordered.

- Occasionally, computed tomography (CT) and magnetic resonance (MR) imaging are performed on patients with vitreous hemorrhage, for example, in Terson's syndrome to evaluate for intracranial hemorrhage.
- If sickle cell retinopathy is suspected, a hemoglobin electrophoresis is indicated.

30.9 Prognosis and Management

The prognosis of vitreous hemorrhage depends on the underlying disease. In general, patients with underlying diseases that have low tendency of recurrent bleeding, such as a vessel tear associated with a posterior vitreous detachment, will have a good prognosis for resolution of the hemorrhage and visual acuity. Patients with vitreous bleeding secondary to diabetic retinopathy have the worst prognosis for resolution of the vitreous hemorrhage and vision, with visual acuity worsening in up to 42 % of eyes. Vitreous hemorrhage secondary to age-related macular degeneration also has a poor prognosis. In patients with retinal vein obstruction, patients with branch retinal vein occlusion generally have the best prognosis, while patients with central retinal vein occlusion have the worst prognosis. Photocoagulation has reduced the incidence of vitreous hemorrhage secondary to diabetic retinopathy, branch retinal vein occlusion, and sickle cell retinopathy over the last 30 years, yet many patients still develop vitreous hemorrhage. Observation is safe and reasonable in most cases in which the underlying cause of vitreous hemorrhage does not threaten the health of the eye, and the fellow eye has functional visual acuity. Strict enforcement of positioning with elevation of the head is somewhat controversial. If after several months the hemorrhage has failed to clear, the established treatment option is pars plana vitrectomy. Patients with nondiabetic vitreous hemorrhage have a better visual prognosis than patients with diabetic vitreous hemorrhage after vitrectomy, with improvement of visual acuity ranging between 77 and 94 %.

30.10 Follow-Up

If an etiology of the hemorrhage cannot be established, then the patient should be followed weekly, with indirect ophthalmoscopy or serial ultrasounds if no view into the fundus, to look for possible retinal detachment. Patients should be educated about symptoms of retinal detachment, including flashing lights and loss of visual field. Diabetic patients who have vitreous hemorrhage and who have not had previous panretinal photocoagulation (PRP) are at greater risk for progression of their proliferative disease and tractional retinal detachment. In these patients, if there has been no improvement after 2 or 3 months, vitrectomy and PRP should be considered (Fig. 30.1).

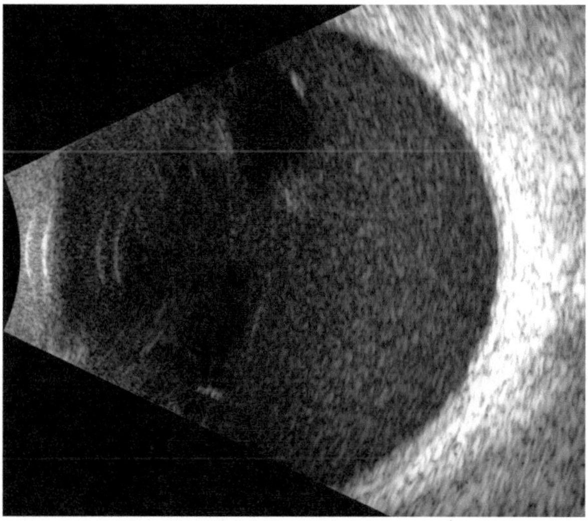

Fig. 30.1 B-scan ultrasonography with vitreous hemorrhage. Note absence of retinal detachment or breaks

Reference and Suggested Reading

1. A randomized clinical trial of early panretinal photocoagulation for ischemic central vein occlusion. The Central Vein Occlusion Study Group N report. Ophthalmology. 1995;102(10):1434–44.
2. Cordido M, et al. Natural evolution of massive vitreous hemorrhage in diabetic retinopathy. Retina. 1988;8(2):96–101.
3. Dana MR, et al. Spontaneous and traumatic vitreous hemorrhage. Ophthalmology. 1993;100(9):1377–83.
4. Early vitrectomy for severe vitreous hemorrhage in diabetic retinopathy. Four-year results of a randomized trial: diabetic Retinopathy Vitrectomy Study Report 5. Arch Ophthalmol. 1990;108(7):958–64.
5. el Baba F, et al. Massive hemorrhage complicating age-related macular degeneration. Clinicopathologic correlation and role of anticoagulants. Ophthalmology. 1986;93(12):1581–92.
6. Eller A. Diagnosis and management of vitreous hemorrhage. In: Focal points. Clinical modules for ophthalmologists. San Francisco: The Foundation of The American Academy of Ophthalmology; 2000. p. 1–14.
7. Li C, Gao R. Vitrectomy for nondiabetic vitreous hemorrhage. Yan Ke Xue Bao. 1991;7(2):95–7.
8. Lindgren G, Sjodell L, Lindblom B. A prospective study of dense spontaneous vitreous hemorrhage. Am J Ophthalmol. 1995;119(4):458–65.
9. Oya kawa RT, Michels RG, Blase WP. Vitrectomy for nondiabetic vitreous hemorrhage. Am J Ophthalmol. 1983;96(4):517–25.
10. Spraul CW, Grossniklaus HE. Vitreous hemorrhage. Surv Ophthalmol. 1997;42(1):3–39.

Chapter 31
Asteroid Hyalosis and Amyloidosis

Angelica Ortiz and Carlos A. Medina

31.1 Definition

- Asteroid hyalosis (AH) is a common degenerative condition in which calcium-lipid complexes are suspended by the network of collagen fibrils of the vitreous humor.
- Amyloidosis involving the vitreous is generally associated with the transthyretin-related familial amyloidosis and is rarely observed in nonfamilial cases. The amyloid deposits consist of delicate fibrils made of protein from various origins, depending on the form of amyloidosis.

31.2 Symptoms

Patients with asteroid hyalosis are usually asymptomatic, but they may complain of decreased visual acuity, glare, and floaters.

Patients with systemic amyloidosis may initially present with slowly progressive visual deterioration due to vitreous opacities. They may have non-ocular manifestations of the disease including upper and lower extremity polyneuropathy and central nervous system abnormalities. Varying systemic manifestations may result from amyloid deposited in multiple organs including the heart, skin, and the gastrointestinal tract.

A. Ortiz, MD • C.A. Medina, MD (✉)
Department of Ophthalmology, Bascom Palmer Eye Institute,
University of Miami, 900 NW 17th Street, Miami, FL 33136, USA
e-mail: camedina2020@gmail.com

C.A. Medina et al. (eds.), *Manual of Retinal Diseases: A Guide to Diagnosis and Management*, DOI 10.1007/978-3-319-20460-4_31

31.3 Signs

Minute white opacities, termed asteroid bodies, are found in the otherwise normal vitreous in asteroid hyalosis (Fig. 31.1).

Amyloid deposits in the vitreous body are gray or yellowish white, appearing granular with wispy fringes initially, but then developing a "cotton- or glass-wool"-like appearance as they enlarge and aggregate (Fig. 31.2). Deposits are bilateral in most cases, but they can be asymmetric or unilateral.

Abnormalities of the eyelids, orbit, extraocular muscles, conjunctiva, iris, and cornea may also present in amyloidosis.

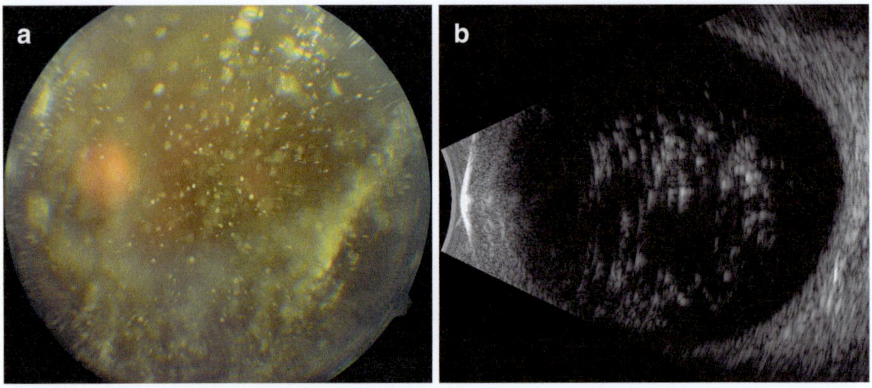

Fig. 31.1 Asteroid hyalosis. Fundus photograph showing yellow white suspended opacities in the vitreous cavity (**a**). B-scan ultrasonography reveals multiple discrete opacities (**b**) (Courtesy of Brandy Lorek BS, Cleveland, OH)

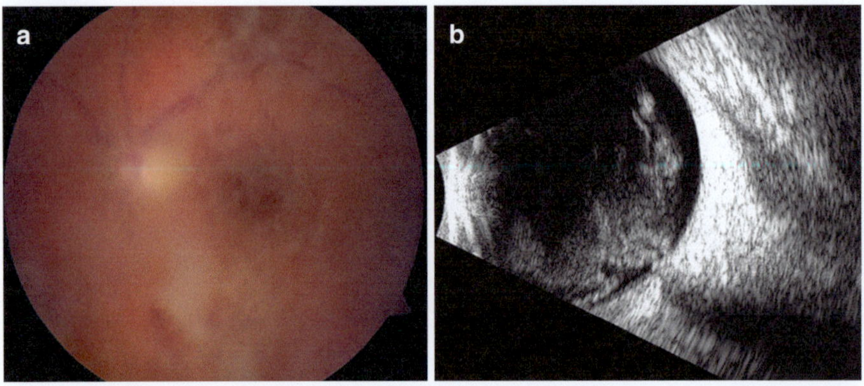

Fig. 31.2 Vitreous amyloidosis can mimic the clinical appearance of vitreoretinal lymphoma (**a**). The vitreous deposits are amorphous, predominantly in the posterior vitreous and overlying the posterior pole (**b**) (Reproduced with permission from: Ahluwalia MS, Dahiya S, Aronow ME, Peereboom D, Singh AD. Chapter 7: Primary central nervous system and retinal lymphoma. In: Singh AD, Murphree AL, Damato BE, editors. Clinical ophthalmic oncology. Retinal tumors. 2nd ed. Springer; 2015. p. 75–90)

Retinal findings may include exudates, cotton-wool spots, hemorrhages, and peripheral retinal neovascularization.

Amyloid deposition may occur in the choroid, trabecular meshwork, and retinal vasculature.

31.4 Epidemiology

Asteroid hyalosis most commonly occurs unilaterally (75 %) in patients greater than 50 years and has an incidence of approximately 1 in 200 persons in the general population. The condition has no sex or race predisposition.

Amyloidosis involving the vitreous is generally hereditary and has been described from many different countries with the largest number of patients from Japan, Portugal, and Sweden.

31.5 Predisposing Conditions

Systemic conditions such as diabetes mellitus, systemic hypertension, and atherosclerotic vascular disease have been associated with asteroid hyalosis. However, no systemic or ocular condition has been consistently linked to the condition.

Amyloidosis of the vitreous is especially linked to some of the hereditary neuropathies associated with the amyloid protein transthyretin.

31.6 Differential Diagnosis

The differential diagnosis for amyloidosis and asteroid hyalosis includes conditions in which vitreous opacities are present, including chronic dehemoglobinized vitreous hemorrhage, uveitis (vitritis), and ocular or systemic lymphoma. Synchysis scintillans or cholesterolosis presents as numerous highly refractile yellowish white, gold, or multicolored cholesterol crystals in the vitreous and/or anterior chamber. Cholesterol deposits tend to deposit inferiorly unlike the evenly distributed opacities in asteroid hyalosis. Careful examination under the slit lamp may help elucidate the cause.

31.7 Etiology

The etiology of asteroid hyalosis is not yet clear and may be caused by exogenous cell products, such as from inflammation, hemorrhage, or leakage from adjacent vessels. Systemic hypertension, diabetes mellitus, and atherosclerosis can predispose retinal vessels to damage and subsequent leakage. The higher prevalence of asteroid hyalosis in patients greater than 50 years of age may be due to the increasing vascular and microvascular changes that occur during this time period.

Vitreous amyloidosis is most often seen in transthyretin-related familial amyloidosis with polyneuropathy. This condition is inherited in an autosomal dominant mode and is caused by deposition of mutant transthyretin (TTR) protein in different tissues and organs, including the eyes, as amyloid fibrils.

31.8 Workup/Testing

- Ocular Examination
  - Slit-lamp examination is necessary for evaluation of vitreous opacities.
  - Examination for afferent pupillary defect (APD) should be performed.
  - A high intraocular pressure (IOP) in amyloidosis may indicate secondary glaucoma.
  - Fundus examination should be performed in suspected cases of amyloidosis.
  - Fluorescein angiography may be helpful in examining the retina if the opacities are dense and the view via indirect ophthalmoscopy is insufficient.
- Histologic examination of removed vitreous may show material with a fibrillar appearance and a characteristic Congo red staining with birefringence in amyloidosis.
- Biopsy and electron microscopic studies are confirmatory in systemic amyloidosis.

31.9 Prognosis and Management

Asteroid hyalosis has an excellent prognosis and rarely causes a significant decrease in visual acuity. Vitrectomy may be necessary to remove visually significant opacities if there is no other causal ocular pathology. Other indications for pars plana vitrectomy include better visualization of the fundus for diagnostic purposes, prolapse of asteroid body-laden vitreous into the anterior chamber during or after cataract extraction, and inability to perform laser treatment of the posterior segment. Asteroid hyalosis may cause an artifactual lowering of axial length measurement, leading to significant error in calculation of intraocular lens power, which must be considered prior to cataract surgery.

Familial amyloidosis is a systemic disease with a poor prognosis. Patients with amyloidosis may require a pars plana vitrectomy for vitreous opacities when there is progression of visual impairment. Recurrence can occur, requiring repeat vitrectomy, particularly when there is incomplete vitreous removal.

31.10 Follow-Up

In patients with asymptomatic asteroid hyalosis, the therapeutic approach should be conservative and follow-up can be extended. Patients with amyloidosis should have regular follow-up to assess for gradual deterioration of visual acuity and to monitor other ocular manifestations.

References and Suggested Reading

1. Beirao JM, Malheiro J, Lemos C, Beirao I, Costa P, Torres P. Ophthalmological manifestations in hereditary transthyretin (ATTR V30M) carriers: a review of 513 cases. Amyloid. 2015;22(2):117–22.
2. Beirao NM, Matos E, Beirao I, Costa PP, Torres P. Recurrence of vitreous amyloidosis and need of surgical reintervention in Portuguese patients with familial amyloidosis ATTR V30M. Retina. 2011;31(7):1373–7.
3. Bergren RL, Brown GC, Duker JS. Prevalence and association of asteroid hyalosis with systemic diseases. Am J Ophthalmol. 1991;111(3):289–93.
4. Ciulla TA, Tolentino F, Morrow JF, Dryja TP. Vitreous amyloidosis in familial amyloidotic polyneuropathy. Report of a case with the Val30Met transthyretin mutation. Surv Ophthalmol. 1995;40(3):197–206.
5. Feist RM, Morris RE, Witherspoon CD, Blair NP, Ticho BH, White Jr MF. Vitrectomy in asteroid hyalosis. Retina. 1990;10(3):173–7.
6. Hitchings RA, Tripathi RC. Vitreous opacities in primary amyloid disease. A clinical, histochemical, and ultrastructural report. Br J Ophthalmol. 1976;60(1):41–54.
7. Sandgren O. Ocular amyloidosis, with special reference to the hereditary forms with vitreous involvement. Surv Ophthalmol. 1995;40(3):173–96.
8. Topilow HW, Kenyon KR, Takahashi M, Freeman HM, Tolentino FI, Hanninen LA. Asteroid hyalosis. Biomicroscopy, ultrastructure, and composition. Arch Ophthalmol. 1982;100(6):964–8.
9. Winkler J, Lunsdorf H. Ultrastructure and composition of asteroid bodies. Invest Ophthalmol Vis Sci. 2001;42(5):902–7.
10. Yazar Z, Hanioglu S, Karakoc G, Gursel E. Asteroid hyalosis. Eur J Ophthalmol. 2001;11(1): 57–61.

Chapter 32
Hereditary Vitreoretinopathies

Brian Goldhagen and Audina Berrocal

32.1 Definition

Congenital vitreous abnormalities and associated retinal changes

32.2 Common Features

Cataract, increased risk of retinal detachment, additional ocular/systemic findings; variable expression

32.3 Types

1. Snowflake vitreoretinal degeneration
   - Inheritance: AD, KCNJ13 gene
   - Vision: typically good, visual field constriction
   - Ocular findings: corneal guttae, disk pallor, fibrillar vitreous degeneration, small snowflake-like opacities in peripheral retina, sheathing and obliteration of peripheral retinal vessels, cataract, increased incidence of retinal detachments
   - Systemic findings: none

B. Goldhagen, MD (✉) • A. Berrocal, MD
Department of Ophthalmology, Bascom Palmer Eye Institute,
University of Miami Miller School of Medicine,
900 NW 17th Street, Miami, FL 33136, USA
e-mail: bxg150@miami.edu

C.A. Medina et al. (eds.), *Manual of Retinal Diseases: A Guide to Diagnosis and Management*, DOI 10.1007/978-3-319-20460-4_32

2. Wagner syndrome

   - Inheritance: AD, 5q13-14 (chondroitin sulfate proteoglycan 2 gene)
   - Vision: vision loss as cataract and chorioretinal atrophy progress, nyctalopia, difficulty with dark adaption
   - Ocular findings: optically empty vitreous with strands and veils, moderate myopia, early "dotlike" cataracts, chorioretinal degeneration with atrophy, foveal ectopia (positive angle kappa), perivascular pigmentary changes; retinal detachment is not common
   - Systemic findings: none
   - Related syndromes:

3. Jansen syndrome: increased incidence of retinal detachments
4. Erosive vitreoretinopathy: increased incidence of retinal detachments (>50 %)
5. Enhanced S-cone syndrome/Goldmann-Favre vitreotapetoretinal degeneration

   - Inheritance: AR, NR2E3 gene (retinal nuclear receptor subfamily 2, group E, member 3)
   - Vision: poor due to retinoschisis, night blindness
   - Ocular findings: vitreous liquefaction with strands and veils, peripheral bone spicule-like pigmentary changes, peripheral retinoschisis that may involve the macula, cataract, abnormal ERG response
   - Systemic findings: none

6. Stickler syndrome

   - Inheritance: AD

   - Type 1: COL2A1 (collagen 2 alpha 1 gene), most common type
   - Type 2: COL11A1 (collagen 11 alpha 1)

   - Vision: typically good
   - Ocular findings: high myopia, cataract, membranous or optically empty vitreous (type 1), vitreous with beaded and fibrillary appearance (type 2), perivascular pigmentary changes, retinal detachment with multiple and/or posterior tears (50 %), ocular hypertension or glaucoma (Fig. 32.1)
   - Systemic findings: cleft palate, Pierre Robin sequence, flat midface, hearing loss, epiphyseal dysplasia, arthritis
   - Related syndromes:

     – Marshall syndrome: hypertelorism, ectodermal dysplasia, thickened calvarium and meningeal calcifications, absence of frontal sinuses
     – Kniest dysplasia: short stature, kyphoscoliosis, flat midface, cleft palate, hearing loss
     – Knobloch syndrome: occipital encephalocele
     – Weissenbacher-Zweymuller: micrognathia, midfacial hypoplasia, rhizomelic limb shortening, dumbbell-shaped femora and humeri, hearing loss

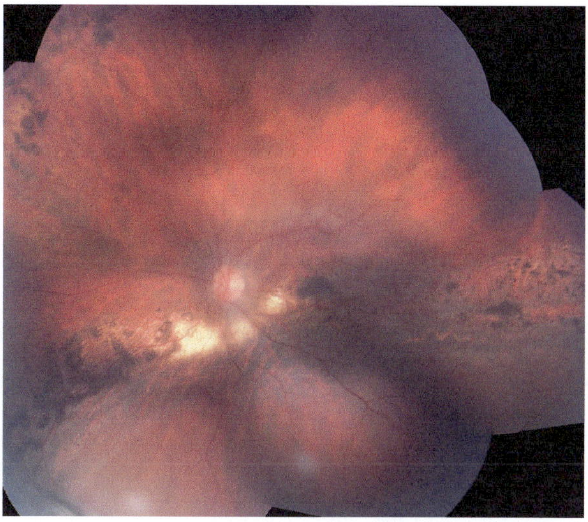

Fig. 32.1 Stickler syndrome. Typical fundus appearance of perivascular pigmentary changes

7. Autosomal dominant vitreoretinochoroidopathy (ADViRC)/autosomal dominant neovascular inflammatory vitreoretinopathy (ADNIV)
   - Ocular findings: cystoid macular edema, peripheral retinal neovascularization, retinal pigmentary changes (both hyper and hypo), vitreous cells and hemorrhage, and cataracts
   - ADViRC: distinct circumferential band of pigmentary change; complications are uncommon
   - ADNIV: asymptomatic until 20s; ERG abnormalities; neovascular glaucoma, tractional retinal detachments
8. Lattice degeneration
9. X-linked retinoschisis
10. Familial exudative vitreoretinopathy

32.4 Management

Regular eye screening: including education of symptoms of retinal detachment.

Genetic counseling: consider prenatal testing given autosomal dominant inheritance of most types of vitreoretinopathies.

Refractive error: correct with glasses or contact lenses.

Cataract: early onset; surgery is difficult to due lack of vitreous support; consider pars plana infusion to assist in maintaining intraocular pressure.

Glaucoma: monitor for development and manage accordingly.

Prophylactic retinopexy: no established guidelines; may be of benefit to those types of vitreoretinopathies with increased risk of retinal detachment.

Retinal detachment: monitor for and manage using established methods.
Retinoschisis: prophylactic treatment of outer layer retinal breaks associated with retinoschisis is not recommended.
Systemic complications: symptomatic treatment of systemic findings.

References and Suggested Reading

1. Brown DM, Weingeist TA. Disorders of the Vitreous and Vitreoretinal Interface. In: Wright KW, Spiegel PH, Thompson LS, editors. Handbook of pediatric retinal disease. New York: Springer Science+Business Media, Inc; 2006. p. 178–200.
2. Edwards AO. Clinical features of the congenital vitreoretinopathies. Eye (Lond). 2008;22(10):1233–42.
3. Robin NH, Moran RT, Ala-Kokko L. (Updated November 26, 2014). Stickler syndrome. In: *GeneReviews* at GeneTests Medical Genetics Information Resource (database online). Copyright, University of Washington, Seattle. 1997–2013. Available at http://www.genetests.org. Accessed 1 June 2015.
4. Shuler MF, Sullivan JM, Hurley BR, McNamara JA. Vitreoretinal dystrophies. In: Reynolds JD, Olitsky SE, editors. Pediatric retina. New York: Springer; 2011. p. 315–44.
5. Tang S, Ding X, Luo Y. Hereditary vitreoretinal degenerations. In: Ryan SJ, editor. Retina. 5th ed. London: Saunders; 2013. p. 836–51.

Section V
Uveal Tumors and Associated Conditions

Mary E. Aronow

Chapter 33
Choroidal Nevus

Maria J. Suarez

33.1 Definitions

Choroidal nevi are benign melanocytic lesions. The Collaborative Ocular Melanoma Study (COMS) defined nevi by having ≤5 mm in greatest basal diameter and ≤1 mm in thickness.

33.2 Symptoms

In general, nevi are asymptomatic and are discovered as an incidental finding on routine dilated fundus examination. Associated choroidal neovascularization, photoreceptor atrophy, or associated exudative retinal detachment may cause decreased visual acuity.

33.3 Signs

The majority of nevi (91 %) occur posterior to the equator. Clinically, they appear as flat to minimally elevated, brown to greenish lesions within the choroid. Overlying drusen is common feature and suggests chronicity (Fig. 33.1). Histopathologically, choroidal nevi are characterized by benign melanocytic proliferation of spindle-shaped cells with bland nuclei (Fig. 33.2).

M.J. Suarez, MD
Ophthalmic Pathology, Wilmer Eye Institute, Johns Hopkins School of Medicine,
400 N Broadway, Suite 4070, Baltimore, MD 21231, USA
e-mail: msuarez9@jhmi.edu

C.A. Medina et al. (eds.), *Manual of Retinal Diseases: A Guide to Diagnosis and Management*, DOI 10.1007/978-3-319-20460-4_33

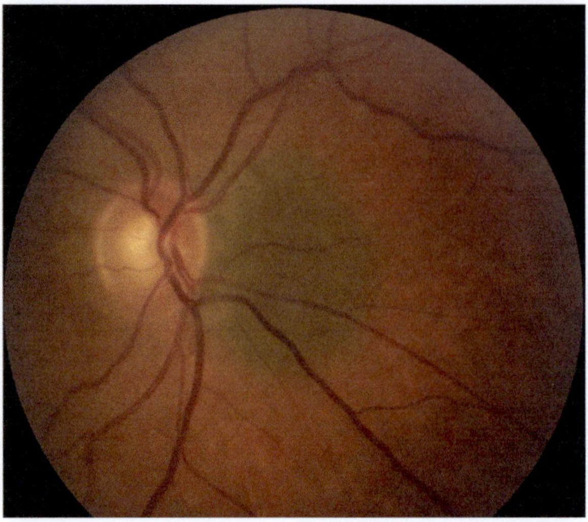

Fig. 33.1 Flat, juxtapapillary choroidal nevus in the right eye. Note is made of the absence of orange pigment or overlying subretinal fluid

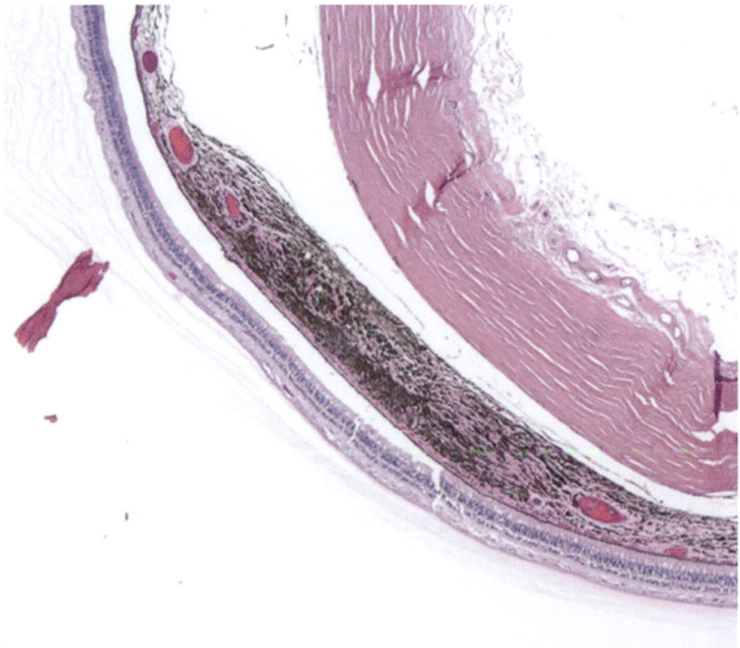

Fig. 33.2 Histopathology of choroidal nevus demonstrating melanocytic proliferation between Bruch's membrane and the sclera (hematoxylin and eosin, 40×) (Courtesy of Charles G. Eberhart, MD, PhD and Michael J. Mines, MD)

33.4 Predisposing Conditions

Choroidal nevi are common and occur in approximately 7 % of adults [3]. Nevi of the choroid have no gender predilection. The risk of malignant transformation in the general population is estimated to be 1 in 8,845. Seven clinical features predictive of growth of nevi and transformation to uveal melanoma include tumor thickness >2 mm, posterior tumor margin close to the optic nerve, presence of visual symptoms, overlying orange pigment, associated subretinal fluid, ultrasonographic hollowness, and absence of halo.

33.5 Inheritance

Choroidal nevi are a common incidental finding; no pattern of inheritance has been described.

33.6 Differential Diagnosis

The differential diagnosis includes choroidal melanoma, congenital hypertrophy of the RPE, macular degeneration, hemangioma, metastasis, and melanocytoma.

33.7 Etiology

There is no known etiology for this condition.

33.8 Workup/Testing

A detailed dilated fundus examination should be performed to document the appearance of the nevus. Color fundus photography should be used for documentation. Further characterization of dimensions (including thickness in minimally elevated lesions) and reflectivity can be assessed by B-scan and A-scan ultrasonography. Enhanced depth imaging (EDI) SD-OCT of small choroidal lesions, which are undetectable by ultrasound, can be used to objectively measure and follow thickness. OCT can also confirm the presence or absence of features such as subretinal fluid and overlying drusen. For indeterminate lesions, fluorescein angiography (FA) and indocyanine green angiography (ICG) can be helpful in detecting intrinsic vascularization which is more suggestive of choroidal melanoma.

33.9 Prognosis and Management

Choroidal nevi are benign lesions with an excellent prognosis. The vast majority require no medical or surgical therapy.

33.10 Follow-Up

Serial fundus photography and ultrasonography (for minimally elevated lesions) are recommended to document the appearance over time. In cases of newly noted choroidal nevi or indeterminate melanocytic lesions, close follow-up (every 3 months) may be warranted to document either stability or growth of lesion. Documented significant growth over a short interval is more suggestive of melanoma for which treatment is recommended.

References and Suggested Reading

1. Group COMS. COMS manual of procedures: accession no. PBS 179693. Springfield: National Technical Information Service; 1995.
2. Yanoff M, Sassani JW. Ocular pathology, text and atlas. 6th ed. UK: Mosby Elsevier Ch. 17; 2009. p. 697–702.
3. Shields CL, Furuta M, et al. Choroidal nevus transformation into melanoma: analysis of 2514 consecutive cases. Arch Ophthalmol. 2009;127(8):981–7.
4. Singh AD. Tumors of the uvea: benign melanocytic tumors. In: Singh AD, editor. Clinical ophthalmic oncology. Philadelphia: WB Saunders Company; 2007. p. 185–97.
5. Kaiserman I, Kaiserman N, Pe'er J. Long term ultrasonic follow up of choroidal naevi and their transformation to melanomas. Br J Ophthalmol. 2006;90:994–8.
6. Torres VL, Brugnoni N, Kaiser PK, Singh AD. Optical coherence tomography enhanced depth imaging of choroidal tumors. Am J Ophthalmol. 2011;151(4):586–93.

Chapter 34
Melanocytoma

Ahmadreza Moradi

34.1 Definitions

Melanocytoma (magnocellular nevus) is a benign, congenital hamartoma arising from melanocytes.

34.2 Symptoms

The majority (86 % of cases) are asymptomatic. A small proportion of patients may experience symptoms including decreased visual acuity, floaters, and/or flashes of light.

34.3 Signs

Melanocytoma appears clinically as a dark brown to black lesion, often with feathery margins, which frequently occurs at the optic nerve head. The lesion sometimes extends into the peripapillary retina and choroid (Fig. 34.1). Melanocytoma is nearly always unilateral. Associated findings may include relative afferent pupillary defect (RAPD) in the affected eye and visual field defects including enlargement of the blind spot. Ophthalmologists should be aware of rare complications of melanocytoma such as retinal edema, retinal exudation, associated hemorrhage, and vascular occlusion.

A. Moradi, MD
Wilmer Eye Institute, Johns Hopkins Hospital,
600 N Wolfe Street, B-20, Baltimore, MD 21287, USA
e-mail: amoradi1@jhmi.edu

C.A. Medina et al. (eds.), *Manual of Retinal Diseases: A Guide to Diagnosis and Management*, DOI 10.1007/978-3-319-20460-4_34

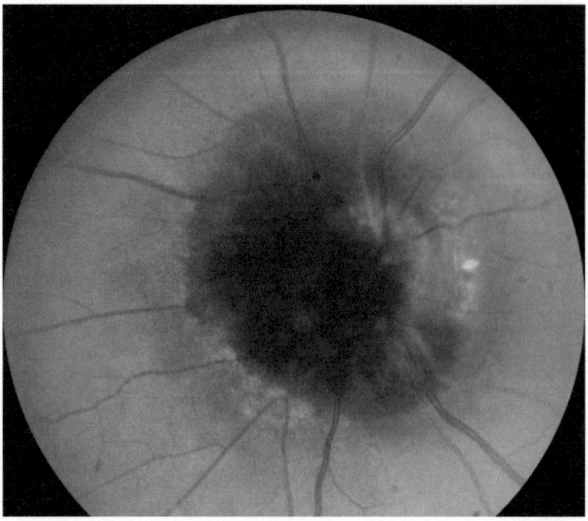

Fig. 34.1 Optic disk melanocytoma demonstrating a uniformly dark mass with feathery borders involving the surrounding retina and choroid. Deposition of calcium is observed

34.4 Epidemiology

The mean age of diagnosis is 50 years. There is a slight predilection for females (female/male ratio = 3/2) and a racial predisposition, with approximately one-third to one-half occurring in persons of African ancestry. Caucasian individuals with melanocytoma are more commonly of Hispanic or Italian descent.

34.5 Predisposing Conditions

Melanocytoma has no strong association with systemic disease and is generally considered to occur sporadically. There have been reports of optic disc melanocytoma occurring with intracranial meningioma and ocular melanocytosis.

34.6 Differential Diagnosis

Choroidal melanoma is the most important entity to consider in the differential diagnosis of melanocytoma. Other diagnoses include choroidal nevus, congenital hyperplasia of the retinal pigment epithelium (CHRPE), combined hamartoma of the retina and RPE, RPE adenoma, and juxtapapillary subretinal hemorrhage.

34.7 Etiology

These lesions occur sporadically. The etiology of optic disc melanocytoma is unknown.

34.8 Workup/Testing

The diagnosis of a melanocytoma of the optic disc is generally straightforward and can be made with dilated ophthalmoscopic examination alone. Formal visual field testing and fundus photography should be performed at the time of diagnosis to document baseline characteristics. Ancillary imaging can also be helpful:

- Optical coherence tomography (OCT): useful in detecting microscopic extension of the tumor into the retrolaminar portion of the optic nerve as well as in determining the extent of subretinal fluid and macular edema which may not be apparent with ophthalmoscopy alone [8].
- Fluorescein and indocyanine green angiography (FA and ICG): useful for differentiating melanocytoma from melanoma, as the former demonstrates dense hypofluorescence corresponding to the location of the tumor. In contrast to uveal melanoma, intrinsic vasculature is not present.
- Ultrasonography (B/A scan): reveals an acoustically solid mass (Fig. 34.2) with high internal reflectively.

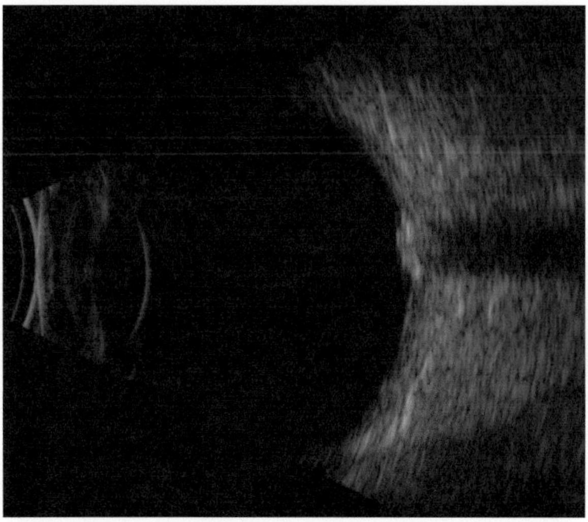

Fig. 34.2 B-scan ultrasonography reveals a solid, dome-shaped, regularly structured lesion overlying the optic disc. Maximal elevation measures 1.6 mm. There is adjacent orbital shadowing secondary to calcification

34.9 Prognosis and Management

An initial tumor thickness of ≥1.5 mm is a risk factor for growth. A small fraction, 1–2 % percent of optic nerve melanocytoma, transforms to malignant melanoma. Rapid visual loss may result from central retinal vascular occlusion, ischemic optic neuropathy associated with tumor necrosis, or malignant transformation. If the vision loss is accompanied by progressive growth, malignant transformation should be suspected and treatment should be initiated. Unfortunately, there are no current therapies to prevent growth of optic nerve melanocytoma.

34.10 Follow-Up

For typical, asymptomatic melanocytoma, annual dilated fundus examination with fundus photography and formal visual field testing is recommended. When melanocytoma demonstrates atypical features, patients should be followed at closer intervals to exclude the possibility of malignant transformation.

References and Suggested Reading

1. Zimmerman LE, Garron LK. Melanocytoma of the optic disk. Int Ophthalmol Clin. 1962;2:431–40.
2. Joffe L, Shields JA, Osher RH, et al. Clinical and follow-up studies of melanocytomas of the optic disc. Ophthalmology. 1979;86:1067–83.
3. Shields JA, Demirci H, Mashayekhi A, et al. Melanocytoma of optic disc in 115 cases: the 2004 Samuel Johnson Memorial Lecture, part 1. Ophthalmology. 2004;111:1739–46.
4. Shields JA, Demirci H, Mashayekhi A, Eagle RC, Shields CL. Melanocytoma of the optic disk: a review. Surv Ophthalmol. 2006;51:93–104.
5. Turell ME, Singh AD. Nonvascular hamartomas. In: Wright KW, Spiegel PH, editors. Pediatric ophthalmology and strabismus, vol. 1. 3rd ed. New York: Springer; 2012. p. 928–37.
6. Walsh TJ, Packer S. Bilateral melanocytoma of the optic nerve associated with intracranial meningioma. Ann Ophthalmol. 1971;3:885–8.
7. Shinoda K, Hayasaka S, Nagaki Y, et al. Melanocytoma of the left optic nerve head and right retrobulbar optic neuropathy compressed by a tuberculum sellae meningioma. Ophthalmologica. 2000;214:161–3.
8. Shields CL, Perez B, Benavides R, Materin M, Shields JA. Optical coherence tomography of optic disk melanocytoma in 15 cases. Retina. 2008;28(3):441–6.

Chapter 35
Choroidal Melanoma

Nazlee Zebardast

35.1 Definition

Choroidal melanoma is a neoplasm of melanocytes and represents the most common primary intraocular malignancy in adults.

35.2 Symptoms

Patients may be asymptomatic, or depending on proximity to the macula, individuals may report metamorphopsia, visual field defects, floaters, and photopsias. Decreased visual acuity may occur secondary to exudative retinal detachment. Pain is rare.

35.3 Signs

Typically presents as an elevated, dome-shaped, choroidal mass. Pigmentation may vary from brown to green to amelanotic. There is frequently overlying orange pigment and subretinal fluid (Fig. 35.1). In some cases, absence of drusen (Drusen imply chronicity and are frequently associated with choroidal nevi) may help to distinguish between long-standing choroidal nevi and melanoma. Classically, ultrasonography reveals a mushroom-shaped choroidal mass with low to medium internal reflectivity, choroidal excavation, and orbital shadowing.

N. Zebardast, MD, MSc
General Eye Services B-20, Wilmer Eye Institute, Johns Hopkins University School of Medicine, 600 N Wolfe Street, Baltimore, MD 21287-9277, USA
e-mail: nzebard1@jhmi.edu

C.A. Medina et al. (eds.), *Manual of Retinal Diseases: A Guide to Diagnosis and Management*, DOI 10.1007/978-3-319-20460-4_35

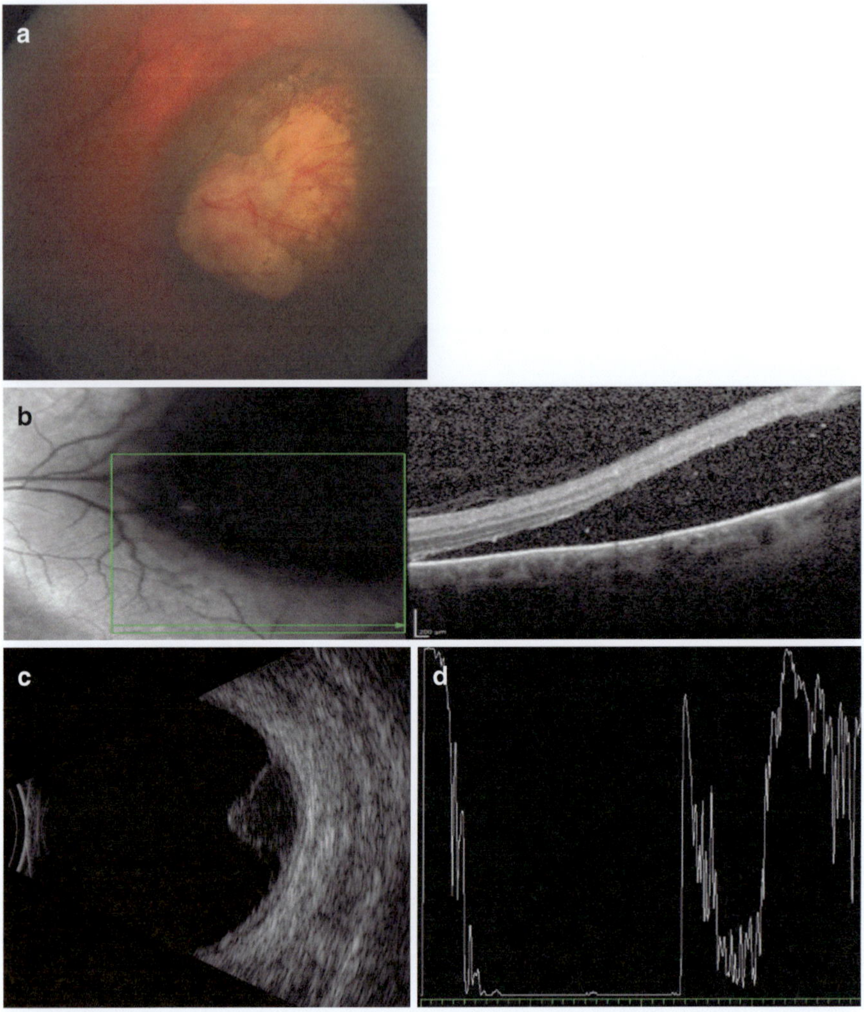

Fig. 35.1 A 54-year-old Caucasian male presented with choroidal melanoma in the left eye. Note the orange pigment along the superior margin, overlying subretinal fluid, focus of retinal invasion, and the intrinsic vasculature (**a**). OCT confirms overlying subretinal fluid (**b**). B-scan ultrasonography demonstrates a collar button-shaped lesion measuring 6.3 mm in maximal thickness and 10.1 mm by 9.8 mm in base (**c**). A-scan ultrasonography reveals that the tumor has moderate to low reflectivity (**d**)

35.4 Predisposing Conditions

The incidence is approximately 5.1 per million population. White race has the strongest association (rare in nonwhite populations). Choroidal melanoma may arise from preexisting nevi. In patients with oculodermal melanocytosis (nevus of Ota), the lifetime risk of choroidal melanoma is approximately 1 in 400. Other

Table 35.1 Differential diagnosis of choroidal melanoma

Choroidal nevus
Choroidal metastasis
Circumscribed choroidal hemangioma
Melanocytoma
Choroidal hemorrhage
Disciform lesion/peripheral exudative hemorrhagic chorioretinopathy
Posterior nodular scleritis
Congenital hypertrophy of the retinal pigment epithelium

predisposing conditions include: familial atypical mole and melanoma (FAM-M) syndrome, neurofibromatosis type 1 (NF-1), and Li-Fraumeni syndrome. Familial occurrence is rare.

35.5 Differential Diagnosis

The differential includes: choroidal nevus, choroidal metastasis, circumscribed choroidal hemangioma, melanocytoma, choroidal hemorrhage, disciform lesions/ peripheral exudative hemorrhagic chorioretinopathy (PEHCR), posterior nodular scleritis, and congenital hypertrophy of the retinal pigment epithelium (Table 35.1).

35.6 Etiology

Unknown. The association between ultraviolet sun exposure and uveal melanoma is uncertain.

35.7 Workup/Testing (Table 35.2)

- External/slit lamp examination for melanocytosis, sentinel vessels, iris heterochromia
- Indirect ophthalmoscopy with fundus photography: classic features include presence of orange pigment and overlying subretinal fluid. Drusen may be present or absent
- Optical coherence tomography (Fig. 35.1b): helpful in confirming the presence of overlying subretinal fluid
- B/A scan ultrasonography (Fig. 35.1c, d)
- Fluorescein angiography (FA) and indocyanine green angiography (ICG) may demonstrate classic "double circulation sign"

Table 35.2 Ancillary imaging studies in choroidal melanoma

Imaging study	Result
Ultrasonography B-Scan	Mushroom or collar button shape Choroidal excavation, orbital shadowing Vascularity within the lesion
Ultrasonography A-Scan	Low to medium internal reflectivity
OCT	Overlying subretinal fluid (some cases)
FA	Double circulation sign
ICG	Double circulation sign

- Systemic evaluation: laboratory studies such as liver function tests and systemic imaging (CT, MRI, PET) are useful for detection of metastases. Hematogenous spread is preferential to the liver (>90%). The American Joint Committee on Cancer (AJCC) has established Tumor-Node-Metastasis (TNM) staging criteria.
- Tumor biopsy (e.g., fine-needle aspiration biopsy or enucleation tissue) can provide both diagnostic confirmation and be used for prognostication

35.8 Prognosis and Management

The Collaborative Ocular Melanoma Study (COMS) defined melanoma size as small (>1.5 to <2.5 mm in height, 5–16 mm greatest basal diameter), medium (2.5–10 mm in height, ≤16 mm greatest basal diameter), and large (>10 mm in height or >16 mm greatest basal diameter). The cumulative melanoma-related mortality rates 25 years following treatment of the primary tumor were 18%, 52%, and 59% for small, medium, and large tumors, respectively. Treatment depends upon factors such as the size and location of the tumor, visual acuity of the affected and fellow eye, and patient preference. Periodic observation may be warranted for some small, indeterminate lesions. Treatment options for small and medium tumors include plaque brachytherapy using COMS dosing (85 Gy to the apex of the tumor) and proton beam radiotherapy. Enucleation is recommended for large tumors, tumors encircling the optic nerve, or in eyes with poor visual potential. Transpupillary thermotherapy (TTT) may be used in combination with radiotherapy (so-called sandwich therapy). Other forms of stereotactic radiotherapy and tumor resection are performed in some oncology centers.

35.9 Follow-Up

Patients with choroidal melanoma should be followed closely by both an experienced ophthalmic oncologist and a medical oncologist. Periodic systemic surveillance is generally performed, particularly imaging and/or laboratory studies of the liver, as this is the most common site of metastasis.

References and Suggested Reading

1. Bedikian AY, Legha SS, Mavligit G, et al. Treatment of uveal melanoma metastatic to the liver: a review of the M.D. Anderson Center experience and prognostic factors. Cancer. 1995;76(9):1665–70.
2. Edge SB, Byrd DR, Compton CC, Fritz AG, Greene FL, Trotti A. American Joint Committee on Cancer (AJCC) cancer staging manual. 7th ed. Chicago: Springer; 2010.
3. Kujala E, Makitie T, Kivela T. Very long-term prognosis of patients with malignant uveal melanoma. Invest Ophthalmol Vis Sci. 2003;44:4651–9.
4. Shields CL, Kaliki S, Livesey M, et al. Association of ocular and oculodermal melanocytosis with the rate of uveal melanoma metastasis analysis of 7872 consecutive eyes. JAMA Ophthalmol. 2013;131(8):993–1003.
5. Singh AD, Shields CL, Potter D, et al. Familial uveal melanoma: clinical observations on 56 patients. Arch Ophthalmol. 1996;114:392–9.
6. Singh AD, Turell ME, Topham AK. Uveal melanoma: trends in incidence, treatment, and survival. Ophthalmology. 2011;118:1881–5.

Chapter 36
Congenital Hypertrophy of the Retinal Pigment Epithelium

Sherveen S. Salek

36.1 Definitions

Congenital hypertrophy of the retinal pigment epithelium (CHRPE)
Familial adenomatous polyposis (FAP)
Pigmented ocular fundus lesions (POFLs)
Retinal detachment (RD)

36.2 Symptoms

Usually asymptomatic but can present with decreased vision, especially if lesion involves the fovea

36.3 Signs (Table 36.1)

36.3.1 Solitary CHRPE

- Flat, round, hyperpigmented lesion (Fig. 36.1).
- Well demarcated with smooth or scalloped margins.
- Color varies from light gray, brown, to black.

S.S. Salek, MD
Wilmer Eye Institute, Johns Hopkins Hospital,
600 N Wolfe Street, B-20, Baltimore, MD 21205, USA
e-mail: ssalek1@jhmi.edu

C.A. Medina et al. (eds.), *Manual of Retinal Diseases: A Guide to Diagnosis and Management*, DOI 10.1007/978-3-319-20460-4_36

Table 36.1 Clinical features of CHRPE, grouped CHRPE, and POFLs [1]

Feature	CHRPE	Grouped CHRPE	POFLs
Shape	Round	Variable	Ovoid
Size	0.2–1.3 mm	Variable	0.15–4.5 mm
Laterality	Unilateral	Uni- or bilateral	Bilateral
Hypopigmentation	Lacunae	Absent	Comet tail
Number	Solitary	Grouped	≥4
Growth behavior	Minimal, slow	Unknown	Unknown
Systemic association	None	None	FAP

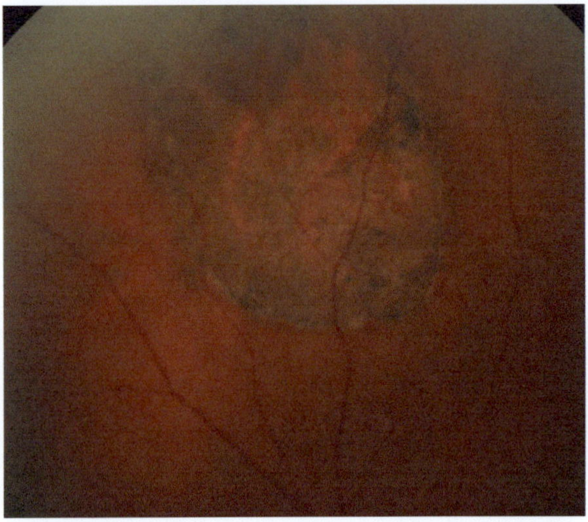

Fig. 36.1 Solitary CHRPE lesion in superior midperiphery of left eye

- Overlying retina appears normal and may have focal intraretinal hyperpigmentation near margin.
- Rare associated vascular abnormalities – microaneurysms, intraretinal A-V anastomoses, and neovascularization.
- Predominantly located in superotemporal or equatorial region
- Majority slowly enlarges over time and can involve fovea and become symptomatic.
- Not associated with FAP.

36.3.2 *Grouped CHRPE*

- Commonly referred to as "bear tracks" (Fig. 36.2) or "polar bear tracks" if amelanotic
- Clusters of flat, well-demarcated lesions, with about 3–30 lesions in each cluster, and increasing size and pigmentation anteriorly toward fundus periphery; likely reflects migration of RPE cells during embryogenesis

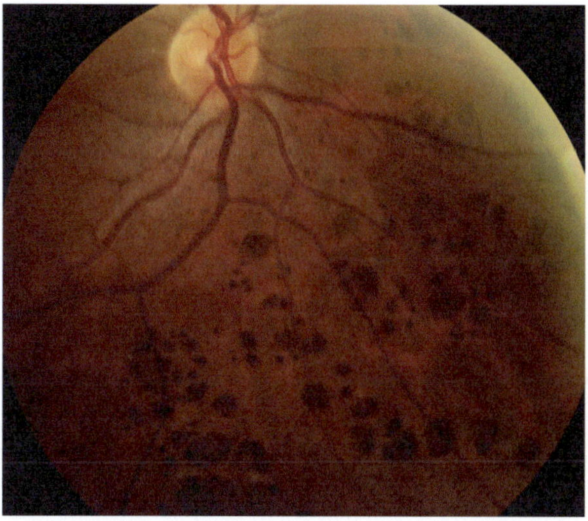

Fig. 36.2 Grouped pigmented CHRPE (so-called bear tracks) in the inferonasal quadrant of the right eye

- Associated with "cutaneous lines of Blaschko" ipsilateral to affected eye
- No association with FAP

36.3.3 POFLs

- Associated with FAP, found in 70–80 % of patients with FAP.
- Multiple, bilateral, ovoid/schistocyte shape, comet/fishtail oriented toward posterior pole.
- Retinal invasion and glial, capillary, and pigment epithelial proliferation and hypertrophy may be seen.

36.4 Predisposing Conditions

The prevalence of CHRPE is as low as 1.25%. The median age of diagnosis is 45 years for solitary CHRPE. There are no predisposing conditions for solitary, unilateral CHRPE. Grouped CHRPE is associated with cutaneous lines of Blaschko. FAP is found in approximately 1 in 7000–22,000 individuals. POFLs are associated with Gardner syndrome (FAP with extracolonic manifestations including skeletal hamartomas, epidermoid cysts, fibromas, and lipomas) and Turcot syndrome (FAP with brain tumors such as astrocytoma, ependymoma, and medulloblastoma). For FAP, inheritance is typically autosomal dominant and caused by mutation in the *APC* gene. FAP can also be caused by autosomal recessive mutation in *MUTYH*.

36.5 Differential Diagnosis

- Choroidal melanoma
- Choroidal nevus
- Melanocytoma
- Sunburst lesions in sickle cell retinopathy
- Chorioretinal scar secondary to injury, infection, inflammation, or drug toxicity

36.6 Etiology

Solitary and grouped CHRPE consist of a single layer of hypertrophied RPE cells packed with large round pigment granules consisting of macromelanosomes. There is associated thickening of Bruch's membrane, normal inner retinal layers, and vasculature. POFLs demonstrate both hyperplasia and hypertrophy of RPE cells, with retinal invasion and more vascular features. POFLs may be elevated and involve the full thickness of the retina.

36.7 Workup/Testing

- Dilated fundus exam.
- Color photographs for documentation, including wide-field Optomap.
- Fundus autofluorescence may identify smaller lesions.
- SD-OCT: thinning of neurosensory retina, absence of RPE in lacunae
- POFLs: prompt evaluation for FAP, periodic colonoscopy, screening of family members

36.8 Prognosis and Management

Generally excellent; the vast majority of patients are asymptomatic. If the lesion enlarges or extends toward macula or subretinal fluid threatens vision, one can consider laser photocoagulation. If lesion causes wrinkling in macular region, one can consider vitrectomy with membrane peel.

36.9 Follow-Up

Periodic eye examinations, typically annually unless symptomatic or threatening central vision

References and Suggested Reading

1. Traboulsi EI, Heur M, Singh AD. Tumors of the retinal pigment epithelium. In: Singh AD, Damato BE, Pe'er J, et al., editors. Clinical ophthalmic oncology. Philadelphia: Saunders-Elsevier; 2007. p. 358–65.
2. Turell ME, Leonardy NJ, Singh AD. A unique presentation of grouped congenital hypertrophy of the retinal pigment epithelium. Ophthalmic Genet. 2011;32(3):162–4.
3. Turell ME, Singh AD. Nonvascular hamartomas. In: Wright KW, Spiegel PH, editors. Pediatric ophthalmology and strabismus, vol. 1. 3rd ed. New York: Springer; 2012. p. 928–37.
4. Meyer CH, Gerding H. Congenital hypertrophy of the retinal pigment epithelium. In: Ryan SJ, editor. Retina. 5th ed. London: Saunders-Elsevier; 2013.
5. Shields CL, Mashayekhi A, Ho T, et al. Solitary congenital hypertrophy of the retinal pigment epithelium. Ophthalmology. 2003;110:1968–76.
6. Shields JA, Shields CL. Intraocular tumors: an atlas and textbook. Philadelphia: Lippincott Williams & Wilkins; 2008.

Chapter 37
Combined Hamartoma of the Retina and Retinal Pigment Epithelium

Ian C. Han

37.1 Definitions

CHR-RPE: combined hamartoma of the retina and retinal pigment epithelium is a benign hamartoma first described by Gass.

37.2 Symptoms

Decreased vision, distortion, and strabismus. Painless vision loss is secondary to direct involvement of the optic nerve, the papillomacular bundle, or the fovea.

37.3 Signs

Gray-green/brown-black discoloration and elevation of retina/RPE, fibrosis, tortuous vessels, epiretinal membrane formation with foveal dragging, retinal exudation, and/or edema (Fig. 37.1).

I.C. Han, MD
Deparment of Ophthalmology, Wilmer Eye Institute, Johns Hopkins University, 600 N. Wolfe Street, 272 Woods Building, Baltimore, MD 21287, USA
e-mail: ihan@jhmi.edu

C.A. Medina et al. (eds.), *Manual of Retinal Diseases: A Guide to Diagnosis and Management*, DOI 10.1007/978-3-319-20460-4_37

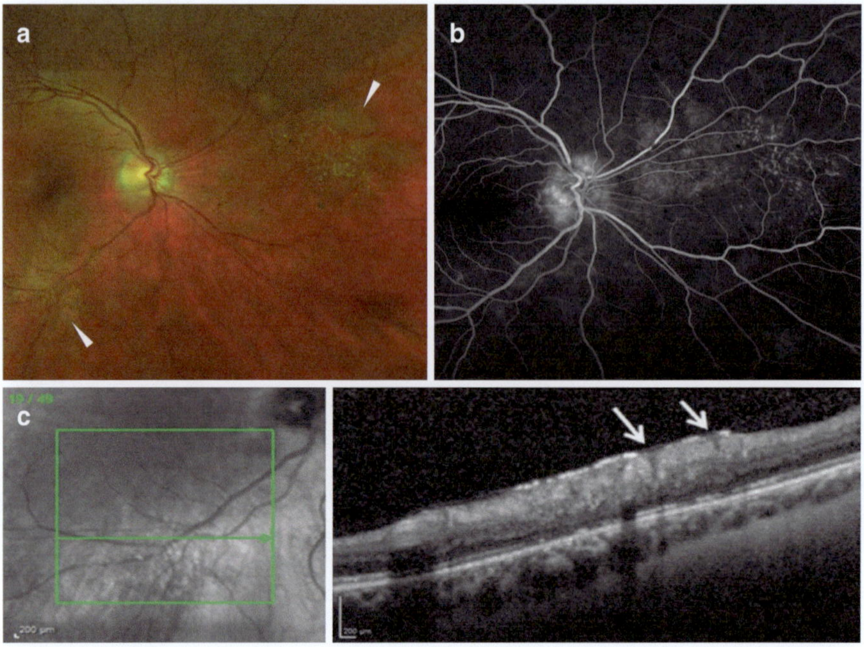

Fig. 37.1 Grayish-green discoloration of the retina nasal to the optic nerve and along the inferotemporal arcade consistent with CHR-RPE (**a**, *arrows*) (Image courtesy of Ian Han, MD, and Majed Alkharashi, MBBS). Fluorescein angiogram showing fine intrinsic vasculature and mild leakage (**b**). Spectral-domain optical coherence tomography line scan through the CHR-RPE along the inferotemporal arcade showing thickening and disorganization of the inner retinal layers, characteristic sawtooth inner retinal folds (*arrows*), and epiretinal membrane formation (**c**)

37.4 Predisposing Conditions

Rare tumor, most commonly diagnosed in children or young adults, typically unilateral, but can be bilateral. Generally considered sporadic, no known inheritance pattern. Possible association with neurofibromatosis type I and type II.

37.5 Differential Diagnosis

Retina/RPE origin: retinoblastoma, astrocytic hamartoma, and toxocariasis
Choroidal origin: choroidal nevus, melanoma, and hemangioma

37.6 Etiology

Not well understood. Histopathologic studies show disorganization and thickening of the optic nerve/retina with dysplastic glial tissue and redundant folds of RPE.

37.7 Workup/Testing

- Fluorescein angiography (FA): fine intrinsic vascularity of retinal tumor with mild leakage, vascular tortuosity (Fig. 37.1b)
- Optical coherence tomography (OCT): thickening/irregularity of retinal layers, sawtooth pattern of folded inner retinal layers, highlights epiretinal membrane and areas of retinal edema or traction (Fig. 37.1c)

37.8 Prognosis and Management

No proven therapy. Extramacular hamartomas are typically asymptomatic. Macular tumors may cause vision loss <20/200 in about half of cases secondary to epiretinal membrane formation, progressive traction, amblyopia/strabismus, or, rarely, exudation/choroidal neovascularization. Pars plana vitrectomy with epiretinal membrane peel may relieve traction in select cases where delineation between membrane and tumor is clear and where the retinal architecture is relatively preserved. CHR-RPE does not undergo malignant transformation.

37.9 Follow-Up

Monitor changes in epiretinal membrane and traction with OCT, with frequency based on severity of findings.

References and Suggested Reading

1. Cotlier E. Café-au-lait spots of the fundus in neurofibromatosis. Arch Ophthalmol. 1977;95:1990–2.
2. Gass JDM. An unusual hamartoma of the pigment epithelium and retina simulating choroidal melanoma and retinoblastoma. Trans Am Ophthalmol Soc. 1973;71:171–83.

3. Schachat AP, Shields JA, Fine SL, Sanborn GE, Weingeist TA, Valenzuela RE, Brucker AJ. Combined hamartomas of the retina and retinal pigment epithelium. Ophthalmology. 1984;91(12):1609–15.
4. Shields CL, Mashayekhi A, Dai VV, Materin MA, Shields JA. Optical coherence tomographic findings of combined hamartoma of the retina and retinal pigment epithelium in 11 patients. Arch Ophthalmol. 2005;123(12):1746–50.
5. Shields CL, Thangappan A, Hartzell K, Valente P, Pirondini C, Shields JA. Combined hamartoma of the retina and retinal pigment epithelium in 77 consecutive patients visual outcome based on macular versus extramacular tumor location. Ophthalmology. 2008;115(12):2246–52.
6. Traboulsi EI, Heur M, Singh AD. Tumors of the retinal pigment epithelium. In: Singh AD, Damato BE, Pe'er J, et al., editors. Clinical ophthalmic oncology. Philadelphia: Saunders-Elsevier; 2007. p. 358–65.
7. Tsai P, O'Brien JM. Combined hamartoma of the retina and retinal pigment epithelium as the presenting sign of neurofibromatosis-1. Ophthalmic Surg Lasers. 2000;31:145–7.
8. Turell ME, Singh AD. Nonvascular hamartomas. In: Wright KW, Spiegel PH, editors. Pediatric ophthalmology and strabismus, vol. 1. 3rd ed. New York: Springer; 2012. p. 928–37.

Chapter 38
Assessment of Amelanotic Choroidal Mass

Tahreem A. Mir and Mary E. Aronow

38.1 Definitions

Amelanotic choroidal mass includes a variety of benign and malignant conditions.

38.2 Symptoms

Decreased vision, flashes/floaters, visual field defects, and metamorphopsia. Some patients may be asymptomatic with amelanotic choroidal mass identified on dilated fundus examination as an incidental finding.

38.3 Signs

Amelanotic (white, yellow, or orange) choroidal mass (Fig. 38.1a), margins (sharp or ill-defined), intrinsic vessels, drusen, retinal pigment epithelial (RPE) changes, subretinal fluid (SRF), orange pigmentation, vitreous cells (may indicate inflammatory etiology, e.g., tuberculous/sarcoid granuloma), subretinal hemorrhage (suggestive of secondary choroidal neovascular membrane), lipid exudation (vascular incompetence), and choroidal folds (some cases) are clinical features that provide valuable diagnostic information.

Tahreem A. Mir, MD • M.E. Aronow, MD (✉)
Wilmer Eye Institute, Johns Hopkins University School of Medicine,
600 N Wolfe Street, Baltimore, MD 21287-9277, USA
e-mail: maronow1@jhmi.edu

C.A. Medina et al. (eds.), *Manual of Retinal Diseases: A Guide to Diagnosis and Management*, DOI 10.1007/978-3-319-20460-4_38

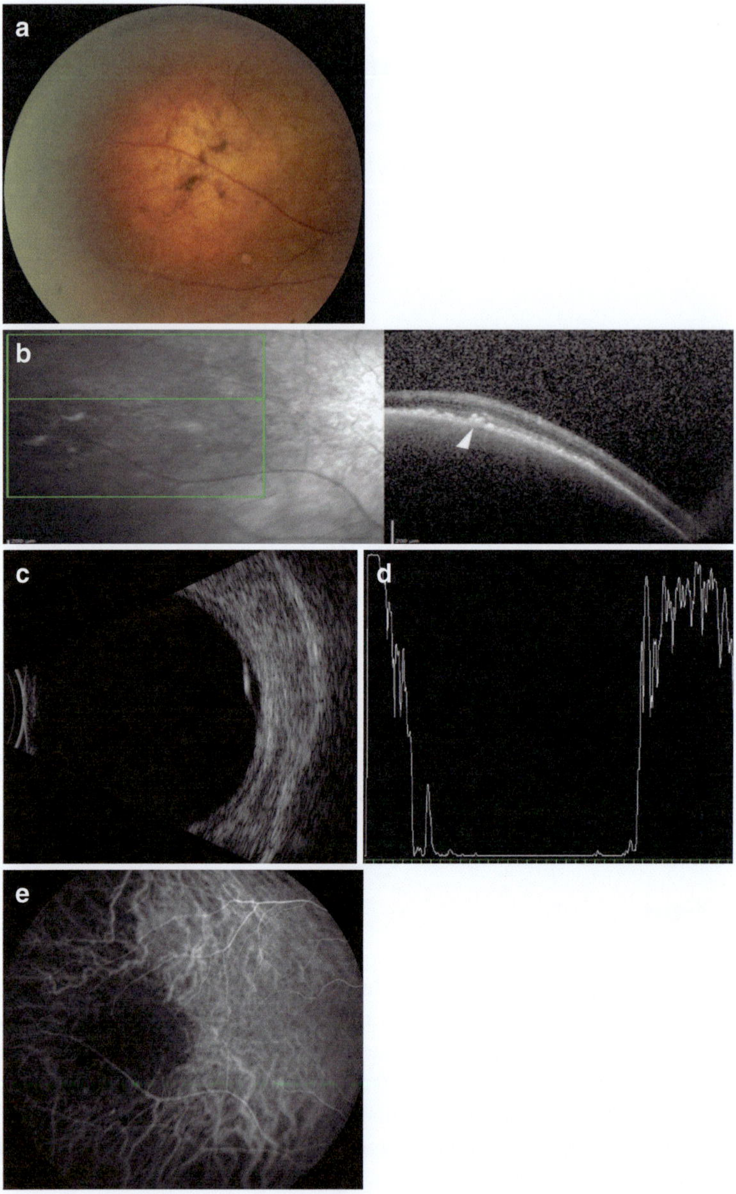

Fig. 38.1 A 65-year-old Caucasian female presented with an amelanotic choroidal mass in the right eye. There were overlying drusen and RPE changes. Orange pigment, intrinsic vascularity, and overlying subretinal fluid were absent (**a**). OCT confirms the presence of overlying drusen (*arrow*) and absence of subretinal fluid (**b**). B-scan ultrasonography demonstrates a small choroidal lesion measuring 1.4 mm in maximal thickness by 7.6 mm by 6.3 mm in base (**c**). A-scan ultrasonography reveals high internal reflectivity (**d**). ICG angiography shows blockage in the area of the clinically observed choroidal mass and absence of a "double circulation" sign (**e**). Ancillary imaging was helpful in establishing the diagnosis of presumed amelanotic choroidal nevus. Periodic observation was recommended

38.4 Predisposing Conditions

Known systemic malignancy (may indicate choroidal metastasis), fair complexion, and blue eyes (more common in nevus and melanoma)

38.5 Differential Diagnosis

Broad and includes both benign and malignant conditions (Table 38.1).

38.6 Etiology

- Neoplastic (metastasis, melanoma, hemangioma, osteoma, schwannoma)
- Inflammatory (posterior scleritis)
- Infectious (sarcoid, tuberculosis)

38.7 Workup/Testing (Table 38.2)

38.7.1 History

- Last dilated fundus examination and history of any prior noted lesions
- Past medical history (cancer, inflammatory, autoimmune disease)
- Review of systems (constitutional, infectious symptoms)
- Prevention/cancer screening: metastasis, one-third have no cancer history
- Social history (tobacco use, foreign travel, or high-risk exposures)

Table 38.1 Differential diagnosis of amelanotic choroidal mass

Choroidal metastasis
Amelanotic melanoma
Amelanotic nevus
Choroidal hemangioma (circumscribed)
Inflammatory granuloma (i.e., sarcoid, tuberculosis)
Posterior scleritis
Osteoma
Schwannoma

Table 38.2 Clinical features and ancillary studies for amelanotic choroidal mass

Diagnosis	Clinical features	Ancillary studies
Choroidal metastasis (lung, breast, prostate)	Multiple, bilateral, SRF, "leopard spot" RPE changes	USG: high reflectivity OCT: extensive SRF
Amelanotic melanoma (5.1 per million)	Mushroom-shaped orange pigment, SRF, vascularity, lack of drusen	USG: low-medium reflectivity, vascularity ICG/FA: double circulation sign
Amelanotic nevus (nevi occur in 5–8 % of white population)	Flat/slightly elevated, drusen, SRF rare	USG: high-medium reflectivity OCT: no SRF in most
Hemangioma (circumscribed)	Orange-red color, indistinct margins, SRF, absence of intrinsic vessels	USG: high reflectivity, homogenous, no intrinsic vascularity FA/ICG: early hyperfluorescence, variable late leakage, late-phase washout
Granuloma (TB or sarcoid)	Whitish lesions (active), yellowish-gray (inactive)	USG: medium-low reflectivity, heterogenous ICG: hypofluorescence, late hyperfluorescence Labs/imaging: chest CT, ACE, tuberculin test, Quantiferon gold
Posterior scleritis (associated with inflammatory disease)	Yellowish mass, diffuse choroidal thickening, choroidal folds, SRF	USG: medium-low reflectivity, "T" sign FA: heterogeneous hyperfluorescence
Osteoma (predominantly females)	Whitish-yellow, distinct, scalloped borders, may have associated neovascular membrane	USG: medium-high reflectivity, orbital shadowing/calcification FA/ICG: early hyperfluorescence, late staining
Schwannoma	Suprachoroidal mass, orange pigment and drusen absent	USG: medium reflectivity, no vascularity

38.7.2 Examination

- Visual acuity, intraocular pressure measurement, pupil reactions
- External
- Slit lamp biomicroscopy
- Dilated fundus examination: size, location of mass
- Extraocular motility examination
- Confrontation to visual fields

38.7.3 Ancillary Testing

- Fundus photography (document size, location, borders, clinical features)
- Optical coherence tomography (OCT): subretinal fluid, macular edema, drusen, and RPE changes. Ideal for small lesions (<1 mm thick) that are difficult to detect on USG (Fig. 38.1b)

- Ultrasonography (USG): dimensions, reflectivity, intrinsic vascularity, presence/absence of SRF, and extraocular extension (Fig. 38.1c, d)
- Fluorescein angiography (FA): hypo-/hyperfluorescence, leakage
- Indocyanine green angiography (ICG): intrinsic vasculature (Fig. 38.1e)
- Systemic imaging to identify primary neoplasm

38.8 Prognosis and Management

The management of amelanotic choroidal mass varies widely and is based on the underlying diagnosis, symptoms, size, location, and documented growth. Choroidal metastases can be treated with multiple modalities including chemotherapy, external beam radiotherapy, brachytherapy, or proton therapy.

For choroidal melanoma, the most widely used therapies are brachytherapy or proton therapy for small- and medium-sized tumors and enucleation for large tumors or in cases in which visual prognosis is poor.

Choroidal nevi should be carefully documented and observed. Nevi without suspicious features can be observed every 6–12 months. Indeterminate lesions should be followed closely every 3 months initially, and then every 6 months after stability is documented.

Asymptomatic choroidal hemangioma can be observed, but for cases with exudative retinal detachment threatening the fovea, treatment options include photodynamic therapy, brachytherapy, laser photocoagulation, cryotherapy, and transpupillary thermotherapy. Systemic evaluation in patients with circumscribed choroidal hemangioma is not indicated; however, a thorough systemic evaluation, including neuroimaging, is warranted in individuals with diffuse hemangioma due to the association with Sturge-Weber syndrome.

Granuloma secondary to sarcoidosis may be treated with topical, periocular, or oral steroids, while granuloma caused by tuberculosis is managed with multidrug therapy (common drugs include ethambutol, isoniazid, pyrazinamide, rifabutin, rifampin, and rifapentine).

Posterior scleritis can be treated with corticosteroids and immunomodulatory agents particularly when associated with systemic disease.

Osteoma may be observed; however, laser photocoagulation, photodynamic therapy, and anti-angiogenic agents should be considered if vision threatening choroidal neovascularization is present.

Schwannoma can be observed, unless large or vision threatening. Many cases are diagnosed upon enucleation for suspected choroidal melanoma. If the correct diagnosis is made preoperatively, uveal-sparing excision can be performed.

38.9 Follow-Up

Indeterminate lesions should be followed closely (every 3 months), whereas stable lesions can be followed at longer intervals accordingly.

References and Suggested Reading

1. Medina CA, Aronow ME, Singh AD. Amelanotic choroidal mass. Advanced Ocular Care. 2012;3:33–5.
2. Shields CL, Shields JA, Gross NE, Schwartz GP, Lally SE. Survey of 520 eyes with uveal metastases. Ophthalmology. 1997;104(8):1265–76.
3. Shields CL, Shields JA, De Potter P. Patterns of indocyanine green videoangiography of choroidal tumours. Br J Ophthalmol. 1995;79(3):237–45.
4. Sobottka B, Kreissig I. Ultrasonography of metastases and melanomas of the choroid. Curr Opin Ophthalmol. 1999;10(3):164–7.
5. Verbeek AM, Thijssen JM, Cuypers MH, Brink H, Deutman AF. Echographic classification of intraocular tumours. A 15-year retrospective analysis. Acta Ophthalmol (Copenh). 1994;72(4):416–22.

Chapter 39
Choroidal Hemangioma

Suzanne van Landingham and Mary E. Aronow

39.1 Definitions

Choroidal hemangioma is a benign hamartoma of the choroid. These can be classified into two distinct forms:

- Circumscribed (localized)
- Diffuse

39.2 Circumscribed Choroidal Hemangioma

39.2.1 Symptoms

- May be asymptomatic.
- Exudative retinal detachment may cause metamorphopsia, photopsias, and/or reduction in vision.

S. van Landingham, MD
Wilmer Eye Institute, Johns Hopkins University School of Medicine, Baltimore, MD, USA

M.E. Aronow, MD (✉)
Wilmer Eye Institute, Johns Hopkins University School of Medicine,
744 Maumenee Building, 600 N Wolfe Street, Baltimore, MD 21287-9277, USA
e-mail: maronow1@jhmi.edu

C.A. Medina et al. (eds.), *Manual of Retinal Diseases: A Guide to Diagnosis and Management*, DOI 10.1007/978-3-319-20460-4_39

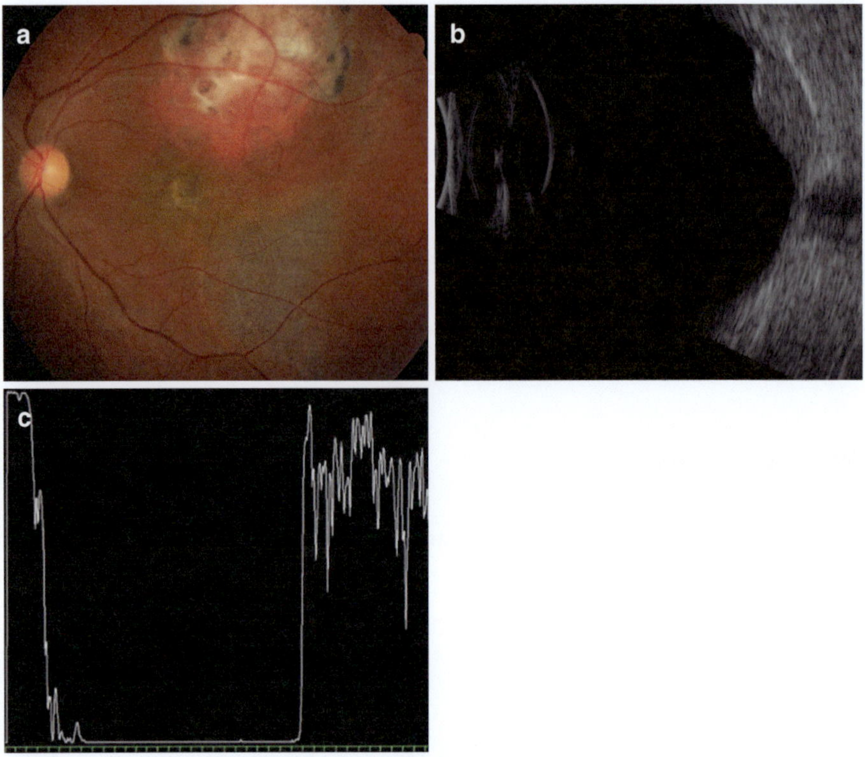

Fig. 39.1 Color fundus photograph of the left eye demonstrating circumscribed choroidal hemangioma previously treated with laser ablation (**a**, Courtesy of Jim Handa, MD). B-scan ultrasonography reveals a dome-shaped choroidal mass with a smooth contour typical of circumscribed hemangioma (**b**, Courtesy of Ellen Greenberg, COT). A-scan ultrasonography demonstrates high internal reflectivity of the choroidal hemangioma (**c**, Courtesy of Ellen Greenberg, COT)

39.2.2 Signs

Ophthalmoscopy reveals an orange to reddish tumor with indistinct margins that blend into the surrounding choroid (median diameter 6.0 mm, thickness 3.1 mm in one large case series) (Fig. 39.1a). These tumors are typically located in the posterequatorial region, often in the macula. Feeding arterioles and draining venules are not typically observed. More than 80 % of cases develop overlying exudative retinal detachment at some point in the disease course.

39.2.3 Predisposing Conditions

- Occur sporadically in the absence of systemic disease.
- Usually present in the second to fourth decade.

- No sex predilection.
- Most reported cases are in Caucasians.

39.2.4 Differential Diagnosis

Includes amelanotic choroidal melanoma, choroidal metastasis, choroidal osteoma, choroidal granuloma (tuberculosis or sarcoid), posterior scleritis, and atypical central serous choroidopathy.

39.2.5 Etiology

Unknown/sporadic

39.2.6 Workup/Testing

Characteristic findings on fundus examination (described above) are key to diagnosis. Ancillary imaging studies can help to differentiate these benign lesions from malignancies and to assess the health of the overlying retina:

- Fluorescein angiography (FA): lacy vascular network with early hyperfluorescence and variable late leakage.
- Indocyanine green (ICG) angiography: Early hyperfluorescence within the tumor with a characteristic late "washout" effect.
- Optical coherence tomography (OCT): may demonstrate secondary changes of the overlying retina, such as shallow subretinal fluid or cystoid macular edema.
- Ultrasonography: B-scan demonstrates a dome-shaped choroidal mass with smooth contours, and A-scan reveals high internal reflectivity (Fig. 39.1b, c).

39.2.7 Prognosis and Management

Asymptomatic cases require no treatment and may be managed with periodic observation. Treatment of symptomatic cases is aimed at inducing tumor atrophy and resolution of subretinal fluid. Therapeutic options include photodynamic therapy, laser photocoagulation, transpupillary thermotherapy, and radiotherapy. Oral propranolol has also been proposed as a treatment for circumscribed choroidal hemangioma, but preliminary studies have not demonstrated consistent or clinically significant impact. The use of intravitreal anti-VEGF agents has been reported for associated choroidal neovascularization; however, these medications have not been formally studied in large series. Visual prognosis is guarded due to the likelihood of development of subretinal fluid, cystoid macular edema, and the side effects of treatment. In one large case series, 37 % of patients had a final visual acuity of 20/40 or better while 52 % had 20/200 or worse.

39.2.8 Follow-Up

Periodic surveillance at intervals is determined by disease activity. Evaluation should occur more frequently if symptoms develop.

39.3 Diffuse Choroidal Hemangioma

39.3.1 Symptoms

- May be asymptomatic.
- Exudative retinal detachment may cause metamorphopsia, photopsias, and/or reduced vision.
- May have anisometropia due to hyperopic shift in the affected eye.

39.3.2 Signs

Ophthalmoscopy reveals a diffuse, orange to reddish thickening of the fundus ("tomato ketchup fundus") (Fig. 39.2a.) There may be associated exudative retinal detachment. Diffuse choroidal hemangioma occurs in association with Sturge-Weber syndrome, which also characteristically features *nevus flammeus* (port-wine stain), mental retardation/developmental delay, and seizure disorder due to leptomeningeal hemangiomatosis. Glaucoma, ipsilateral to the diffuse choroidal hemangioma and port-wine stain, occurs in approximately 70 %.

39.3.3 Predisposing Conditions

- Almost all cases occur in association with Sturge-Weber syndrome (neuro-oculocutaneous hemangiomatosis).
- Typically evident at birth.

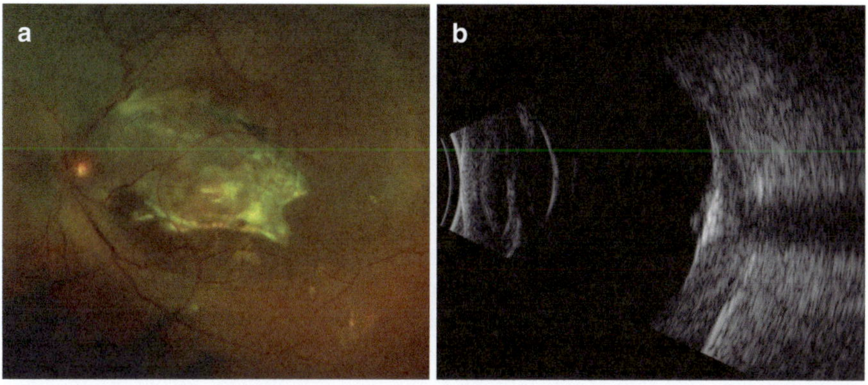

Fig. 39.2 Optos wide-angle image of the left fundus in a patient with Sturge-Weber syndrome. There is diffuse choroidal thickening and a macular scar secondary to prior exudative retinal detachment (**a**, Image courtesy of Peter Campbell, MD). B-scan ultrasonography demonstrates diffusely thickened choroid (**b**, Courtesy of Peter Campbell, MD)

39.3.4 Differential Diagnosis

The diagnosis is straightforward in the setting of typical Sturge-Weber syndrome.

39.3.5 Etiology

Sturge-Weber syndrome occurs sporadically.

39.3.6 Workup/Testing

Testing may be useful to distinguish ambiguous cases of diffuse choroidal hemangioma, particularly in the absence of typical Sturge-Weber syndrome.

- FA: early diffuse hyperfluorescence that persists in the late phases. Leakage is less common than in circumscribed choroidal hemangioma.
- ICG angiography: rapid diffuse filling with persistence of intense hyperfluorescence.
- OCT: may demonstrate secondary changes of the overlying retina, such as shallow subretinal fluid or cystoid macular edema.
- Ultrasonography: B-scan demonstrates a diffusely thicken choroid. A-scan shows high internal reflectivity (Fig. 39.2b).

39.3.7 Prognosis and Management

As with circumscribed choroidal hemangioma, asymptomatic cases require no treatment and may be managed with periodic observation. Vision loss may occur due to refractive error, glaucoma, and exudative retinal detachment. In addition to the correction of refractive error and medical or surgical management of associated glaucoma, symptomatic cases may be treated with low-dose lens-sparing external beam radiotherapy and photodynamic therapy [7]. Oral propranolol has been used in some cases with apparent reduction in exudative retinal detachment; however, robust data for this treatment approach is limited. Anti-VEGF agents have been used for diffuse choroidal hemangioma complicated by exudative retinal detachment; however, the role of this therapy is not well established. Visual prognosis is guarded to poor.

39.3.8 Follow-Up

Periodic follow-up depending upon the presence of associated glaucoma. Periodic evaluation is appropriate in the absence of symptoms or known complications.

References and Suggested Reading

1. Arevalo JF, Arias JD, Serrano MA. Oral propranolol for exudative retinal detachment in diffuse choroidal hemangioma. Arch Ophthalmol. 2011;129(10):1373–5.
2. Aronow MD, Singh AD, Bergstrom C. Uveal vascular tumors. In: Grossniklaus HE, editor. Pocket guide to ocular oncology and pathology. Berlin: Springer; 2013. p. 323–31.
3. Querques G, Forte R, Querques L, Souied EH. Intravitreal ranibizumab for choroidal neovascularization associated with circumscribed choroidal haemangioma. Clin Experiment Ophthalmol. 2011;39(9):916–8.
4. Shields CL, Honavar SG, Shields JA, Cater J, Demirci H. Circumscribed choroidal hemangioma: clinical manifestations and factors predictive of visual outcome in 200 consecutive cases. Ophthalmology. 2001;108(12):2237–48.
5. Tanabe H, Sahashi K, Kitano T, Tomita Y, Saito AM, Hirose H. Effects of oral propranolol on circumscribed choroidal hemangioma: a pilot study. JAMA Ophthalmol. 2013;131(12):1617–22.
6. Thapa R, Shields CL. Oral propranolol therapy for management of exudative retinal detachment from diffuse choroidal hemangioma in Sturge-Weber syndrome. Eur J Ophthalmol. 2013;23(6):922–4.
7. Turell ME, Singh AD. Vascular tumors of the retina and choroid: diagnosis and treatment. Middle East Afr J Ophthalmol. 2010;17(3):191–200.

Chapter 40
Choroidal Metastases

Maria J. Suarez

40.1 Definitions

Choroidal metastasis is the most common intraocular malignancy in adults. These tumors spread via a hematogenous or lymphatic route to the uveal tract. The most common location of uveal metastasis is the choroid, followed by the iris and the ciliary body.

40.2 Symptoms

Patients may present with blurred vision, floaters, scotoma, and progressive hypermetropia, or they may be asymptomatic.

40.3 Signs

Choroidal metastasis typically appears as yellow or creamy, dome or plateau-shaped choroid mass that often has associated exudative retinal detachment (Fig. 40.1a). Tumors are often bilateral and multifocal. Choroidal metastasis is located in the posterior pole in the majority (92 %) of cases. Less than 10 % of uveal metastatic tumors involve the iris and/or ciliary body.

M.J. Suarez, MD
Ophthalmic Pathology, Wilmer Eye Institute, Johns Hopkins School of Medicine,
400 N Broadway, Suite 4070, Baltimore, MD 21231, USA
e-mail: msuarez9@jhmi.edu

C.A. Medina et al. (eds.), *Manual of Retinal Diseases: A Guide to Diagnosis and Management*, DOI 10.1007/978-3-319-20460-4_40

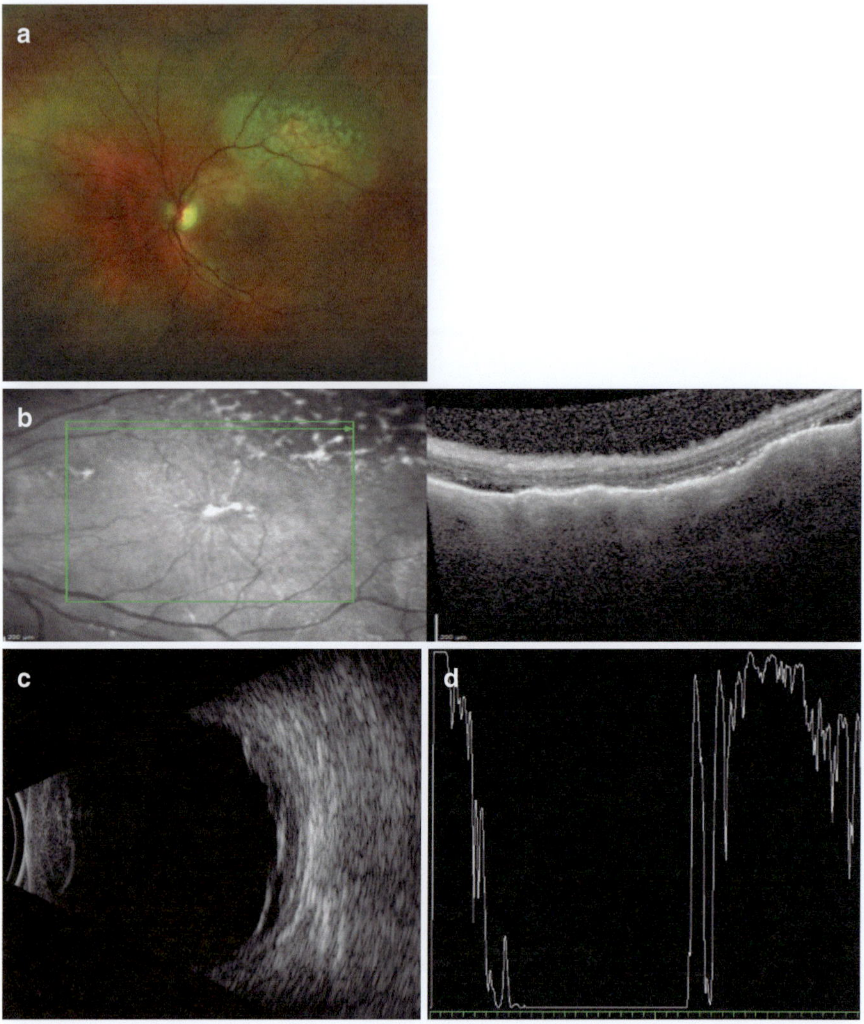

Fig. 40.1 A 69-year-old female with known metastatic breast cancer presented with painless, gradual decrease in vision. Optos wide-angle imaging of the left eye shows multiple areas of amelanotic choroidal thickening with overlying RPE changes and associated exudative retinal detachment consisting of choroidal metastases (**a**). OCT confirms choroidal thickening and overlying subretinal fluid (**b**). B-scan ultrasonography shows thickened and irregular choroid diffusely with overlying exudative detachment (**c**). A-scan ultrasonography demonstrates high internal reflectivity (**d**)

40.4 Predisposing Conditions

The majority of choroidal metastases arise in the setting of known preexisting primary malignancy in distant organs. Approximately one-third of the patients with choroidal metastasis have no prior history of cancer.

Table 40.1 Differential diagnosis of choroidal metastasis

Amelanotic melanoma
Amelanotic nevus
Lymphoma
Choroidal hemangioma (circumscribed)
Osteoma
Granuloma (tuberculosis and sarcoid)
Posterior scleritis

40.5 Differential Diagnosis

The differential diagnosis includes amelanotic melanoma, amelanotic nevus, lymphoma, choroidal hemangioma, choroidal osteoma, choroidal granuloma, and posterior scleritis (Table 40.1).

40.6 Etiology

The most common primary tumors which metastasize to the choroid are breast (47 %) in females and lung carcinoma (21 %) in males. Less frequent sites of the primary malignancy include gastrointestinal tract (4 %), kidney (4 %), skin (2 %), prostate (2 %), and other (uterus, thyroid, pancreas, bladder, ovary, bile duct, testes, bone, and adrenal gland) tumors (4 %). Primary tumors of unknown etiology can also metastasize (16 %).

40.7 Workup/Testing

A complete past medical history should be obtained including documentation of prior malignancy, age-appropriate cancer screening, and social history, particularly tobacco use. A thorough examination should include slit lamp biomicroscopy and dilated fundus examination.

Ancillary studies can be useful in differentiating choroidal metastasis from other simulating lesions:

- Fluorescein angiography (FA): blockage of choroidal flush and hyperfluorescence in the late venous phase, slightly later than typical choroidal melanoma or hemangioma.
- Optical coherence tomography (OCT): may confirm overlying exudative retinal detachment (Fig. 40.1b).
- Ultrasonography: B-scan demonstrates a dome to plateau-shaped choroidal lesion, while A-scan shows high to medium internal reflectivity (Fig. 40.1c, d).

- Magnetic resonance imaging (MRI): reveals a lower T1 signal intensity than choroidal melanoma.
- Fine needle aspiration biopsy with cytopathologic evaluation with or without immunohistochemical techniques may be a necessary definitive diagnosis

40.8 Prognosis and Management

The overall prognosis of patients with choroidal metastasis is guarded, but improving in response to other advances in cancer therapy. Mean survival is approximately 9–10 months [2]. Patients with choroidal metastasis secondary to breast carcinoma have a more favorable prognosis compared to patients with metastatic lung cancer or melanoma. Treatment for choroidal metastasis consists of systemic chemotherapy, hormonal therapy in some cases, and local therapies such as external beam radiotherapy, plaque brachytherapy, transpupillary thermotherapy, and photodynamic therapy. In cases where the eye becomes painful or unresponsive to treatment, enucleation may be considered.

40.9 Follow-Up

Periodic follow-up visits are recommended to assess the clinical outcomes to the implemented systemic or local therapy and to evaluate for necessary further steps in management.

References and Suggested Reading

1. Shields JA, Shields CL. Metastatic tumors to the uvea, retina, and optic disc. In: Shields JA, Shields CL, editors. Intraocular tumors: an atlas and textbook. 2nd ed. Philadelphia: Lippincott Williams & Wilkins; 2008. p. 198–9.
2. Eagle RC, editor. Eye pathology an atlas and text. 2nd ed. Philadelphia: Lippincott Williams & Wilkins; 2011.
3. Chung YH, Singh AD, Bergstrom C, Grossniklaus HE. Uveal metastatic tumors. In: Grossniklaus HE, editor. Pocket guide to ocular oncology and pathology. Berlin/Heidelberg: Springer; 2013. p. 317–21.
4. Intraocular Inflammation and Uveitis. Chapter 9: American Academy of Ophthalmology basic and clinical science course. San Francisco, CA: American Academy of Ophthalmology; 2011–2012. p. 286–7.
5. Weng Sehu K, WR Lee. Chapter 11: Ophthalmic pathology: an illustrated guide for clinicians. Oxford, UK: Blackwell Publishing; 2005. p. 250.
6. Shields CL, Shields JA, Gross NE, et al. Survey of 520 eyes with uveal metastases. Ophthalmology. 1997;104:1265–76.

Chapter 41
Choroidal Osteoma and Calcification

Jithin Yohannan and Mary E. Aronow

41.1 Definitions

Choroidal osteoma (CO)
Idiopathic sclerochoroidal calcification (ISCC)

41.2 Symptoms

Usually asymptomatic. Can present with gradual vision loss, metamorphopsia, and visual field defects corresponding to tumor location and associated choroidal neovascularization in some cases.

41.3 Signs

CO is a flat to minimally elevated, yellow-white choroidal lesion frequently located in the juxtapapillary or macular location. Small vascular tufts that emerge on the tumor surface are pathognomonic. Generally, these have an oval to round shape with well-defined, geographic or scalloped borders. CO is typically solitary but can be multifocal. There is often mottling of overlying RPE.

J. Yohannan, MD, MPH
Wilmer Eye Institute, Johns Hopkins University School of Medicine, Baltimore, MD, USA

M.E. Aronow, MD (✉)
Wilmer Eye Institute, Johns Hopkins University School of Medicine,
744 Maumenee Building, 600 N Wolfe St, Baltimore, MD 21287-9277, USA
e-mail: maronow1@jhmi.edu

C.A. Medina et al. (eds.), *Manual of Retinal Diseases: A Guide to Diagnosis and Management*, DOI 10.1007/978-3-319-20460-4_41

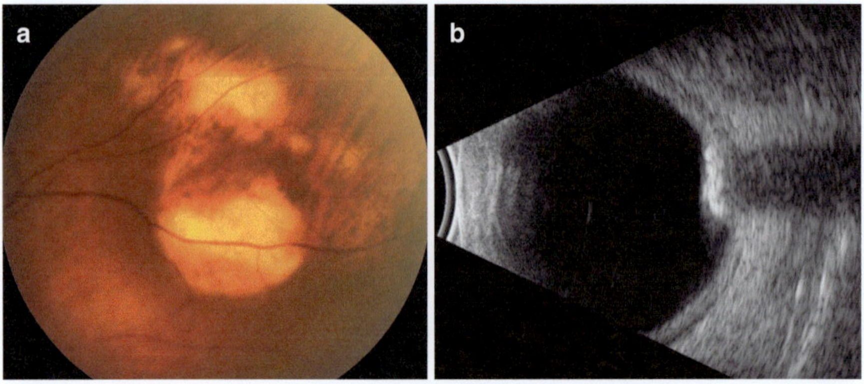

Fig. 41.1 Idiopathic sclerochoroidal calcification demonstrating typical yellow-white nodules with ill-defined margins located in the midperiphery (**a**). B-scan ultrasonography demonstrates orbital shadowing consistent with calcium deposition (**b**)

ISCC is the abnormal deposition of calcium in the sclera and adjacent choroid in elderly individuals. The typical appearance is bilateral, yellow-white nodules with ill-defined margins, which are often multiple, and located in the midperiphery (Fig. 41.1a). These are frequently located along the superotemporal arcades and may be minimally elevated and associated with overlying RPE atrophy.

41.4 Predisposing Conditions

CO is a benign choristoma. The vast majority, 90 %, occur in females with a mean age of presentation of 21 years. Approximately 75 % of cases are unilateral. ISCC occurs as an age-related change. Rarely, abnormal calcium deposition within the choroid may be secondary to an underlying disorder including Bartter syndrome, Gitelman syndrome, hyperparathyroidism, or hypomagnesaemia.

41.5 Differential Diagnosis

Entities to consider in the differential of CO include choroidal metastasis, amelanotic choroidal melanoma, amelanotic choroidal nevus, choroidal hemangioma, and choroidal granuloma. Nevus sebaceous of Jadassohn is a condition that presents with midline facial skin lesions; seizures; mental retardation; chondroid choroidal choristomas (nearly identical to typical CO); subretinal neovascularization; conjunctival lipodermoid; colobomas of the eyelids, iris, disc, and choroid; and angiomas of the orbit.

41.6 Etiology

CO is a benign choristoma composed of cancellous bone. Histopathology shows interconnected bony trabeculae with large vascular spaces. Cytopathology shows populations of osteocytes and osteoblasts as well as occasional osteoclasts.

41.7 Workup/Testing

Diagnosis is clinical and based on the classic appearance of the lesion on ophthalmoscopy. The following imaging modalities may be helpful in supporting the diagnosis:

- Ultrasonography: B-scan shows orbital shadowing consistent with calcium deposition (Fig. 41.1b). A-scan shows sharp high-intensity spike from anterior tumor surface and high internal reflectivity.
- Fluorescein angiography (FA): Early patchy hyperfluorescence and late staining. Leakage secondary to associated choroidal neovascularization may be apparent.
- OCT: Platelike regions of high signal intensity in tumor, fluid spaces in tumor, elevation of overlying retina, and reflectivity of tissues posterior to tumor.
- CT: Radiopaque lesion consistent with calcification at the level of the choroid

41.8 Prognosis and Management

At 10 years, 51 % of patients with CO have tumor growth and 56 % of patients have visual acuity less than or equal to 20/200. Poor visually acuity outcomes are associated with development of choroidal neovascularization (occurs in 50 % of patients by 10 years follow-up), decalcification (occurs in 46 % of patients at 10 years follow-up), subretinal hemorrhage, subretinal fluid, and RPE alterations. Asymptomatic or stable CO can be observed. If vision-threatening neovascularization is present, laser photocoagulation, photodynamic therapy, and antiangiogenic therapy can be considered.

41.9 Follow-Up

Patients should be evaluated at regular intervals to assess for the development of treatable choroidal neovascularization which can lead to permanent vision loss.

References and Suggested Reading

1. Aylward GW, Chang TS, Pautler SE, Gass JD. A long-term follow-up of choroidal osteoma. Arch Opthalmol. 1998;116:1337–41.
2. Blaise P, Duchateau E, Comhaire Y, Rakic JM. Improvement of visual acuity after photodynamic therapy for choroidal neovascularization in choroidal osteoma. Acta Ophthalmol Scand. 2005;83:515–6.
3. Lambert HM, Sipperley JO, Shore JW, et al. Linear nevus sebaceous syndrome. Ophthalmology. 1987;94(3):278–82.
4. Rose SJ, Burke JF, Brockhurst RJ. Argon laser photoablation of a choroidal osteoma. Retina. 1991;11:224–8.
5. Shields CL, Sun H, Demirci H, Shields JA. Factors predictive of tumor growth, tumor decalcification, choroidal neovascularization, and visual outcome in 74 eyes with choroidal osteoma. Arch Ophthalmol. 2005;123:1658–66.
6. Song JH, Bae JH, Rho MI, Lee SC. Intravitreal bevacizumab in the management of subretinal fluid associated with choroidal osteoma. Retina. 2010;30:945–51.
7. Turell ME, Singh AD. Nonvascular hamartomas. In: Wright KW, Spiegel PH, editors. Pediatric ophthalmology and strabismus, vol. 1. 3rd ed. New York: Springer; 2012. p. 928–37.

Chapter 42
Inflammatory Granuloma

Sumayya Ahmad

42.1 Definitions

Granuloma: An organized collection of macrophages (histiocytes)

42.2 Symptoms

Decreased vision, photosensitivity, floaters, photopsias, pain, redness

42.3 Signs

Yellow to white (amelanotic) choroidal mass, which can be solitary or multiple. Overlying subretinal fluid may be present. There may also be associated anterior, intermediate, or posterior uveitis and/or vasculitis (Fig. 42.1a).

42.4 Predisposing Conditions

History of exposure to tuberculosis, African American race (sarcoidosis), exposure to dogs (toxocariasis)

S. Ahmad, MD
Wilmer Eye Institute, Johns Hopkins Hospital,
600 N Wolfe St, B-20, Baltimore, MD 21205, USA
e-mail: sahmad16@jhmi.edu

C.A. Medina et al. (eds.), *Manual of Retinal Diseases: A Guide to Diagnosis and Management*, DOI 10.1007/978-3-319-20460-4_42

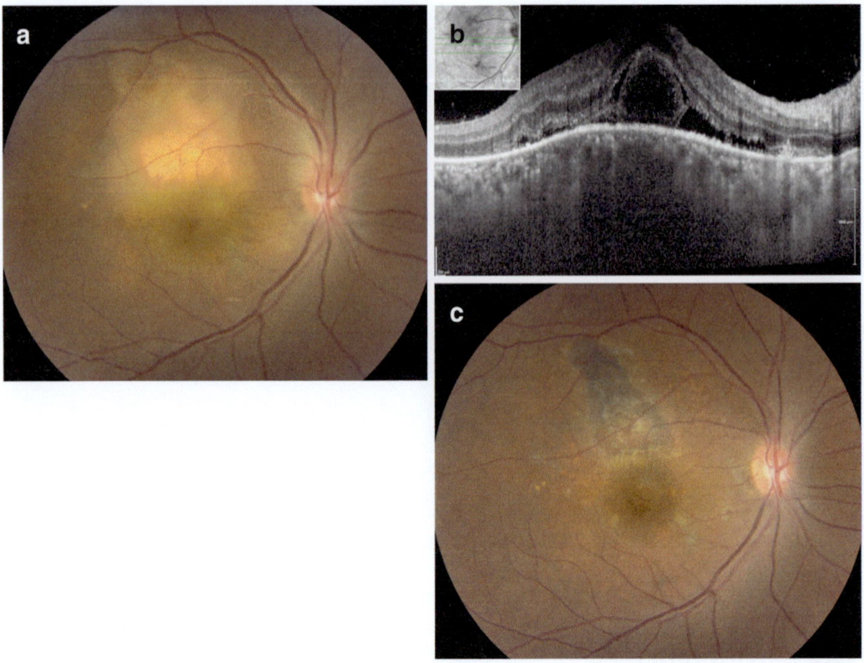

Fig. 42.1 Choroidal granuloma in a 31-year-old African female who complained of painless decrease in vision (best corrected visual acuity was 20/80). Dilated fundus examination of the right eye revealed 1+ vitreous cells and a creamy yellow-white choroidal mass with overlying exudative detachment (**a**). OCT demonstrating a choroidal mass corresponding to the clinically observed granuloma with overlying subretinal fluid (**b**). Quantiferon gold testing was positive. The patient was treated with multidrug tuberculosis therapy (pyrazinamide, isoniazid, rifampin, and ethambutol). One month following initiation of four-drug tuberculosis therapy, there was near complete interval resolution of the choroidal granuloma (**c**). Her vision returned to 20/25 in the right eye

42.5 Differential Diagnosis

Choroidal granuloma appears as an amelanotic choroidal mass. The differential diagnosis includes amelanotic choroidal melanoma, amelanotic choroidal nevus, circumscribed choroidal hemangioma, choroidal metastasis, and posterior nodular scleritis. The two major systemic causes of infectious/inflammatory choroidal granuloma are tuberculosis and sarcoidosis. Rarely, ocular toxocariasis can produce infectious choroidal granuloma.

42.6 Etiology

Collection of inflammatory cells within the choroid, often secondary to systemic disease

42.7 Workup/Testing

Laboratory studies and systemic imaging are recommended to diagnosis underlying systemic conditions:

- Tuberculosis: tuberculin skin test or quantiferon gold
- Sarcoidosis: serum angiotensin converting enzyme (ACE) and lysozyme, chest x-ray, or chest CT if strong suspicion and chest x-ray is negative
- Toxocariasis: excretory-secretory antigen (TES-ELISA); Goldmann-Witmer coefficient >3.0

42.7.1 Ophthalmic Imaging

- Color fundus photography to document size/margins of granuloma
- OCT to evaluate granuloma height and degree of overlying subretinal fluid (Fig. 42.1b)
- Ultrasonography: to measure dimensions; high internal reflectivity
- Fluorescein angiography (FA): multifocal choroiditis or periphlebitis indicative of ocular sarcoidosis

A complete dilated fundus examination should be performed to assess the degree anterior, intermediate, and/or posterior uveitis. Rare cases of granuloma associated with toxocariasis have characteristic features such as a fibrocellular band running from the peripheral granuloma to the optic nerve or posterior retina.

42.8 Prognosis and Management

The key is early recognition, diagnosis of underlying systemic condition, and treatment for the prevention of permanent visual sequelae.

- Tuberculosis: multidrug therapy consisting of isoniazid (300 mg daily), rifampin (600 mg daily), pyrazinamide (2 g daily), and ethambutol (1200 mg daily) for at least 2 months and/or rifampin and isoniazid for 4 months (Fig. 42.1c).
- Sarcoidosis: For unilateral disease, topical, periocular, intravitreal, or oral steroids; for systemic disease, mainstay of treatment is oral corticosteroids (0.5–0.1 mg/kg/day) or steroid sparing immunomodulatory agents.
- Ocular Toxocariasis: albendazole 800 mg/day for adults and 400 mg/day for children for 2–4 weeks along with oral steroids 0.5 mg/kg day.

42.9 Follow-Up

After the underlying etiology/systemic condition is established, patients should be monitored according to severity of symptoms. If there is a bilateral panuveitis, they should be monitored closely after initiation of appropriate therapy to ensure improvement. Most causes of granuloma are related to systemic disease, which requires prolonged systemic or local treatment.

References and Suggested Reading

1. Herbort CP, Rao NA. Mochizuki M; Members of scientific committee of first international workshop on ocular sarcoidosis. International criteria for the diagnosis of ocular sarcoidosis: results of the first international workshop on ocular sarcoidosis (IWOS). Ocul Immunol Inflamm. 2009;17(3):160–9.
2. Jamilloux Y, Kodjikian L, Broussolle C, Sève P. Sarcoidosis and uveitis. Autoimmun Rev. 2014;13(8):840–9.
3. Rubinsky-Elefant G, Hirata CE, Yamamoto JH, Ferreira MU. Human toxocariasis: diagnosis, worldwide seroprevalences and clinical expression of the systemic and ocular forms. Ann Trop Med Parasitol. 2010;104(1):3–23.

Chapter 43
Uveal Lymphoma

Roomasa Channa and Mary E. Aronow

43.1 Definitions

Uveal lymphoma occurs as a primary neoplasm of the uveal tract or as a secondary neoplasm in the setting of known systemic lymphoma. Primary uveal lymphoma is typically a low-grade, non-Hodgkin's, B-cell lymphoma and can be further classified:

- Choroidal lymphoma (most common)
- Iridal lymphoma (very rare)
- Ciliary body lymphoma (very rare)

43.2 Symptoms

Blurred vision, orbital fullness, diplopia, metamorphopsia, foreign body sensation, conjunctival salmon patch, and eye pain secondary to elevated intraocular pressure in some cases. Patients may be asymptomatic at the time of presentation.

R. Channa, MD
Wilmer Eye Institute, Johns Hopkins Hospital, Baltimore, MD, USA

M.E. Aronow, MD (✉)
Wilmer Eye Institute, Johns Hopkins University,
600 North Wolfe Street, Maumenee 744, Baltimore, MD 21287, USA
e-mail: maronow1@jhmi.edu

C.A. Medina et al. (eds.), *Manual of Retinal Diseases: A Guide to Diagnosis and Management*, DOI 10.1007/978-3-319-20460-4_43

43.3 Signs

Solitary or multiple yellow to white, creamy choroidal infiltrates or placoid choroidal infiltrates (Fig. 43.1a). The vitreous is clear as there is absence of cellular reaction. In some cases, there is diffuse thickening of the uveal tract. There can be associated exudative retinal detachment. Episcleral extension can appear as a non-mobile "salmon" patch.

43.4 Predisposing Conditions

- Systemic lymphoma
- Possible association with infection (i.e., *C. psittaci* and *H. pylori*) (3)

43.5 Differential Diagnosis (Table 43.1)

- Uveal effusion syndrome
- Uveal metastases
- Posterior scleritis
- Birdshot chorioretinopathy
- Diffuse amelanotic uveal melanoma
- Acute multifocal placoid pigment epitheliopathy (AMPPE)

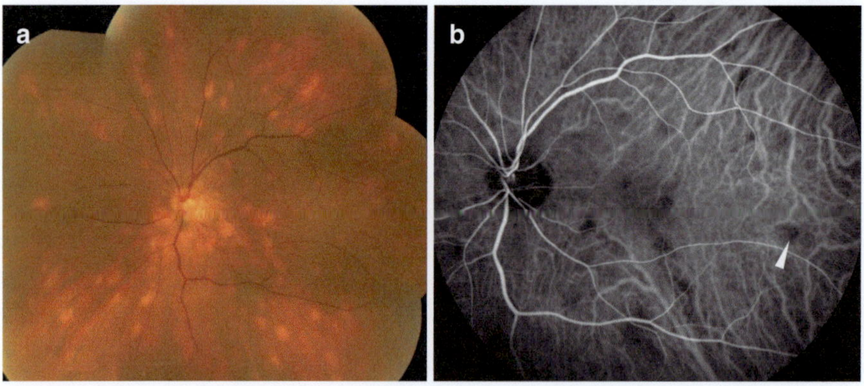

Fig. 43.1 A 72-year-old Caucasian female presented with bilateral, multiple *yellow to white*, creamy choroidal infiltrates (**a**, *left fundus shown*). ICG angiography of the left eye shows filling defects (*arrowhead*) corresponding to the clinically observed choroidal infiltrates (**b**). Prior HLA-A29 testing (for birdshot chorioretinopathy) was negative. Systemic imaging including CT of the neck, chest, abdomen, and pelvis was unremarkable. The clinical diagnosis was primary choroidal lymphoma. She was treated with low-dose (24 Gy) intensity-modulated radiotherapy

Table 43.1 Differential diagnosis for choroidal lymphoma: distinguishing features

Diagnosis	Key distinguishing features
Uveal effusion syndrome	More common in hyperopic, middle-aged men
Diffuse malignant melanoma	Faster growth rate, nodularity, intrinsic vasculature
Choroidal metastases	Mottled RPE changes, medium to high reflectivity on ultrasonography, history of systemic malignancy
Posterior Scleritis	Unilateral, high internal reflectivity, and "T-sign" on ultrasonography
Birdshot chorioretinopathy	ERG changes, HLA-A29 association
AMPPE	Bilateral, placoid, responds to steroids

43.6 Etiology

While an infection/inflammation/mutation (IMM) model of lymphomagenesis has been proposed, no definitive link has been established between uveal lymphoma and predisposing factors.

43.7 Workup/Testing

Uveal lymphoma can coexist with ocular adnexal lymphoma. Therefore, a complete bilateral ophthalmic examination, including dilated fundus examination should be performed. Ancillary testing includes:

- Ultrasonography: can detect choroidal thickening and occult extrascleral extension. Ultrasonographic features include diffuse choroidal thickening (most typical), low reflectivity, crescentic thickening outside the posterior scleral margin, discrete mass, and subretinal fluid (rarely).
- Fluorescein angiography: early hyperfluorescence, choroidal folds, and hypofluorescent foci corresponding to clinically observed choroidal infiltrates.
- Indocyanine green angiography: hypofluorescent foci corresponding to clinically observed choroidal infiltrates (Fig. 43.1b).
- Neuroimaging: computed tomography (CT) or magnetic resonance imaging (MRI) of the brain and orbits is important for detection of extraocular involvement.

Tissue biopsy is required for definitive diagnosis. This could be extraocular (e.g., a peripheral lymph node) or ocular. Pathology reveals monomorphous cells with a thin cytoplasmic rim and indistinct nucleoli. Immunohistochemical studies show predominantly B lymphocytes and expression of B-cell antigens (such as CD20) in the majority of cases.

43.8 Prognosis and Management

Uveal lymphoma is a variant of ocular adnexal lymphoma (OAL) and has a better prognosis when compared with vitreoretinal lymphoma, which is a more aggressive lymphoma. Similar to OAL, the majority of uveal lymphoma are of the extranodal marginal zone lymphoma (EMZL) subtype. EMZL is characterized by slow progression and excellent response to treatment including radiation, chemotherapy, and monoclonal antibody therapy.

Ocular-only disease can be treated with intensity-modulated radiotherapy (IMRT) alone (dose ranges from 23 to 36 Gy). When there is systemic disease, patients can be treated with chemotherapy or monoclonal antibody therapy (rituximab). Chemotherapy with combination rituximab, cyclophosphamide, doxorubicin, vincristine, and prednisone (RCHOP) is reserved for widespread systemic disease and more aggressive subtypes of lymphoma.

43.9 Follow-Up

Patients should be monitored by both an ophthalmologist familiar with ocular lymphoma and a medical oncologist to screen for the development of systemic disease. This includes periodic surveillance with systemic imaging.

References and Suggested Reading

1. Aronow ME, et al. Uveal lymphoma: clinical features, diagnostic studies, treatment selection, and outcomes. Ophthalmology. 2014;121(1):334–41.
2. Mashayekhi A, et al. Choroidal lymphoma: clinical features and association with systemic lymphoma. Ophthalmology. 2014;121(1):342–51.
3. Coupland SE (2014) Uveal lymphoproliferative tumors. In: Clinical ophthalmic oncology. Heidelberg: Springer; p. 341–54
4. Ferreri AJ, Guidoboni M, Ponzoni M, et al. Evidence for an association between Chlamydia psittaci and ocular adnexal lymphomas. J Natl Cancer Inst. 2004;96(8):586–94.
5. Chan CC, Smith JA, Shen DF, et al. Helicobacter pylori (H. pylori) molecular signature in conjunctival mucosa-associated lymphoid tissue (MALT) lymphoma. Histol Histopathol. 2004;19(4):1219–26.
6. Fuller ML, Sweetenham JM, Schoenfield LR, Singh AD. Uveal lymphoma: a variant of ocular adnexal lymphoma. Leuk Lymphoma. 2008;49(12):2393–7.

Section VI
Retinal Tumors and Associated Conditions

Abdul Hassan Aziz

Chapter 44
Retinoblastoma

Hadi Kaakour and Eric D. Hansen

44.1 Definitions

Retinoblastoma (RB) is a rare but rapidly progressive malignant tumor of the retina, most commonly afflicting young children.

44.2 Symptoms

Leukocoria,[1] strabismus, red and painful eye, and diminished visual acuity are the most frequently reported symptoms.

44.3 Signs

Anterior segment: Examining the anterior chamber is difficult in this population, but under anesthesia, findings such as iris neovascularization, hyphema, pseudohypopyon, and/or anterior chamber invasion by the tumor may be appreciated.

[1]Young children with leukocoria should be considered to have retinoblastoma until proven otherwise.

H. Kaakour (✉)
Bascom Palmer Eye Institute, University of Miami Miller School of Medicine, 1600 NW 10th Ave, Miami, FL 33136, USA
e-mail: akaakour@med.miami.edu

E.D. Hansen
Bascom Palmer Eye Institute, University of Miami, Miami, FL, USA

C.A. Medina et al. (eds.), *Manual of Retinal Diseases: A Guide to Diagnosis and Management*, DOI 10.1007/978-3-319-20460-4_44

Posterior segment: Indirect ophthalmoscopy is most critical for diagnosis and can lead to visualization of the lesion. RB may take on a variety of growth patterns [2].

- *Endophytic*: Upon penetration of the internal limiting membrane, a white-to-cream fluffy mass is observed and often results in vitreous seeding, simulating endophthalmitis or iridocyclitis (Fig. 44.1).
- *Exophytic*: A lesion may spread into the subretinal space, commonly resulting in retinal detachment. Invasion of Bruch's membrane and spread to blood vessels or ciliary nerves may occur.
- *Diffuse infiltrating*: Least common type and slowest growing. The infiltrating retinal lesion appears flat, without a discrete tumor mass.

44.4 Epidemiology

There are 250–350 new cases diagnosed annually in the USA, with one case in 18,000–30,000 live births worldwide. On average, patients are diagnosed at 18 months of age: bilateral cases are found before 12 months, while unilateral cases are discovered later in life, at 24 months.

44.5 Predisposing Conditions

RB is a childhood disease, and most cases are diagnosed before 5 years of age. No predilection for any race or gender has been found, although clear genetic mechanisms have been elucidated.

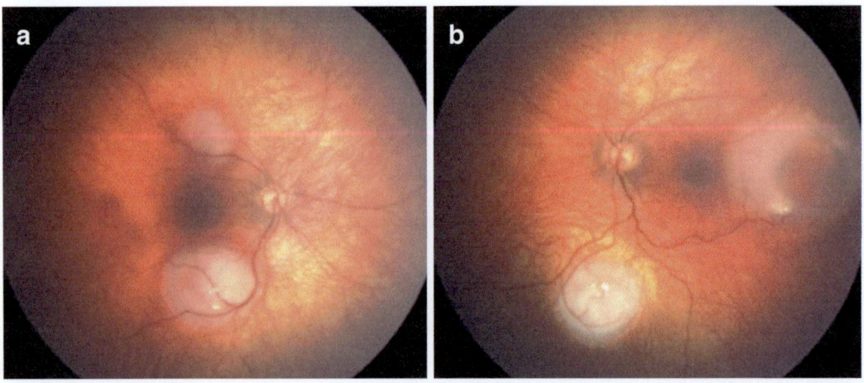

Fig. 44.1 Color fundus photo of (**a**) right eye and (**b**) left eye showing white retinal tumors with associated calcification present in the posterior pole with a cystic component in the macular tumor in the left eye

44.6 Inheritance

Retinoblastoma can occur as either a hereditary (30–40 % of cases) or non-hereditary tumor. The *RB1* tumor suppressor gene on chromosome 13 (autosomal dominant gene with 90 % penetrance) has been implicated as the prototypical *two-hit hypothesis* of RB pathogenesis. In heritable manifestations, the first "hit" is inherited as a germline mutation; the second "hit" follows after conception during development. In non-hereditary sporadic RB, it is understood that two separate somatic *RB1* mutation events occur in a single retinal progenitor cell. Distinctions can be made in the presentation of RB based on the mechanism of *RB1* mutation (Table 44.1).

Whether familial or sporadic, a germline carrier has a 26 % chance of developing a non-ocular tumor within 30 years and a 40–45 % chance of passing the gene onto progeny. In these patients, genetic counseling is indicated.

44.7 Differential Diagnosis

Retinoblastoma has many classical and pathognomonic features, but in cases with an opaque view of intraocular contents, forming a concise differential may become difficult (Table 44.2). The three most common differentials are PHPV, Coats' disease, and ocular toxocariasis.

Table 44.1 Distinguishing features between heritable and nonheritable RB [7]

	Nonheritable RB	Heritable RB
Laterality	~100 % unilateral	~85 % bilateral and ~15 % unilateral
Age of onset	~24 months on average	≤12 months generally
Risk of second malignancy	No increased risk	Trilateral RB (pineal gland neoplasm), melanoma, osteosarcoma, etc.
Offspring inheritance	Somatic, 0 % risk	40–45 % of progeny will inherit *RB1* mutation

Table 44.2 Differential diagnosis of retinoblastoma

Congenital and acquired pseudoretinoblastomas	
Persistent fetal vasculature	Coats' disease
Toxocariasis	Retinopathy of prematurity
Vitreous hemorrhage	Retinochoroidal coloboma
Astrocytic hamartoma	Uveitis (pars planitis)
Familial exudative vitreoretinopathy (FEVR)	Retinal angiomatosis
Choroidal hemangioma	Norrie's disease
Incontinentia pigmenti	Leukemia

44.8 Workup/Testing

Indirect ophthalmoscopy continues to be the most useful diagnostic tool, as most diagnoses of RB may be secured by detection of salient clinical features, without a need for biopsy. Ultrasonography is another valuable tool that typically reveals an intraocular mass with high internal reflectivity and intralesional calcification.

Birth, medical, and family histories are useful, and confirmation with diagnostic imaging (such as fluorescein angiography, OCT, ultrasonography, CT, and MRI) may aid in ruling out other pseudoretinoblastomas.

44.9 Prognosis and Management

Historically, RB resulted in a nearly 100 % mortality rate, but in contemporary developed nations, RB is cured in 95–98 % of children. Patients who are diagnosed before 2 years of age or after 7 years of age experience the greatest survival [3].

In treating RB, the foremost goal is to preserve the patient's life, followed by the patient's vision. Various treatment options exist and depend on similar tumor prognostication parameters: size, shape, location, laterality, and metastasis. The decision to pursue a treatment modality should be considered in conjunction with a pediatric oncologist and a geneticist. Options include chemoreduction, local consolidation therapies, radiation, and surgery (Table 44.3) [5, 6].

44.10 Follow-Up

If the patient is undergoing a chemotherapeutic regimen, follow-up examinations should occur every 3 weeks. Under other focal therapies, examinations may be extended to a 4–8-week period until complete tumor regression is achieved.

Table 44.3 Treatment options for retinoblastoma

Radiation therapy	External beam
	Proton beam
	Brachytherapy
Chemotherapy	Local (intravitreal or sub-tenon)
	Intra-arterial
	Systemic
Local therapy	Cryotherapy
	Laser photocoagulation
	Thermotherapy
Surgical therapy	Enucleation
	Exenteration (for advanced disease)

Once the complete tumor regression has been achieved, the patient should be followed every 3 months for the first year and then every 6 months for 3 years afterward or until the patient reaches the age of six. Subsequently, annual examinations are indicated.

References and Suggested Reading

1. Abramson DH, Frank CM, Susman M, Whalen MP, Dunkel IJ, Boyd 3rd NW. Presenting signs of retinoblastoma. J Pediatr. 1998;132(3 Pt 1):505–8.
2. Balmer A, Munier F. Differential diagnosis of leukocoria and strabismus, first presenting signs of retinoblastoma. Clin Ophthalmol (Auckland, NZ). 2007;1(4):431–9.
3. Rodriguez-Galindo C, Orbach DB, VanderVeen D. Retinoblastoma. Pediatr Clin North Am. 2015;62(1):201–23.
4. Villegas VM, Hess DJ, Wildner A, Gold AS, Murray TG. Retinoblastoma. Curr Opin Ophthalmol. 2013;24(6):581–8.
5. Chintagumpala M, Chevez-Barrios P, Paysse EA, Plon SE, Hurwitz R. Retinoblastoma: review of current management. Oncologist. 2007;12(10):1237–46.
6. Kaliki S, Shields CL. Retinoblastoma: achieving new standards with methods of chemotherapy. Indian J Ophthalmol. 2015;63(2):103–9.
7. Pandey AN. Retinoblastoma: an overview. Saudi J Ophthalmol. 2014;28(4):310–5.

Chapter 45
Coats' Disease

Hadi Kaakour and Eric D. Hansen

45.1 Definitions

Coats' disease (CD), *also known as* exudative retinopathy or retinal telangiectasias, can be defined as developmental retinal exudative vasculopathy.

45.2 Symptoms

Painless unilateral decreased vision, leukocoria, and strabismus

45.3 Signs

External: Leukocoria, due to yellow subretinal cholesterol exudation
Anterior segment: Although typically clear in early CD, advanced stages may demonstrate ischemic and inflammatory sequelae including:

- Cataract
- Aqueous cells and flare
- Hyphema
- Neovascularization of the iris and/or angle

H. Kaakour (✉)
Bascom Palmer Eye Institute, University of Miami Miller School of Medicine, 1600 NW 10th Ave, Miami, FL 33136, USA
e-mail: akaakour@med.miami.edu

E.D. Hansen
Bascom Palmer Eye Institute, University of Miami, Miami, FL, USA

C.A. Medina et al. (eds.), *Manual of Retinal Diseases: A Guide to Diagnosis and Management*, DOI 10.1007/978-3-319-20460-4_45

Table 45.1 Staging and corresponding management in Coats' disease

Stage	Findings	Management
1	Retinal vessel telangiectasia and aneurysms	Observation, photocoagulation
2a	Exudate, extra-foveal	Photocoagulation, cryotherapy
2b	Exudate, foveal	
3a	Subtotal exudative retinal detachment	Cryotherapy, surgical reattachment, photocoagulation
3b	Total exudative retinal detachment	Vitreoretinal surgery
4a	Secondary glaucoma, painful	Surgical enucleation
5	End stage (pre-phthisis disease), no pain	Observation

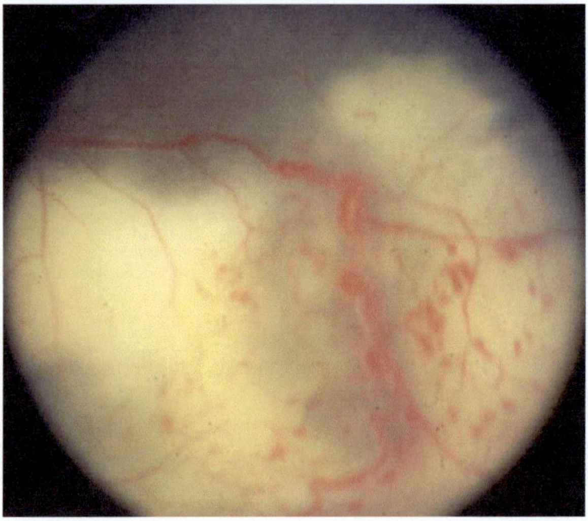

Fig. 45.1 Color fundus photo of the left eye showing retinal telangiectasia with sausage-like dilatation of the blood vessels and associated exudation (Courtesy Jonathan Sears, MD, Cleveland, OH)

Posterior segment: Findings on fundoscopy are variable based on stage of disease (Table 45.1). The vitreous is clear, offering unimpeded visualization of underlying retinal pathology; vessels are visible across the retina and do not disappear. Irregular sausage-like dilation of retinal vasculature is seen in all stages of disease, and the macula may contain xanthochromic cholesterol exudation with no feeding vessels (Fig. 45.1). Localized to total exudative retinal detachment may be associated with the disease process.

45.4 Epidemiology

- *Male* (3:1 or greater ratio male/female)
- *Young* (60–70 % of cases manifest in the first decade of life)
- *Unilateral leukocoria* (>75 % of patients have unilateral disease)

45.5 Predisposing Conditions

Not yet known; currently idiopathic

45.6 Inheritance

Unclear hereditary component. Somatic mutations are being investigated given the unilateral and nonfamilial features of the disease.

45.7 Differential Diagnosis

CD is on the differential diagnosis of leukocoria (Table 45.2). The foremost challenge of Coats' disease is to differentiate it from retinoblastoma, as both are characterized by leukocoria, dilated retinal vessels, and exudative retinal detachments. On the other hand, intraocular calcification is frequently present in retinoblastoma but not in CD.

45.8 Etiology

Unknown. It is postulated that abnormal vascular endothelial cells lead to the loss of the blood-retinal barrier and increased vessel permeability. Hematological components such as lipids, lipid-laden macrophages, and cholesterol crystals exude into the retinal and subretinal spaces. This can result in retinal detachment along with secondary neovascularization in both the posterior and anterior chambers.

45.9 Workup/Testing

The diagnosis for Coats' disease can be made noninvasively in an office setting. Birth, medical, and family histories are helpful, and slit lamp examination of the anterior chamber aids in ruling out other diseases as well as assisting in

Table 45.2 Differential diagnosis of leukocoria

Retinoblastoma	Congenital cataract
Persistent fetal vasculature	Toxocariasis
Coats' disease	Retinochoroidal coloboma
Retinopathy of prematurity (stage 4/5)	Uveitis (pars planitis)
Astrocytic hamartoma	Vitreous hemorrhage
Familial exudative vitreoretinopathy (FEVR)	Norrie disease
Retinal angiomatosis	Incontinentia pigmenti

prognostication. All CD patients with elevated IOP must be evaluated with a gonioscope for neovascular glaucoma, particularly if the eye is painful.

Indirect ophthalmoscopy is often sufficient to make the diagnosis as well as staging of the disease. Ocular ultrasonography is useful especially to rule out presence of calcification, and fluorescein angiography enables delineation of irregularly dilated, tortuous, and permeable vessels.

Ancillary testing with CT and MRI have utility and are frequently used, particularly in advanced disease where it may be difficult to distinguish from retinoblastoma.

45.10 Prognosis and Management

The natural history of CD varies but is almost always characterized by slow, progressive vision loss in the affected eye. Patients who present less than 5 years of age can expect a worse prognosis and more rapid advancement, whereas older patients typically experience a milder disease course. Findings in the anterior segment indicate advanced disease and portend a poor prognosis. If total exudative retinal detachment occurs, loss of sight is generally permanent.

Treatment is directed at halting the proliferation of abnormal retinal vasculature as well as the obliteration of abnormal vessels by either cryotherapy or laser photocoagulation. Treatment recommendations vary by disease stage (Table 45.1). Though its safety in children is still unknown, intravitreal anti-VEGF therapy has shown promise. In painful, glaucomatic eyes, enucleation is appropriate.

45.11 Follow-Up

Periodic observation is necessary to check for progression or recurrence of the disease, even after treatment.

References and Suggested Reading

1. Black GC, Perveen R, Bonshek R, et al. Coats' disease of the retina (unilateral retinal telangiectasis) caused by somatic mutation in the NDP gene: a role for norrin in retinal angiogenesis. Hum Mol Genet. 1999;8(11):2031–5.
2. Chang MM, McLean IW, Merritt JC. Coats' disease: a study of 62 histologically confirmed cases. J Pediatr Ophthalmol Strabismus. 1984;21(5):163–8.
3. Edward DP, Mafee MF, Garcia-Valenzuela E, Weiss RA. Coats' disease and persistent hyperplastic primary vitreous. Role of MR imaging and CT. Radiol Clin North Am. 1998;36(6):1119–31, x.

4. Fernandes BF, Odashiro AN, Maloney S, Zajdenweber ME, Lopes AG, Burnier Jr MN. Clinical-histopathological correlation in a case of Coats' disease. Diagn Pathol. 2006;1:24.
5. Ray R, Baranano DE, Hubbard GB. Treatment of Coats' disease with intravitreal bevacizumab. Br J Ophthalmol. 2013;97(3):272–7.
6. Shields JA, Shields CL, Honavar SG, Demirci H, Cater J. Classification and management of Coats disease: the 2000 Proctor Lecture. Am J Ophthalmol. 2001;131(5):572–83.
7. Smithen LM, Brown GC, Brucker AJ, Yannuzzi LA, Klais CM, Spaide RF. Coats' disease diagnosed in adulthood. Ophthalmology. 2005;112(6):1072–8.

Chapter 46
Retinal Astrocytic Hamartoma

Hadi Kaakour and Eric D. Hansen

46.1 Definitions

Retinal astrocytic hamartoma ((RAH) *also known as* retinal astrocytoma or phakoma) is a benign, minimally progressive, neoplastic lesion of the retinal nerve fiber layer caused by proliferation of glial cells.

46.2 Epidemiology

RAH is found in 50–80 % of patients with tuberous sclerosis (TS) and more rarely in patients with neurofibromatosis (NF-1). It can also be detected incidentally as a sporadic and isolated tumor.

46.3 Symptoms

Patients are often asymptomatic, but some patients may report decreased vision or scotomas in their visual field.

H. Kaakour (✉)
Bascom Palmer Eye Institute, University of Miami Miller School of Medicine,
1600 NW 10th Ave, Miami, FL 33136, USA
e-mail: akaakour@med.miami.edu

E.D. Hansen
Bascom Palmer Eye Institute, University of Miami, Miami, FL, USA

C.A. Medina et al. (eds.), *Manual of Retinal Diseases: A Guide to Diagnosis and Management*, DOI 10.1007/978-3-319-20460-4_46

46.4 Signs

RAHs typically present with one of two appearances:

- *Type 1*: Peripheral, flat, semitranslucent plaques that are chalky white to gray in color (Fig. 46.1a).
- *Type 2*: Peripapillary, elevated, multi-lobulated "mulberry" lesions that are yellow with patchy calcifications.

In many cases, RAH lesions may possess traits of both appearances.
Idiopathic cases are typically unilateral and unifocal, whereas RAH associated with TS or NF-1 phakomatoses can present bilateral and multifocal.

46.5 Inheritance

There are three known mechanisms for RAH:

- *Tuberous sclerosis*: Autosomal dominant disorder with two forms, TS-1 and TS-2, resulting from a defect in chromosomes 9 and 16, respectively. Variable expressivity, complete penetrance

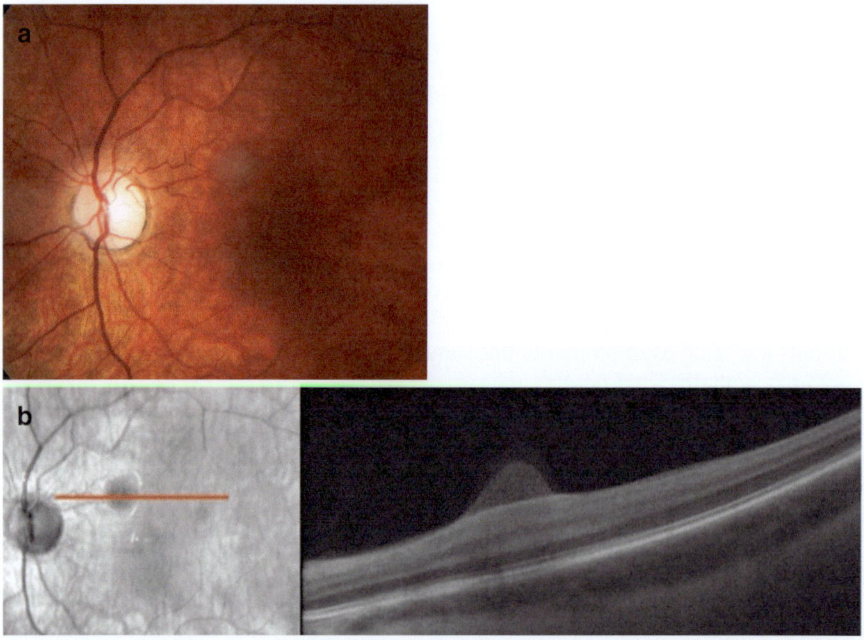

Fig. 46.1 Color fundus photo of the right eye showing a gray, flat, semitranslucent plaque in a perifoveal location (**a**). OCT scan through the lesion showing thickening of the retinal nerve fiber layer (**b**)

- *Neurofibromatosis-1*: Autosomal dominant disorder resulting from a defect in chromosome 17. Highly variable expressivity, complete penetrance
- *Sporadic*: Idiopathic and spontaneous – no inheritance

46.6 Differential Diagnosis

- Retinoblastoma
- Papillitis
- Optic disk drusen
- Retinal granuloma
- Amelanotic melanoma
- Myelinated nerve fibers

46.7 Etiology

Most instances of RAH occur congenitally in association with phakomatoses: principally TS or less frequently NF-1.

46.8 Workup/Testing

All patients who present with RAH must undergo a full neurological examination with neuroimaging as part of evaluation for TS and NF-1. A complete personal and family history should be performed specifically asking about seizures, intellectual disabilities, and characteristic dermatological findings. In patients suspected of having TS, referral for systemic workup should be initiated.

- *Fundoscopy*: Lesions appear more prominent with red-free light.
- *Fluorescein angiography*: The tumor appears hypofluorescent in the early phase and stains intensely in the late phase.
- *OCT*: Shows high reflectivity and elevation of the retinal nerve fiber layer (Fig. 46.1b).
- *B-scan ultrasonography*: Useful in ruling out other diagnoses; the lesion will typically appear as a sharply demarcated ovoid mass with calcification.
- *MRI*: In patients with TS, subependymal hamartomas can be seen.

46.9 Prognosis and Management

Most cases of RAH are asymptomatic and small and exhibit little growth. Periodic observation is recommended for rare complications that can include exudative retinal detachment, traction, hemorrhage, and neovascular glaucoma. Treatments are warranted in these circumstances and might involve photodynamic therapy laser photocoagulation or surgical vitrectomy.

46.10 Follow-Up

Annual examination is recommended to monitor progression and symptoms. Family members should be examined for TS and NF-1 and should receive neurological and genetic consultation when appropriate.

References and Suggested Reading

1. Aronow ME, Nakagawa JA, Gupta A, Traboulsi EI, Singh AD. Tuberous sclerosis complex: genotype/phenotype correlation of retinal findings. Ophthalmology. 2012;119(9):1917–23.
2. Crino PB, Nathanson KL, Henske EP. The tuberous sclerosis complex. N Engl J Med. 2006;355(13):1345–56.
3. Mennel S, Meyer CH, Peter S, Schmidt JC, Kroll P. Current treatment modalities for exudative retinal hamartomas secondary to tuberous sclerosis: review of the literature. Acta Ophthalmol Scand. 2007;85(2):127–32.
4. Prasad S, Kamath GG. Retinal astrocytic hamartoma. Postgrad Med J. 2001;77(911):556.
5. Ulbright TM, Fulling KH, Helveston EM. Astrocytic tumors of the retina. Differentiation of sporadic tumors from phakomatosis-associated tumors. Arch Pathol Lab Med. 1984;108(2):160–3.

Chapter 47
Retinal Hemangioma

Hadi Kaakour and Eric Hansen

47.1 Definitions

Retinal hemangioma (RH) is a benign retinal vascular tumor that is capable of occurring as a solitary lesion but more frequently occurs concurrently as part of von Hippel-Lindau (VHL) disease, a hereditary multi-tumor syndrome.

Also known as retinal hemangioblastoma
Also known as retinal capillary hemangioma
Also known as retinal angiomatosis (when multifocal)

47.2 Symptoms

Decreased visual acuity or visual field loss (if subretinal fluid or lipid exudates involve the macula). Otherwise, patients may be asymptomatic.

47.3 Signs

On fundoscopy, retinal hemangiomas are commonly found in the mid-peripheral retina or the juxtapapillary region and appear as circular, red-orange lesions (Fig. 47.1). Tortuous vessels tracing back to the optic disk sustain the solitary tumor, which may be multifocal in 1/3 of patients with VHL.

H. Kaakour (✉)
Bascom Palmer Eye Institute, University of Miami Miller School of Medicine,
1600 NW 10th Ave, Miami, FL 33136, USA
e-mail: akaakour@med.miami.edu

E. Hansen
Bascom Palmer Eye Institute, University of Miami, Miami, FL, USA

C.A. Medina et al. (eds.), *Manual of Retinal Diseases: A Guide to Diagnosis and Management*, DOI 10.1007/978-3-319-20460-4_47

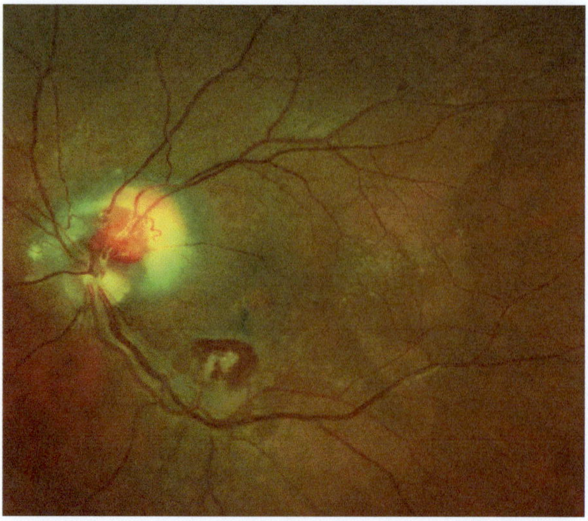

Fig. 47.1 Color fundus photograph of the right eye showing a peripapillary and a macular capillary hemangioma associated with significant retinal edema and exudation

47.4 Epidemiology

VHL occurs in approximately one per 36,000 live births per year, with no gender predilection. The median age for VHL disease-associated RH is 17.6 years, and for sporadic VHL, patients are diagnosed at a median age of 36.1 years.

47.5 Predisposing Conditions

Nearly half of patients with solitary RH are found to have underlying VHL disease, and the risk progressively decreases with increasing age of diagnosis.

47.6 Inheritance

VHL disease occurs when the *VHL* gene, an autosomal dominant tumor suppressor gene with high penetrance, undergoes a germ line mutation. Of note, VHL-associated tumors operate via the two-hit model of tumorigenesis, analogous to the pathogenesis of retinoblastoma. Approximately 80 % of patients with RH have a family history and inherit a mutated allele; other cases result from a de novo mutation.

47.7 Differential Diagnosis

The differential for RH includes other vascular tumors, such as racemose hemangioma, retinal macroaneurysm, or retinal cavernous hemangioma. In patients with severe exudation, RH may be confused with Coats's disease.

47.8 Workup/Testing

Fundoscopy is often sufficient, as the diagnosis for RH can be made noninvasively in the office setting. Additional data can be gathered from fluorescein angiography, enabling delineation of the vascularity that accompanies the lesion. In cases where subretinal fluid is suspected, OCT of the macula or B-scan ultrasonography is a useful confirmatory tool.

47.9 Prognosis and Management

As with many disease entities, an early diagnosis of RH prior to onset of symptoms results in better visual outcomes. With increasing tumor size, multifocality, and degree of subretinal fluid exudation (including retinal detachment), the prognosis generally worsens. Even in eyes that have undergone satisfactory treatment, the prognosis is not entirely optimistic: almost 20 % of eyes cannot see better than 20/100, and over 25 % of eyes permanently lose vision.

In concordance with prognostic factors, the choice of treatment is based upon tumor location, size, degree of subretinal fluid or retinal traction, and impact on visual acuity. Various modalities of treatment exist, including observation, laser photocoagulation, cryotherapy, photodynamic therapy, radiotherapy, and surgical intervention. Of these, observation is typically warranted when the tumor is juxtapapillary in location, is smaller (<0.5 mm), has not affected visual acuity, and has no evidence of exudation. In lesions that are larger, or that have consequences on visual acuity, the mainstays of therapy are laser photocoagulation (91–100 % effective) and cryotherapy. Lesions greater than 4.0 mm and/or resistant to these therapies tend to respond well to radiotherapy.

47.10 Follow-Up

In patients who suffer from VHL syndrome, annual surveillance for new lesions is required, due to the susceptibility to developing multiple lesions bilaterally. Less frequent screening is needed for patients who are older and in whom VHL has been ruled out, as the likelihood of recurrence is low.

References and Suggested Reading

1. Haddad NM, Cavallerano JD, Silva PS. Von Hippel-Lindau disease: a genetic and clinical review. Semin Ophthalmol. 2013;28:377–86.
2. Kreusel KM, Bornfeld N, Lommatzsch A, Wessing A, Foerster MH. Ruthenium-106 brachytherapy for peripheral retinal capillary hemangioma. Ophthalmology. 1998;105:1386–92.
3. Richards FM, Payne SJ, Zbar B, Affara NA, Ferguson-Smith MA, Maher ER. Molecular analysis of De Novo Germline mutations in the Von Hippel-Lindau disease gene. Hum Mol Genet. 1995;4:2139–43.
4. Schmidt D, Natt E, Neumann HP. Long-term results of laser treatment for retinal angiomatosis in Von Hippel-Lindau disease. Eur J Med Res. 2000;5:47–58.
5. Schmidt-Erfurth UM, Kusserow C, Barbazetto IA, Laqua H. Benefits and complications of photodynamic therapy of papillary capillary hemangiomas. Ophthalmology. 2002;109:1256–66.
6. Singh AD, Nouri M, Shields CL, Shields JA, Smith AF. Retinal capillary hemangioma: a comparison of sporadic cases and cases associated with Von Hippel-Lindau disease. Ophthalmology. 2001;108:1907–11.
7. Webster AR, Maher ER, Moore AT. Clinical characteristics of ocular angiomatosis in Von Hippel-Lindau disease and correlation with germline mutation. Arch Ophthalmol. 1999;117:371–8.

Chapter 48
Primary Central Nervous System Lymphoma: Ophthalmic Variant (PCNSL-O)

Hadi Kaakour and Eric D. Hansen

48.1 Definitions

Primary vitreoretinal lymphoma (PVRL) is a rare and aggressive lymphoma. Most PVRL are of the diffuse large B-cell lymphoma cell type that arise either in the retina or the vitreous representing ophthalmic variant of primary central nervous system lymphoma (PCNSL-O)
Also known as primary intraocular lymphoma (PIOL)

48.2 Symptoms

Nonspecific visual symptoms, including floaters, photophobia, blurry vision, red eye, or even painless loss of vision. Patients may experience symptoms in some cases for up to 2 years before lymphoma is suspected [1].

48.3 Signs

External: Often white and quiet.
Anterior segment: Most cases present with few to no findings. Common signs include corneal precipitates and mild aqueous cells and flare. Posterior synechiae are typically absent.

H. Kaakour (✉)
Bascom Palmer Eye Institute, University of Miami Miller School of Medicine, 1600 NW 10th Ave, Miami, FL 33136, USA
e-mail: akaakour@med.miami.edu

E.D. Hansen
Bascom Palmer Eye Institute, University of Miami, Miami, FL, USA

C.A. Medina et al. (eds.), *Manual of Retinal Diseases: A Guide to Diagnosis and Management*, DOI 10.1007/978-3-319-20460-4_48

Posterior segment: The pathognomonic hallmark of PVRL is subretinal pigment epithelium (RPE) deposits with associated choroidal, retinal, or chorioretinal infiltrates, often leading to focal detachments of the RPE (Fig. 48.1a). Vitreous haze is frequently present, consisting of sheets of infiltrating homogenous lymphomatous cells (Fig. 48.1b).

48.4 Epidemiology

- Mean age of diagnosis in immunocompetent individuals is 60 years with a peak incidence in seventh to eighth decade.
- Bilateral involvement in 80–90 % of patients.
- Comorbidities secondary to CNS involvement (up to 85 % develop CNS disease).

48.5 Predisposing Conditions

Immunodeficient individuals (particularly AIDS) are at greater risk for developing PVRL. Moreover, 25 % of patients diagnosed with ocular lymphoma occur in the context of PCNSL.

48.6 Differential Diagnosis

PVRL follows an insidious natural history, commonly masquerading as inflammatory or infectious conditions (posterior uveitis/retinitis), frequently resulting in a 21-month mean delay in diagnosis. Differential should include intraocular lymphomas (Table 48.1), as well as nonneoplastic diseases of the uvea (Table 48.2).

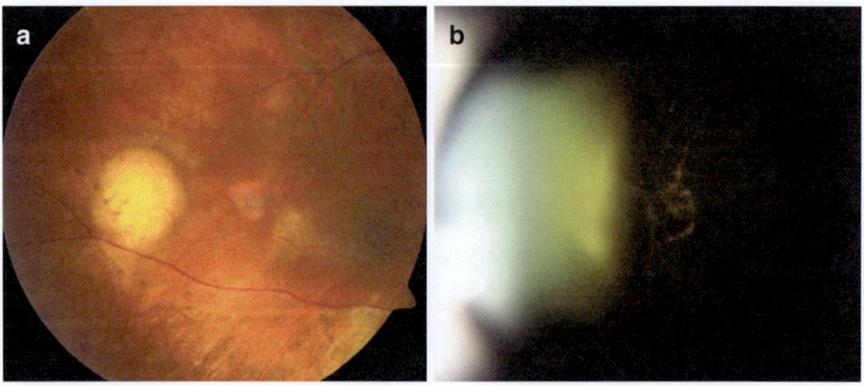

Fig. 48.1 Color fundus photo of the right eye showing subretinal yellow lesions (**a**). Slit lamp photo of the right eye showing vitreous haze and vitreous cellular condensations (**b**)

Table 48.1 Clinical features of intraocular lymphomas

Lymphoma	Subtype	Laterality	Location	Clinical features
Primary vitreoretinal lymphoma	Diffuse large B-cell lymphoma (DLBCL)[a]	Frequently bilateral	Generally subretinal	Vitreous cells CNS involvement Retinal infiltrates
Primary uveal lymphoma	Extranodal marginal zone B-cell lymphoma (EMZL)	Usually unilateral	Choroid (iris rare)	Clear vitreous Exudative retinal detachment
Secondary intraocular lymphoma	Dependent on systemic NHL	Unilateral or bilateral	Usually choroid	*Variable*: pseudohypopyon, iris infiltrates, choroidal thickening, vitreous cells

[a]Rarely, T-cell lymphomas

Table 48.2 Differential diagnosis of PCNSL-O

Tuberculosis	Sarcoidosis	Syphilis
Toxoplasmosis	Serpiginous choroiditis	Cytomegalovirus retinitis
Herpes zoster ophthalmicus	Frosted branch angiitis	Acute retinal necrosis
Birdshot choroidopathy	Multifocal chorioretinitis	Retinal vasculitis
Acute posterior multifocal placoid pigment epitheliopathy		
Branch retinal artery obstruction with coexistent multifocal chorioretinal scars		

48.7 Etiology

Yet to be elucidated, studies propose infectious agents as pathogenic factors in immunocompetent patients (HHV-8, EBV), with more compelling evidence of a viral mechanism (EBV) in AIDS-associated disease. This is hypothesized to involve clonal duplication of malignant lymphocytes undergoing additional secondary mutations, localizing to the CNS.

48.8 Workup/Testing

A high clinical suspicion should be retained for elderly patients presenting with a noninfectious uveitis nonresponsive to anti-inflammatory therapies. Although physical examination and ocular imaging (OCT, fluorescein angiography) are useful adjuncts, biopsy of malignant tissues and detection of malignant PVRL cells remain the gold standard for diagnosis. This may include:

- Aqueous aspiration
- Diagnostic vitrectomy
- Diagnostic retinal or chorioretinal biopsy

It is critical to deliver the specimen to an experienced pathologist promptly after of surgery, as PVRL cells easily undergo necrosis. Cytologically, PVRL cells are pleomorphic: the large atypical lymphoid cells contain scanty basophilic cytoplasm with large, irregular nuclei and prominent nucleoli. To further distinguish benign intraocular inflammatory entities from PVRL, cytokine ratios (of IL-10/IL-6) and immunophenotyping have been used as well, most useful in initial diagnosis and in follow-up for recurrences. Neurological imaging and CSF analysis are indicated in all PVRL patients due to the high likelihood of CNS involvement.

48.9 Prognosis and Management

Given the rarity of PVRL, it has been difficult to establish a protocol for management. Most cases in the literature employ combinations of available therapies, and there are no comparative studies of significant power to date.

Treatments are generally grouped into local or systemic therapies.

Localized therapies: With PVRL patients in whom a neurologic workup is non-revealing, local therapies are introduced to eliminate intraocular disease and prevent any ensuing spread to the CNS. Table 48.3 summarizes the three main modalities of local therapies, outcomes, and the commonly reported side effects.

Systemic therapies: Systemic therapies include whole brain radiation therapy (WBRT), intrathecal chemotherapy, or systemic chemotherapies generally directed toward DLBCL, with methotrexate as a mainstay. Coordination of care with a neuro-oncologist is critical to obtain optimal results.

48.10 Follow-Up

In many situations periodic observation is necessary to check for progression or recurrence of the disease, even after treatment.

Table 48.3 Localized therapies with prognosis for PVRL

Local therapy	Prognosis and outcomes	Toxicity
External beam radiation	95 % local control and 89 % overall survival at 3 years of follow-up [2]	Cataract, punctate keratopathy, optic neuropathy, neovascular glaucoma
Intravitreal methotrexate	95 % of eyes reached clinical remission after ≤13 injections. High rate of resistance	Cataracts, corneal epitheliopathy, vitreous hemorrhage, optic atrophy, sterile endophthalmitis
Intravitreal rituximab	64.6 % of eyes achieved complete remission after a median of three injections	Long-term studies of pending

References and Suggested Reading

1. Aziz HA, Peereboom DM, Singh AD. Primary central nervous system lymphoma. Int Ophthalmol Clin. 2015;55(1):111–21.
2. Chan CC, Rubenstein JL, Coupland SE, et al. Primary vitreoretinal lymphoma: a report from an International Primary Central Nervous System Lymphoma Collaborative Group symposium. Oncologist. 2011;16(11):1589–99.
3. Coupland SE, Heimann H, Bechrakis NE. Primary intraocular lymphoma: a review of the clinical, histopathological and molecular biological features. Graefes Arch Clin Exp Ophthalmol. 2004;242(11):901–13.
4. Read RW, Zamir E, Rao NA. Neoplastic masquerade syndromes. Surv Ophthalmol. 2002;47(2):81–124.
5. Coupland SE. Vitreous biopsy: specimen preparation and interpretation. Monogr Clin Cytol. 2012;21:61–71.
6. Hanson JA, Alexandru D, Bota DA. The evaluation and treatment of primary intraocular lymphoma. J Cancer Ther Res. 2013;2:1.
7. Mikami R, Nakayama H, Goto H, et al. Preliminary results of radiotherapy for primary intraocular non-Hodgkin lymphoma. Leuk Lymphoma. 2013;54(10):2181–4.

Section VII
Retinal Detachments and Associated Diseases

Christopher R. Henry

Chapter 49
Peripheral Retinal Abnormalities

Thalmon R. Campagnoli and William E. Smiddy

49.1 Definitions

Peripheral retinal abnormalities are common and usually not consequential, but might obfuscate patient management. Most are asymptomatic, incidentally found during regular eye exams, and do not confer risk for retinal detachment. A small percentage, however, are associated with retinal detachment (RD), especially in the context of visual symptoms. This chapter reviews the most common abnormalities and their potential to lead to retinal detachment.

49.2 Symptoms

- Photopsia
- Vitreous floaters
- Scotoma (especially associated with retinal detachment)

T.R. Campagnoli, MD • W.E. Smiddy, MD (✉)
Department of Ophthalmology, University of Miami, Bascom Palmer Eye Institute, 900 NW 17th St., Miami, FL 33136, USA
e-mail: wsmiddy@med.miami.edu

C.A. Medina et al. (eds.), *Manual of Retinal Diseases: A Guide to Diagnosis and Management*, DOI 10.1007/978-3-319-20460-4_49

49.3 Signs

49.3.1 Variations from Normal Anatomy

Meridional folds (*prevalence 26 %*): radially oriented, linear elevation of retina crossing the ora serrata, aligned with dentate process, whiter than surrounding retina; and cystoid degeneration is often found in the fold. If the fold is aligned with a ciliary process, it is called *meridional complex*, in which retinal excavation is particularly common posteriorly to the fold. Both are commonly found bilaterally (55 %).

Irregular oral bays (*prevalence 6 %*): posterior extension of a large oral bay into the normal curve of the ora serrata may be partially or completely surrounded by two adjacent dentate processes (*partially* or *completely enclosed oral bays*, respectively). These structures are covered by ciliary epithelium from the pars plana and should not be confused with retinal holes.

Pars plana cysts (*prevalence 18 %*): clear and smooth bullous elevations of the non-pigmented ciliary epithelium, resembling blisters on the pars plana. Roughly one third of the cases are bilateral.

Non-cystic retinal tuft (*prevalence 33 %*): thin fibroglial projections of tissue into vitreous, often in clusters.

Cystic retinal tuft (*prevalence 5 %*): dense deposition of thin cystic projections of chalky-white fibroglial tissue into the vitreous, sometimes with scant pigmentation. Bilateral in approximately 40 % of cases.

Zonular traction tuft (*prevalence 15 %*): whitish strand of tissue in the anterior retina continuous with the apex of a thickened zonule. Mostly unilateral.

White with/without pressure: geographic whitish area in the peripheral retina viewed with or without scleral indentation. Suspected to be caused by exaggerated vitreoretinal adhesion. Predominantly bilateral.

49.3.2 Degenerations

Cobblestone (*paving stone*) *pigmentation*: multiple rounded punched out areas of choroidal and (probably ischemic) outer retina atrophy. Usually yellow-white in color and one to several disk diameters in size. Frequently bilateral.

Typical peripheral cystoid degeneration (*TPCD*): small bubbles or vacuoles in the peripheral retina, near the ora serrata, giving a uniformly stippled appearance to the retina. Located most commonly in the outer plexiform layer. Present in 100 % of the eyes to some degree.

Reticular peripheral cystoid degeneration: cystoid spaces in the inner plexiform layer, usually contiguous with (and posterior to) TPCD areas. May be impossible to differentiate from TPCD, but classically has smoother (fine-stippled) surface appearance.

Retinal lattice degeneration: demarcated area of retinal thinning near the equator, usually circumferentially oriented, with black or brown clumps of RPE within the lesion, and frequently interlaced white lines (atrophic vessels) and flecks (glial hyperplasia). Round holes are frequently present within the lesion. Liquefied vitreous over the lesion and prominent vitreoretinal adhesion surrounding the margins are common and may be seen clinically. Often bilateral. Onset is in the second and third decades.

49.4 Epidemiology

- *Cystic retinal tuft*: as many as 10 % of clinical RDs with associated posterior vitreous detachment are reported to occur in the eyes with retinal tears at sites of cystic retinal tufts, but any etiologic role is debated.
- *Zonular traction tuft*: incidence around 16 % and about 4 % associated anatomically with retinal hole.
- *Lattice degeneration*: present in approximately 6–8 % of the population and in 30 % of phakic RD cases. This is the only peripheral retinal abnormality believed to predispose to retinal detachment, yet, less than 1 % (over an average of 11 years) of RD cases are thought to be due to lattice degeneration in a nonfellow RD eye.

49.5 Predisposing Conditions for Peripheral Retinal Findings

- High myopia
- Fellow eye involvement
- Genetic disorders: Stickler syndrome = > latticelike degeneration, retinal detachment, 5q syndromes (Wagner/Jansen)

49.6 Differential Diagnosis

The main disease processes to be evaluated in an eye presenting with peripheral retinal abnormalities include:

- Retinal holes
- Retinal tears
- Localized retinal detachment

49.7 Workup/Testing

Indirect ophthalmoscopy of the retinal periphery with scleral indentation is the gold standard to diagnose and follow up peripheral retinal abnormalities. Shallow, posterior retinal detachment might escape definitive determination with indirect ophthalmoscopy, and optical coherence tomography might be helpful in establishing the diagnosis.

49.8 Prognosis and Management

Generally, peripheral retinal abnormalities are quiescent and do not require treatment. Absence of visual symptoms leads one only to observation of retinal holes or tears associated with peripheral retina degenerations, and even very limited retinal detachment areas may be observed if a close follow-up is feasible (especially if signs of chronicity such as a demarcation line are present).

Symptomatic retinal breaks should be considered for urgent treatment. Symptomatic horseshoe tear or progressive retinal detachment is a universally accepted indication for treatment.

There is not a consensus, but some recommend treatment of eyes with asymptomatic peripheral retinal abnormalities in cases of high myopia, pre-cataract extraction, family history of RD, or fellow eye of RD.

49.9 Follow-Up

Annual ophthalmologic examination is recommended for patients without or unchanged visual symptoms.

Occurrence of new symptoms warrants a closer follow-up examination schedule commensurate with the degree of diagnostic uncertainty or associated findings (e.g., vitreous hemorrhage, status of fellow eye), as trumped by evolving, new symptoms.

References and Suggested Reading

1. American Academy of Ophthalmology Retina/Vitreous Panel. Preferred Practice Pattern® Guidelines. Posterior vitreous detachment, retinal breaks, and lattice degeneration. San Francisco: American Academy of Ophthalmology; 2014. Available at: www.aao.org/ppp.

2. Bell FC, Stenstrom WJ. Peripheral retinal appearances and degenerations. In: Bell FC, Stenstrom WJ, editors. Atlas of the peripheral retina. 1st ed. Philadelphia: Elsevier Saunders; 1983. p. 13–34.
3. Byer NE. Long-term natural history of lattice degeneration of the retina. Ophthalmology. 1989;96(9):1396–401.
4. Byer NE. Rethinking prophylactic therapy of retinal detachment. In: Stirpe M, editor. Advances in vitreoretinal surgery. New York: Ophthalmic Communications Society; 1992. p. 399–411.
5. Folk JC, Arrindell EL, Klugman MR. The fellow eye of patients with phakic lattice retinal detachment. Ophthalmology. 1989;96(1):72–9.

Chapter 50
Retinal Tears

Christopher R. Henry

50.1 Definitions

- Retinal break: A full-thickness defect of the neurosensory retina.
- Horseshoe retinal tear: A type of retinal break where a strip of retina is pulled anteriorly by vitreoretinal traction. Also known as a flap tear.
- Operculated retinal hole: A retinal break in which vitreous traction amputates the flap of the tear from the retinal surface. The separated retina ("operculum") becomes suspended within the posterior hyaloid above the retinal surface, leaving a hole within the retinal surface that is not typically associated with persistent vitreoretinal traction.
- Atrophic retinal hole: A retinal break that is not associated with vitreoretinal traction.
- Giant retinal tear: A retinal break extending circumferentially more than 3 clock hours (90°).
- Retinal dialysis: A circumferential retinal break occurring along the ora serrata.

50.2 Symptoms

Patients will often endorse symptoms of floaters and/or flashing lights [2]. Condition may be asymptomatic if the patient has an operculated hole, atrophic retinal hole, or a retinal dialysis. Visual field loss is a sign that a retinal tear may be progressing to a retinal detachment.

C.R. Henry, MD
Department of Ophthalmology, Bascom Palmer Eye Institute, University of Miami
Miller School of Medicine, 900 NW 17th Street, Miami, FL 33136, USA
e-mail: Chenry2@med.miami.edu

C.A. Medina et al. (eds.), *Manual of Retinal Diseases: A Guide to Diagnosis and Management*, DOI 10.1007/978-3-319-20460-4_50

50.3 Signs

Small clumps of pigment cells may be seen suspended in the vitreous cavity or anterior segment; this is known as "tobacco dust" or a positive Shafer's sign. Retinal tears or breaks can be visualized on ophthalmoscopy (Figs. 50.1 and 50.2). A complete or partial posterior vitreous detachment is most often present. Patients may have associated vitreous hemorrhage.

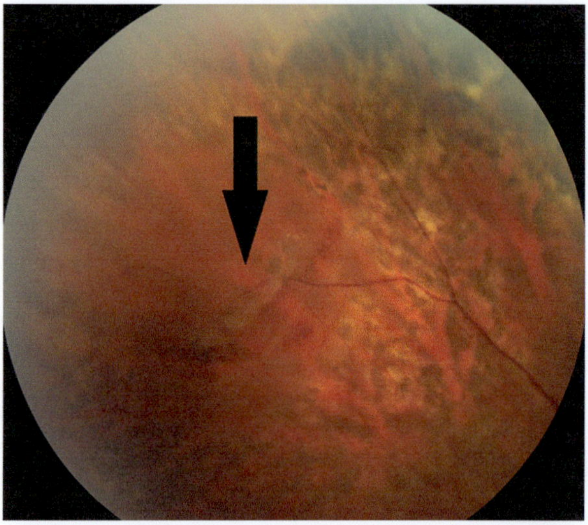

Fig. 50.1 Horseshoe retinal tear (*arrow*) surrounded by laser retinopexy scars

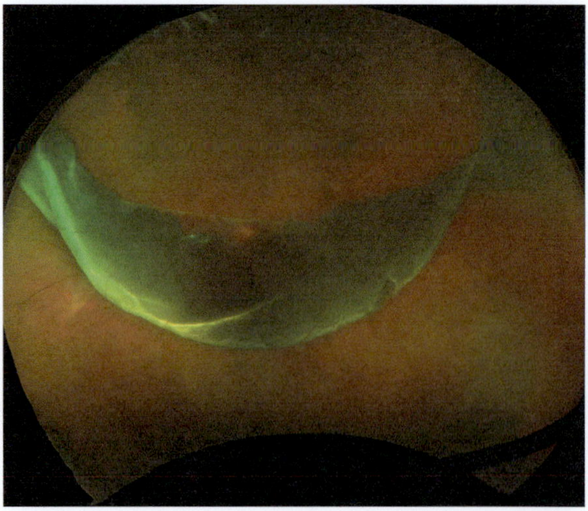

Fig. 50.2 Giant retinal tear

50.4 Predisposing Conditions

- Lattice degeneration
- Posterior vitreous detachment
- Myopia
- Cataract surgery
- Blunt trauma
- Penetrating trauma

50.5 Differential Diagnosis

Horseshoe retinal tear, operculated retinal hole, atrophic retinal hole, giant retinal tear, and retinal dialysis (Table 50.1).

50.6 Etiology

Retinal tears develop as a result of vitreous traction being exerted on an area of preexisting vitreoretinal adhesion, leading to a full-thickness defect of the neurosensory retina. The most common scenario is that a patient develops a posterior vitreous detachment and a flap tear or hole develops as the vitreous exerts traction on and/or separates from the retinal surface. Retinal breaks typically develop at sites of strong vitreoretinal adhesion, commonly at the posterior margin of the vitreous base.

50.7 Workup/Testing

The diagnosis is made clinically from a dilated fundus examination. Wide-field fundus photography can be used to document retinal tears. In the presence of a vitreous hemorrhage or other media opacity, ultrasonography can be used to identify retinal tears that cannot be seen clinically.

Table 50.1 Differential diagnosis of retinal tears

Horseshoe retinal tear or flap tear
Operculated retinal hole
Atrophic retinal hole
Giant retinal tear
Retinal dialysis

50.8 Prognosis and Management

Approximately 6 % of treated retinal tears will still go on to develop into a retinal detachment. In contrast, 30–50 % of untreated horseshoe retinal tears will go on to develop retinal detachment. Symptomatic retinal tears are treated with laser retinopexy or cryopexy surrounding the retinal break. Asymptomatic operculated and atrophic retinal holes are typically observed. Giant retinal tears resulting in retinal detachment require surgical repair.

50.9 Follow-Up

Patients with symptomatic flap tears treated with laser retinopexy or cryopexy are typically followed within 1 week. Asymptomatic and stable operculated retinal holes and atrophic holes can be followed annually.

References and Suggested Reading

1. American Academy of Ophthalmology. Basic and clinical science course. Section 12: Retina. Chapter 11: Peripheral retinal abnormalities. p. 277–301.
2. Tasman WS. Posterior vitreous detachment and peripheral retinal breaks. Trans Am Acad Ophthalmol Otolaryngol. 1968;72:217–24.
3. Robertson DM, Norton EW. Long-term follow-up of treated retinal breaks. Am J Ophthalmol. 1973;75:395–404.
4. Davis MD. Natural history of retinal breaks without detachment. Arch Ophthalmol. 1974;92:183–94.
5. Colyear Jr BH, Pischel DK. Clinical tears in the retina without detachment. Am J Ophthalmol. 1956;41:773–92.

Chapter 51
Degenerative Retinoschisis

Ruwan A. Silva

51.1 Definitions

Splitting of the neurosensory retina to the extent that a recognizable cavity is clinically visible (measuring at least 2 mm^2).

51.2 Symptoms

Asymptomatic (generally), absolute scotoma (rarely).

51.3 Signs

- Typical degenerative retinoschisis: Elevated, stippled inner layer with an attached, beaten-metal-appearing outer layer. Division is at the outer plexiform layer.
- Reticular degenerative retinoschisis: Smooth, translucent, bullous, dome-shaped inner layer with an attached honeycomb-appearing outer layer (Fig. 51.1). More commonly, it has outer retinal holes (often with rolled edges). Division is at the nerve fiber layer.
- The inner retinal layer of both types of retinoschisis may display vessel sheathing and snowflake lesions.

R.A. Silva, MD
Department of Ophthalmology, Byers Eye Institute, Stanford University School of Medicine, 2452 Watson Court, Palo Alto, CA 94303, USA
e-mail: Ruwansilva2002@gmail.com

C.A. Medina et al. (eds.), *Manual of Retinal Diseases: A Guide to Diagnosis and Management*, DOI 10.1007/978-3-319-20460-4_51

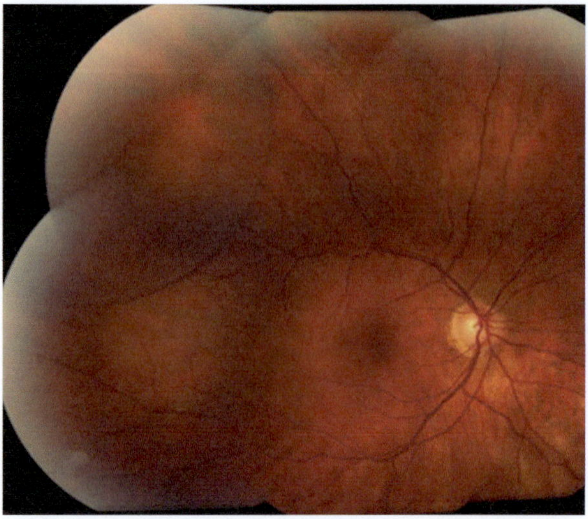

Fig. 51.1 Superotemporal area of bullous retinoschisis

51.4 Epidemiology

Typical degenerative retinoschisis: 3.5 % of the adult population.
Reticular degenerative retinoschisis: 1.6 % of the adult population.
Retinoschisis is bilateral in 50–80 % of patients.
Retinoschisis most commonly involves the inferotemporal quadrant (44 %).

51.5 Predisposing conditions

Typical degenerative cystoid degeneration, reticular degenerative cystoid degeneration, hyperopia.

51.6 Differential Diagnosis

Retinal detachment (rhegmatogenous or serous), choroidal effusion, choroidal mass (Table 51.1).

51.7 Etiology

Largely unknown. Putatively arises from free radical formation (as a consequence of normal retinal function), physiologic peripheral retinal ischemia, and pathologic adherence of the vitreous to the inner retina.

Table 51.1 Differential diagnosis of retinoschisis

Rhegmatogenous retinal detachment
Serous retinal detachment
Choroidal effusion
Choroidal mass

Table 51.2 Differentiation between retinoschisis and retinal detachment

Clinical finding	Retinoschisis	Retinal detachment
Surface	Smooth	Corrugated
Pigment or hemorrhage	Usually absent	Present
Shifting fluid	Absent	Variable
Reaction to photocoagulation	Present	Absent
Scotoma	Absolute	Relative

51.8 Workup/Testing

(Wide-field) fundus photography is recommended for documentation. Optical coherence tomography may be useful to distinguish retinoschisis from subretinal fluid though the peripheral location of the area in question is often limiting (Table 51.2).

51.9 Prognosis and Management

No treatment is indicated unless the retinoschisis is complicated by:

(a) Enlargement of the schisis cavity to involve the macula
(b) A schisis detachment (inner and outer retinal holes)
(c) Symptomatic, increasing subretinal fluid associated with (only) an outer retinal hole

Treatment involves barrier retinopexy (laser photocoagulation or cryo) to demarcate the edge of the schisis cavity or subretinal fluid/schisis-cavity drainage with retinopexy of the outer layer of schisis.

51.10 Follow-Up

Nonprogressive retinoschisis anterior to the equator and without retinal breaks may be followed yearly. Retinoschisis which is symptomatic, is posterior to the equator, or has retinal breaks should initially be followed more closely.

References and Suggested Reading

1. Buch H, Vinding T, Nielsen NV. Prevalence and long-term natural course of retinoschisis among elderly individuals: the Copenhagen City Eye Study. Ophthalmology. 2007;114(4):751–5.
2. Byer NE. Long-term natural history study of senile retinoschisis with implications for management. Ophthalmology. 1986;93(9):1127–37.
3. Byer NE. Perspectives on the management of the complications of senile retinoschisis. Eye (Lond). 2002;16(4):359–64. Review.
4. Schepens CL. Retinal detachment and allied diseases. Philadelphia: WB Saunders Company; 1983. p. 520–42.
5. Straatsma BR. Clinical features of degenerative retinoschisis. Aust J Ophthalmol. 1980;8(3):201–6.
6. Zinn KM. Clinical atlas of peripheral retinal disorder. New York: Springer Verlag; 1988.

Chapter 52
Rhegmatogenous Retinal Detachment

Albert Y. Cheung, Ankoor R. Shah, and Ashkan M. Abbey

52.1 Definitions

Rhegmatogenous retinal detachment (RRD)
Posterior vitreous detachment (PVD)
Proliferative vitreoretinopathy (PVR)

52.2 Symptoms

Flashes, floaters, curtain or shadow defect advancing over field of vision, decreased central and/or peripheral vision.

52.3 Signs

Early: Elevation of the retina from the retinal pigment epithelium (RPE) by clear, accumulated fluid in the subretinal space associated with retinal break(s) or predisposing retinal lesions (see below). The RRD often extends to the ora early with convex borders; the fluid is gravity dependent. The surface appears corrugated and undulated. Other signs include anterior vitreous pigmented cells (Shafer's sign),

A.Y. Cheung, MD • A.R. Shah, MD
A.M. Abbey, MD (✉)
Department of Ophthalmology, William Beaumont Hospital,
3535 W. 13 Mile Road, Suite 344, Royal Oak, MI 48073, USA
e-mail: ashkanabbey@post.harvard.edu

C.A. Medina et al. (eds.), *Manual of Retinal Diseases: A Guide to Diagnosis and Management*, DOI 10.1007/978-3-319-20460-4_52

vitreous hemorrhage, PVD, decreased intraocular pressure in the affected eye, and possibly a mild relative afferent pupillary defect.
Late: Demarcation lines, intraretinal macrocysts, atrophic retina, PVR, subretinal fibrosis, fixed folds. PVR comprises cellular (RPE, glial, etc.) membranes that form on either surface of the retina.

52.4 Predisposing Conditions

- Aphakia/pseudophakia
- Myopia
- Blunt trauma
- Complicated intraocular surgery
- Familial history or detachment in the fellow eye
- Predisposing retinal lesions: lattice degeneration, cystic and zonular vitreoretinal tufts, meridional folds
- Infectious retinitis (e.g., acute retinal necrosis)
- Hereditary vitreoretinal disorders (e.g., Stickler syndrome)
- Glaucoma (especially pigmentary dispersion syndrome)

52.5 Inheritance

Several genetic syndromes are associated with RRD. These include Stickler syndrome, Marshall syndrome, Wagner syndrome, Marfan syndrome, Ehlers-Danlos syndrome, and Knobloch syndrome.

52.6 Differential Diagnosis

Exudative retinal detachment, tractional retinal detachment, retinoschisis, choroidal effusion/detachment, retinal dialysis of the vitreous base, avulsion of the vitreous base, serous detachment associated with optic pit.

52.7 Etiology

While many breaks do not lead to detachment, RRD results from the culmination of certain factors: a full-thickness retinal defect, vitreoretinal traction, and vitreal eddies/currents encouraging fluid to enter the break (Fig. 52.1a). This combination of events overcomes the retinal pigment epithelium's ability to maintain its adhesion with neurosensory retina.

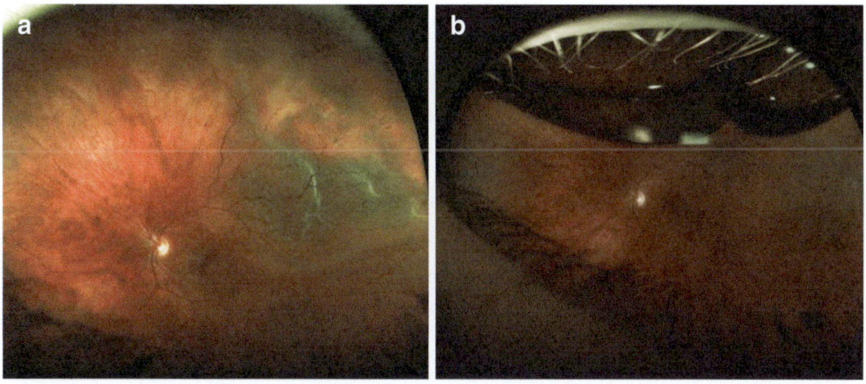

Fig. 52.1 Rhegmatogenous retinal detachment with bullous fluid and a retinal horseshoe tear in the superotemporal quadrant (**a**). Two days after pneumatic retinopexy – note resolving subretinal fluid, intraocular gas, and well-treated retinal tear (**b**)

Table 52.1 Lincoff's rules to find the primary break

Rule	Location of retinal detachment	Location of primary retinal tear
1	Superior temporal/nasal detachment	Within 1.5 clock hours of highest border (98 %)
2	Total or superior detachments that cross the 12 o'clock meridian	Within 1.5 clock hours to either side of 12 o'clock (93 %)
3	Inferior detachment	Primary tear located on the higher side of detachment (95 %)
4	Inferior bullous detachments: subretinal fluid originates from a superior break	Tear on the higher side of the detachment above the horizontal meridian

52.8 Workup/Testing

Diagnosis is often based on clinical funduscopic examination including 360° scleral depression. RRD is confirmed by identification of its characteristic appearance in the setting of a break. A retinal break may be obscured by overlying media opacity (e.g., vitreous hemorrhage) or at times may be too small to see. Utilizing Lincoff's rules can aid in finding a primary break (Table 52.1). If there is a limited view of the fundus, B-scan ultrasonography is essential. Optical coherence tomography may be useful to document the extent of very shallow subretinal fluid.

52.9 Prognosis and Management

Spontaneous complete reattachment is very rare. The natural history of long-standing untreated RRD results in permanent visual loss (typically in the range of light perception to no light perception) as well as anatomic change to the eye, especially cataract, sensory strabismus, hypotony, PVR, and, rarely, phthisis.

Status of the macula will dictate timeliness of repair. Once the macula is detached, a delay of 7–10 days does not appear to affect the visual outcome. However, if the macula is attached at presentation, visual outcomes are better when repair is performed before the macula detaches

Surgical management is indicated for RRD with the goal of identifying and treating/closing all retinal breaks. The retina is usually brought in contact with the RPE/choroid to encourage a chorioretinal adhesion. Available treatment options depending on the clinical setting include pneumatic retinopexy, scleral buckle, vitrectomy, or combined procedures.

Pneumatic retinopexy involves creating a lasting chorioretinal adhesion with cryotherapy or laser combined with closing the break using an internal tamponade of an injected intraocular gas bubble (Fig. 52.1b). Indications for this treatment include identification of all retinal breaks, all breaks confined to the superior 8 clock hours, presence of one retinal break or multiple within 1–2 clock hours, no severe PVR, and clear media. The patient must be able to maintain proper head positioning. Primary success rates range from 64 to 75.5 %. The single operation success rates tend to be higher in phakic rather than pseudophakic patients because the latter group has breaks that are often anterior and small, making them difficult to visualize. The final success rate ranges from 91 to 97.4 %.

Scleral buckling (SB) indents the globe externally with an encircling silicone band and other elements to alter the vitreal eddies/currents and reappose the retina to the RPE in the area of the retinal break after application of cryotherapy/laser to the break. This reduces vitreous traction, changes the intraocular fluidics, and supports the break. Subretinal fluid may be drained externally. SB minimizes the risk of cataract formation, thus reducing its morbidity in phakic patients. SB has shown final anatomic success rates >94 %.

Pars plana vitrectomy involves standard 3-port vitrectomy technique, introducing instruments intraocularly to induce a PVD (if necessary), shaving the peripheral cortical vitreous toward the vitreous base, draining subretinal fluid, and utilizing laser or cryotherapy for retinopexy. If present, PVR is addressed. The single operation success rates of vitrectomy in phakic patients are comparable to SB; however, some reports suggest improved success over SB in pseudophakic patients coupled with reduced morbidity (postoperative pain and refractive changes). Primary success rates range from 71 to 92 %; final success rate is 95 %.

52.10 Follow-Up

Patients are followed postoperatively to monitor for anatomical re-detachment and subsequent retinal tears. PVR is the most common cause of RRD repair failure and occurs in approximately 8–10 % of eyes after primary retinal detachment repair.

References and Suggested Reading

1. Abdullah AS, Jan S, Qureshi MS, Khan MT, Khan MD. Complications of conventional scleral buckling occuring during and after treatment of rhegmatogenous retinal detachment. J Coll Physicians Surg Pak. 2010;20(5):321–6.
2. García-Arumí J, et al. Rhegmatogenous retinal detachment treatment guidelines. Arch Soc Esp Oftalmol. 2013;88(1):11–35.
3. Gupta OP, Benson WE. The risk of fellow eyes in patients with rhegmatogenous retinal detachment. Curr Opin Ophthalmol. 2005;16(3):175–8.
4. Holz ER, Mieler WF. View 3: the case for pneumatic retinopexy. Br J Ophthalmol. 2003;87:787–9.
5. Ivanisević M. The natural history of untreated rhegmatogenous retinal detachment. Ophthalmologica. 1997;211(2):90–2.
6. Leaver PK. Proliferative vitreoretinopathy. Br J Ophthalmol. 1995;79(10):871–2.
7. Lewis H. Peripheral retinal degenerations and the risk of retinal detachment. Am J Ophthalmol. 2003;136(1):155–60.
8. Lincoff H, Gieser R. Finding the hole. Arch Ophthalmol. 1971;85:565–9.
9. Schwartz SG, Flynn HW. Primary retinal detachment: scleral buckle or pars plana vitrectomy? Curr Opin Ophthalmol. 2006;17(3):245–50.
10. Sodhi A, Leung LS, Do DV, Gower EW, Schein OD, Handa JT. Recent trends in the management of rhegmatogenous retinal detachment. Surv Ophthalmol. 2008;53(1):50–67.
11. Soliman MM, Macky TA. Pediatric rhegmatogenous retinal detachment. Int Ophthalmol Clin. 2011;51(1):147–71.

Chapter 53
Exudative Retinal Detachment

Nidhi Relhan, Harry W. Flynn Jr., and Thomas A. Albini

53.1 Definitions

Exudative retinal detachment refers to the separation of the neurosensory retina from the underlying retinal pigment epithelium (RPE) as a result of abnormalities of the normal hydrostatic/osmotic pressure gradients or transport mechanisms that maintain the physical apposition of these two layers or due to excessive production of extracellular fluid. Exudative retinal detachments lack the presence of a retinal break or vitreoretinal traction and generally display a dome or convex configuration. Exudative retinal detachment is usually associated with local ocular or systemic etiology.

53.2 Symptoms

The patient may give history of decreased visual acuity, visual field defects, or metamorphopsia. Hypotony may be observed if there is coexisting ciliary body inflammation or detachment. The patient may also give a history of systemic disease (i.e., metastatic carcinoma).

53.3 Signs

The anterior segment examination may reveal the clues to the diagnosis, such as conjunctival and episcleral injection in scleritis or anterior chamber cell and flare in Vogt-Koyanagi-Harada (VKH) syndrome. The posterior segment shows single or

N. Relhan, MD • H.W. Flynn Jr., MD • T.A. Albini, MD (✉)
Department of Ophthalmology, Bascom Palmer Eye Institute, University of Miami, Miller School of Medicine, Miami, FL, USA
e-mail: TAlbini@med.miami.edu

C.A. Medina et al. (eds.), *Manual of Retinal Diseases: A Guide to Diagnosis and Management*, DOI 10.1007/978-3-319-20460-4_53

multiple foci of dome or convex configuration retinal elevations that vary greatly in extent, from a few disc diameters to the entire retina. In large exudative retinal detachments, shifting subretinal fluid with postural changes may be observed.

53.4 Epidemiology

Epidemiology of exudative retinal detachment depends upon the underlying etiology. Exudative retinal detachment in Coats' disease/retinoblastoma, CSCR, and exudative ARMD are more commonly seen in young, middle-aged, and elderly age groups, respectively. Coats' disease and CSCR have more predilection towards male gender. Vogt-Koyanagi-Harada syndrome appears to be more common in Asians and Hispanics than in Caucasians.

53.5 Pathophysiology

Alterations in choroidal flow (e.g., idiopathic central serous chorioretinopathy, tumors of the choroid and retina, systemic disease with disrupted choroidal blood flow, vasculitis, and autoimmune disease), poor scleral outflow (e.g., posterior scleritis), or breakdown of RPE (e.g., VKH, sympathetic ophthalmia, sarcoidosis, infectious disease, and retinal vascular disease) lead to exudative retinal detachment.

53.6 Differential Diagnosis

Table 53.1 summarizes the differential diagnosis of exudative retinal detachment.

53.7 Etiology: Specific Disease Entities

Idiopathic Central Serous Chorioretinopathy It characteristically presents in the third to fifth decade of life, usually in males, with a unilateral blurred vision and an exudative macular neurosensory detachment. Fluorescein angiography shows a pinpoint focus of dye leakage resulting in pooling of dye at the macula. Most of the cases resolve spontaneously in 4–6 months, but half of these present with recurrent disease. Laser photocoagulation and photodynamic therapy are indicated in chronic, recurrent, or bilateral cases.

Uveal Effusion Syndrome (UES)/Nanophthalmos UES is characterized by spontaneous development of peripheral choroidal and retinal detachments in middle-aged

Table 53.1 Conditions associated with exudative retinal detachment

Choroidal tumors/neoplasms
Melanoma
Hemangioma
Metastases
Lymphoma/leukemia
Inflammation
VKH
Posterior scleritis
Sympathetic ophthalmia
Benign reactive lymphoid hyperplasia
Iatrogenic
Excessive cryopexy during retinal detachment surgery
Postsurgical wound leak and hypotony
Panretinal photocoagulation
Hematologic/vascular
Disseminated intravascular coagulation
Thrombotic thrombocytopenic purpura
Collagen vascular disease (systemic lupus erythematosus)
Wegener's granulomatosis
Organ transplantation/ hemodialysis
Waldenström's macroglobulinemia
Renal failure
Coats' disease
Retinopathy of prematurity
Familial exudative vitreoretinopathy
Arteriovenous fistula/carotid obstruction
Choroidal neovascularization
Hypertensive choroidopathy
Toxemia of pregnancy
Malignant hypertension
Idiopathic
Bullous central serous retinopathy
Idiopathic uveal effusion/nanophthalmos
Surgical or postsurgical
Wound leak
Hypotony
Miscellaneous
Multiple myeloma/immune gammopathies/paraproteinemias
Medication related: interferon (IFN)/ribavirin
Congenital optic nerve anomalies (optic disc pit, morning glory)
Bilateral diffuse uveal melanocytic proliferation (BDUMP)

hyperopic men. Uveal effusion may be caused by surgery, trauma, scleritis, pars planitis, or idiopathic. Ultrasonography shows choroidal thickening, retinal detachment, and short axial length. The subretinal fluid in UES has markedly elevated protein levels (up to three times of serum). Nanophthalmos is an uncommon disorder of ocular development characterized by bilateral, small, hyperopic eyes with small corneal diameter, shallow anterior chamber, high lens-to-eye ratio, thickened sclera, and predisposition to uveal effusion. Along with serous detachments, these patients exhibit dilated conjunctival vessels, shallow anterior chambers, ciliochoroidal effusions, and increased risk of angle-closure glaucoma as a result of the crowded anterior segment. On fluorescein angiography, these patients often demonstrate a diffuse "leopard-spot" pattern which is notably lacking in focal points of leakage. Vortex vein decompression and scleral resection are effective treatment options.

Postsurgical Postoperative hypotony is associated with development of exudative retinal detachment and uveal effusions. The various risk factors are glaucoma, myopia, advanced age, hypertension, arteriosclerosis, and Valsalva maneuvers (coughing during surgery). Exudative retinal detachment and uveal effusions may occur following surgical procedures such as scleral buckle, intraocular procedure, aggressive panretinal photocoagulation, cryotherapy, etc.

Posterior Scleritis Posterior scleritis is inflammation of the sclera and characterized by severe retrobulbar pain, decreased visual acuity, and visual field loss. It may be associated with anterior segment inflammation, optic disc edema, choroidal detachment with surrounding folds, and exudative retinal detachment. The differential diagnosis includes choroidal melanoma, metastatic carcinoma, choroidal hemangioma, and benign reactive lymphoid hyperplasia. The fundus fluorescein angiography shows multiple pinpoint leaks at the level of RPE in middle phases and intense late staining of the exudative retinal detachment. Ultrasonography shows significant sclerochoroidal thickening with overlying retinal detachment and retrobulbar edema. Posterior scleritis can be associated with systemic illness (such as rheumatoid arthritis, granulomatosis with angiitis, systemic vasculitis, systemic lymphoma, or multiple myeloma), infections (herpes zoster or toxoplasmosis), or idiopathic.

Benign Reactive Lymphoid Hyperplasia Benign reactive lymphoid hyperplasia is a rare disorder characterized by diffuse mononuclear infiltration of uveal tract. The disease is typically unilateral and occurs in older adults. The patient may present with salmon-pink conjunctival nodules, anterior chamber cells or secondary angle closure due to ciliary body infiltration, and exudative retinal detachment. Fundus shows a diffuse, yellow-white choroidal mass with RPE pigment mottling. The differential diagnosis includes diffuse malignant melanoma, UES, metastatic carcinoma, posterior scleritis, systemic lymphoma, sarcoidosis, and infectious etiologies.

Vogt-Koyanagi-Harada (VKH) Syndrome and Sympathetic Ophthalmia (SO) VKH is a multisystem inflammatory disease characterized by bilateral exudative retinal detachments with panuveitis and RPE changes. The patient may give history of tinnitus, hearing loss, and flu-like symptoms. The pathologic mechanism is an autoimmune response to melanin-containing tissues, explaining the predilection for the RPE and the highly pigmented choroid. Poliosis, alopecia, perilimbal, and cutaneous vitiligo may develop weeks to months after the development of ocular signs. Fundus fluorescein angiography shows multiple pinpoint leaks at the posterior pole in early phase with eventual pooling of dye in subretinal space with disc staining in later phase of angiogram. Sympathetic ophthalmia (SO) is characterized by an immune reaction to ocular tissue in the presence of a penetrating ocular injury and is rarer but can present a similar pathologic picture.

Infectious Etiologies Various infections can damage the retina, RPE, and choroid, leading to RPE breakdown and exudative retinal detachment. Toxoplasmosis, syphilis, CMV, Lyme disease (*Borrelia burgdorferi*), tuberculosis, histoplasmosis, coccidiomycosis, and cryptococcus have been associated with exudative retinal detachments.

Retinal Vascular Diseases Leakage from abnormal retinal vessels or breakdown of normal vessels leads to exudative retinal detachment. Congenital vascular anomalies in Coats' disease, familial exudative vitreoretinopathy (FEVR), and retinal angiomatosis are associated with exudative RD.

Disseminated Intravascular Coagulation (DIC) DIC is a complex multisystem disorder resulting in widespread thrombosis of small blood vessels with ensuing depletion of clotting factors, platelets, and fibrinogen. It affects the kidneys, heart, brain, and other organs. Ocular involvement is seen as derangement of choroidal vasculature and exudative retinal detachment.

Malignant Hypertension Malignant hypertension develops in 1 % of patients with essential hypertension and can result in a variety of neurologic, cardiac, renal, and gastrointestinal complications. The patients may present with large bilateral exudative retinal detachments, disc edema, and retinal hemorrhages. Fluorescein angiography shows retinal vascular and choroidal vascular leakage and nonperfusion.

53.8 Workup/Testing

The clinical examination is very crucial in the workup of exudative retinal detachment to establish the presence of retinal detachment and associated ocular and systemic abnormalities. Indirect ophthalmoscopy, B-scan ultrasonography, fundus fluorescein angiography (FFA), indocyanine green angiography (ICG), optical coherence tomography (OCT), computed tomography (CT), or magnetic resonance imaging (MRI) are extremely helpful to reach the final diagnosis. Systemic investigations including blood testing (for infections and immune etiologies) and cerebrospinal fluid (CSF) sampling (in VKH) can be useful. Blood workup for Venereal

Disease Research Laboratory (VDRL) test and fluorescein treponema antibody (FTA) test, antineutrophil cytoplasmic antibodies (ANCA), erythrocyte sedimentation rate (ESR), and rheumatoid factor.

53.9 Prognosis and Management

Treatment of exudative retinal detachments must address the underlying local or systemic disease. Systemic treatment with antibiotics (for infectious etiologies) or immunosuppression (for immune etiologies such as posterior scleritis, vasculitides, autoimmune disease, idiopathic frosted branch angiitis) or chemotherapy (for choroidal melanoma, multiple myeloma). Management of exudative retinal detachment may vary greatly depending upon the etiology. Various options include simple observation, laser photocoagulation of focal pathologies (vascular anomalies ad tumors), photodynamic therapy (PDT), external beam radiotherapy, intravitreal anti-VEGF therapy (Coats' disease), intravitreal/peribulbar steroids, creation of scleral windows (uveal effusion syndrome, nanophthalmos), or surgical repair of retinal detachment (chronic unresponsive cases).

Signs of poor prognosis:

- Involvement of macula
- Longer duration of retinal detachment

53.10 Follow-Up

The patients with exudative retinal detachment need to be followed up for complications including neovascular glaucoma and phthisis bulbi.

References and Suggested Reading

1. Cooke MD, Mittra RA, Han DP. Exudative and tractional retinal detachments. In: Scott IU, Regillo CD, Flynn HW Jr, Brown GC, editors. Vitreoretinal disease: the essentials. 2nd ed. New York: Thieme Publishers 2016.
2. Galor A, Davis JL, Flynn Jr HW, et al. Sympathetic ophthalmia: incidence of ocular complications and vision loss in the sympathizing eye. Am J Ophthalmol. 2009;148(5):704–10.
3. Paredes I, Ahmed M, Foster CS. Immunomodulatory therapy for Vogt-Koyanagi-Harada patients as first-line therapy. Ocul Immunol Inflamm. 2006;14:87–90.
4. Spaide RF, Goldbaum M, Wong DW, Tang KC, Iida T. Serous detachment of the retina. Retina. 2003;23(6):820–46; quiz 895–6. Review. PubMed.
5. Thomas BJ, Albini TA. Serous detachments of the neural retina. In: Yanoff M, Duker JS, editors. Ophthalmology. 4th ed. Elsevier Saunders, Philadelphia; 2014.
6. Yang CH, Yeh PT, Lin CP, Yang CM. Non-rhegmatogenous retinal detachment. In: Ryan SJ, editor. 5th ed. Elsevier Saunders, Philadelphia; 2014.

Chapter 54
Tractional Retinal Detachment

Sujit Itty

54.1 Definition

Tractional Retinal Detachment (TRD) Second most common form of retinal detachment (RD) where mechanical forces pull the neurosensory retina away from its attachments to the underlying retinal pigment epithelium without an associated retinal break.

54.2 Symptoms

Vision loss, visual field defect, metamorphopsia, or potentially no symptoms

54.3 Signs

- Localized, concave retinal detachment that usually does not extend to the ora serrata.
- Fibrovascular membranes secondary to proliferative diabetic retinopathy (PDR) or other proliferative retinal vascular disease.
- Cellular and vitreous membranes secondary to proliferative vitreoretinopathy (PVR).

S. Itty, MD
Vitreoretinal Surgery and Retinal Disease, Retina Consultants of Arizona,
1101 E. Missouri Ave, Phoenix, AZ 85014, USA
e-mail: Sujit.itty@gmail.com

C.A. Medina et al. (eds.), *Manual of Retinal Diseases: A Guide to Diagnosis and Management*, DOI 10.1007/978-3-319-20460-4_54

54.4 Etiology

Common PDR, PVR

Rare Retinopathy of prematurity (ROP), penetrating trauma, peripheral proliferative retinal vascular disorders (e.g., familial exudative vitreoretinopathy, incontinentia pigmenti, sickle cell retinopathy), retinal capillary hemangioma, Coats' disease, toxocariasis.

54.5 Pathophysiology

In proliferative retinal vascular disorders (e.g., PDR), contraction of the vitreous gel leads to traction between vitreous attachments at the vitreous base and areas of fibrovascular proliferation usually along the temporal arcades.

In PVR, proliferation and metaplasia of retinal pigment epithelium and glial cells form into contractile membranes that may lead to retinal folds, retinal breaks, or TRDs.

In ROP, vascular endothelial cells proliferate at the junction between avascular and vascularized retina, migrate into formed vitreous network, and then contract, exerting force along the taut posterior hyaloid.

54.6 Differential Diagnosis

Rhegmatogenous Retinal Detachment (RRD) RD associated with a retinal break; usually presents with convex, generalized RD that extends to ora serrata.

Combined Tractional and Rhegmatogenous RD Contraction of fibrocellular membranes leading to the development of a retinal break and a combined mechanism for RD. Appearance is usually convex and extends to the ora serrate similar to a RRD.

54.7 Workup/Testing

Diagnosis is usually made clinically with indirect ophthalmoscopy. B-scan ultrasonography may be necessary if vitreous hemorrhage precludes visualization of the retina. Optical coherence tomography (OCT) may demonstrate the extent of the retinal detachment in the macula.

Table 54.1 Indications for vitrectomy for TRD associated with PDR

Non-clearing vitreous hemorrhage associated with TRD
TRD threatening or involving the fovea
Combined TRD/RRD
Associated macular striae or epiretinal membrane causing vision loss

54.8 Prognosis and Management

A tractional retinal detachment is generally a surgical disease, and there is currently no role for medical therapy. A TRD not threatening the fovea or involving the macula may be observed closely for progression. Extramacular TRD cases may also be treated with panretinal photocoagulation (PRP) that may cause involution of the neovascularization and sometimes release vitreoretinal traction. Cases of TRD that necessitate intervention usually require pars plana vitrectomy with release of tractional membranes. A scleral buckle may be helpful in cases of PVR or in cases of stage 4a ROP. Intravitreal anti-VEGF injections may be helpful as an adjunct to vitrectomy for TRDs associated with PDR. However, surgery should generally be performed within days of injection as delay in surgery may lead to TRD progression (usually less than 10 days) (Table 54.1).

Visual prognosis varies depending on the underlying location, cause of the TRD, and the extent of damage to the retina. The presence of PVR reduces the anatomic success rate for retinal detachment repair to roughly 75 %. The visual outcome after TRD repair is often limited by macular ischemia, and approximately 40 % will end with visual acuity better than 20/100.

References and Suggested Reading

1. Charles S. Vitreous microsurgery. 2nd ed. Baltimore: Williams & Wilkins; 1987.
2. Glaser BM, Cardin A, Biscoe B. Proliferative vitreoretinopathy. The mechanism of development of vitreoretinal traction. Ophthalmology. 1987;94(4):327–32.
3. Kaiser PK, Riemann CD, Sears JE, et al. Macular traction detachment and diabetic macular edema associated with posterior hyaloidal traction. Am J Ophthalmol. 2001;131:44–9.
4. Michels RG. Proliferative diabetic retinopathy: pathophysiology of extraretinal complications and principles of vitreous surgery. Retina. 1981;1:1–17.
5. Moradian S, Ahmadieh H, Malihi M, et al. Intravitreal bevacizumab in active progressive proliferative diabetic retinopathy. Graefes Arch Clin Exp Ophthalmol. 2008;246:1699–705.
6. Rice TA, Michels RG, Rice EF. Vitrectomy for diabetic traction retinal detachment involving the macula. Am J Ophthalmol. 1983;95(1):22–33.
7. Ryan SJ. Chapter 95: Pathogenetic mechanisms of RD. In: Retina. 5th ed. Philadelphia, PA: El Sevier; 2013.
8. Thompson JT, de Bustros S, Michels RG, Rice TA. Results and prognostic factors in vitrectomy for diabetic traction retinal detachment of the macula. Arch Ophthalmol. 1987;105(4):497–502.

Chapter 55
Choroidal Detachments

Luis J. Haddock and Anuj Chawla

55.1 Definition

Choroidal detachments result from an abnormal accumulation of fluid in the suprachoroidal space. There are various terms used interchangeably to describe this finding including choroidal effusion, ciliochoroidal effusion, and ciliochoroidal detachment.

Choroidal detachments can be classified into serous and hemorrhagic. Serous choroidal detachments involve the transudation of serum into the suprachoroidal space. Hemorrhagic choroidal detachment is a hemorrhage in the suprachoroidal space caused by the rupture of choroidal vessels.

When choroidal effusions are appositional, they are termed "kissing choroidals," or "appositional choroidals."

55.2 Symptoms

Small, serous choroidal detachments are often asymptomatic, whereas large detachments can cause decreased vision, a myopic shift, and an absolute scotoma in the corresponding visual field. Appositional choroidal detachments can cause severely decreased vision (patients can be LP). Hemorrhagic choroidal detachments present with abrupt onset of pain, decreased vision, and shadow in vision if large.

L.J. Haddock, MD (✉)
Clinical Ophthalmology, Bascom Palmer Eye Institute, University of Miami Miller School of Medicine, 7101 Fairway Dr., Palm Beach Gardens, FL 33418, USA
e-mail: Ljhaddock@med.miami.edu

A. Chawla, MD
Clinical Ophthalmology, Bascom Palmer Eye Institute, University of Miami Miller School of Medicine, 7101 Fairway Dr., Palm Beach Gardens, FL 33418, USA

C.A. Medina et al. (eds.), *Manual of Retinal Diseases: A Guide to Diagnosis and Management*, DOI 10.1007/978-3-319-20460-4_55

55.3 Signs

Indirect ophthalmoscopy reveals a dome-shaped, smooth, non-undulating elevation in the case of a serous detachment. In larger detachments, the characteristic four-lobed configuration results from attachment of the choroid at the vortex veins which limits the extension (Fig. 55.1). Dilated episcleral vessels, a shallow anterior chamber, and blood in Schlemm's canal viewed on gonioscopy examination may also be present.

B-scan ultrasonography is a useful tool to identify choroidal detachments. Examination will reveal a dome-shaped, smooth elevation with little movement on dynamic ultrasound. A serous detachment will have hyperlucency in the suprachoroidal space, while a hemorrhagic detachment will be hyper-echoic (Fig. 55.2).

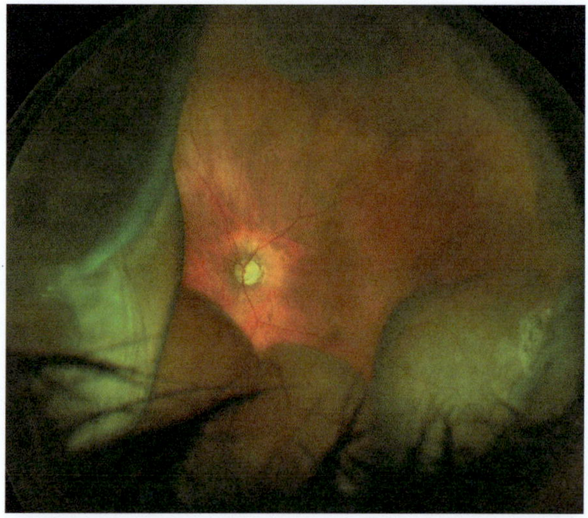

Fig. 55.1 Fundus image showing choroidal detachment most prominent nasally inferior and inferotemporally in patient that developed hypotony after glaucoma surgery

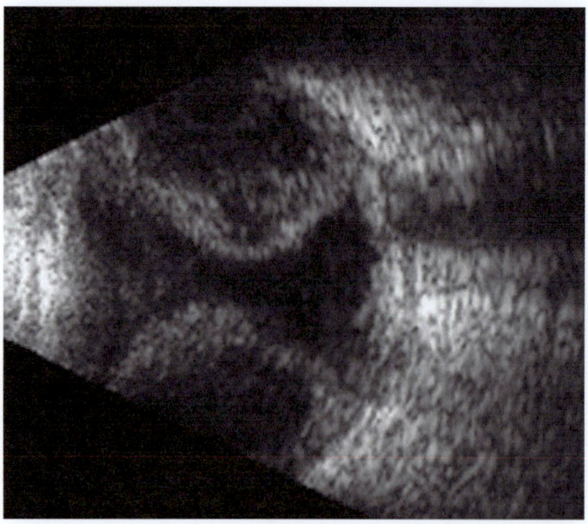

Fig. 55.2 B-scan of a patient with large, hemorrhagic, choroidal detachments following cataract extraction. In this view, the shadow of the optic nerve can be seen with the macula inferior. Note the macula is not affected. This hemorrhage has had ample time to liquefy, which can be seen as alternating areas of hyper- and hypo-echoic signal within the choroidal detachment

When a hemorrhagic choroidal detachment occurs during surgery, the patient will complain of abrupt eye pain, and the red reflex will darken. Usually, this occurs immediately after a patient strains (coughs). The choroidal detachment may be visible to the surgeon, depending on its size. It is important to close all surgical wounds and abort the operation at this time.

55.4 Epidemiology

The incidence of choroidal hemorrhage during cataract surgery has declined with the advent of phacoemulsification techniques and smaller incisions. It has further declined as the use of peri- and retrobulbar block anesthesias has decreased. The most recent data shows approximately 3 % of intracapsular, and 2.2 % of extracapsular cataract surgeries have limited choroidal hemorrhages. Massive choroidal hemorrhage occurs in a very small percentage of patients undergoing phacoemulsification, 0.2 %, and is slightly higher in glaucoma surgery, 0.73 %.

55.5 Predisposing Conditions

Abnormal scleral composition, alterations in hydrodynamic factors, inflammation, and neoplastic conditions are the major causes of choroidal effusions.

Congenital and acquired causes of abnormal scleral composition alter choroidal fluid dynamics and predispose patients to developing choroidal effusions. The most well-known cause is nanophthalmos. Other causes include uveal effusion syndrome, amyloidosis, and mucopolysaccharidosis.

Hydrodynamic factors are influenced by intraocular pressure, with hypotony and elevated episcleral venous pressure causing choroidal detachments. The most common cause of a serous choroidal detachment is hypotony following glaucoma surgery with over-filtration or a bleb leak. The use of mitomycin C in these procedures and the use of aqueous suppressants afterwards are associated with higher rates of prolonged hypotony.

Elevated episcleral venous pressure is seen in Sturge-Weber syndrome, arteriovenous fistulas, and conditions with compression of the vortex veins (e.g., Graves' disease).

Common inflammatory conditions that result in choroidal effusions include postoperative, post-photocoagulation or cryopexy, uveitis, scleritis, and orbital cellulitis. The effusion is a result of increased vascular permeability.

Any metastasis or ocular malignancy can also cause an overlying choroidal detachment.

Medication can also result in inflammation that leads to a choroidal detachment. Sulfa-derived medications are the most commonly implicated, with the most well documented being Topamax. Other medications include tetracyclines, diuretics, and selective serotonin reuptake inhibitors (SSRIs). The effusion typically resolves with discontinuation of the medication.

55.6 Inheritance

Not applicable.

55.7 Differential Diagnosis

Choroidal detachments result from disruption of the normal physiologic state. As described previously, alterations in scleral composition, hydrodynamic factors, inflammation, and neoplasia are all potential causes.

Retinal detachment is the most important entity to differentiate from choroidal effusions. Indirect ophthalmoscopy of a retinal detachment will show a causative break and retinal folds and can span a larger area without the firm attachments at the vortex veins.

Typically these patients will have hypotony or are postsurgical (more commonly seen in those with coughing fits or episodes of Valsalva). It is important to differentiate these from retinal detachments, which will have a causative break and retinal folds and can span a larger area without the firm attachments of the vortex veins.

B-scan ultrasonography is also helpful in differentiating a choroidal detachment from a retinal detachment (Table 55.1). A choroidal detachment will have a

Table 55.1 Comparison between serous choroidal detachment and rhegmatogenous retinal detachment

Feature	Choroidal detachment	Retinal detachment
History	Patient will often have a history of glaucoma-filtering surgery or other intraocular surgeries. This may be acute or remote. They are often asymptomatic or may have mild symptoms related to hypotony (mild decline in visual acuity)	Patients often have an acute history of floaters, flashes, or trauma. In addition, they often complain of a shadow in their vision with preserved central visual acuity (macula on detachment) or loss of central visual acuity, often in the 20/200 range (macula off detachment). There may be an ocular history that predisposes to retinal detachment (high myopia)
Physical appearance	Peripheral, dome shaped, non-undulating with attachments at the vortex veins. There will not be a retinal break	Typically are not dome shaped, but may be bullous and have retinal folds (or PVR if chronic). A corresponding retinal break will be visible (location according to Lincoff rules). Will not have attachments at the vortex veins and can span larger areas
B-scan findings	Dome shaped, hypo-echoic with low reflectivity on A-scan	Concave shape with high reflectivity on A-scan
Treatment	Treatment is aimed at correcting the underling etiology of hypotony. This may require revision of a glaucoma surgery or closure of surgical wounds	Surgical (vitrectomy or scleral buckle) or clinic-based (pneumatic or laser demarcation) intervention to seal the break and drain the subretinal fluid

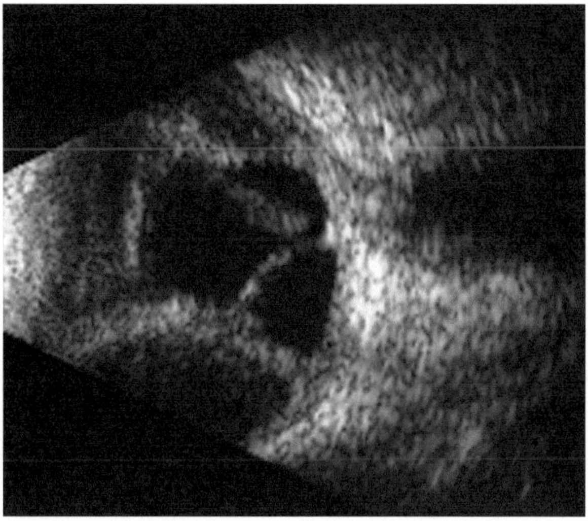

Fig. 55.3 B-scan of a patient with large choroidal detachments and a total retinal detachment. Note the choroidal detachments take on a dome-shaped appearance, whereas the retinal detachment is concave and attached at the nerve

dome-shaped, convex appearance, whereas a retinal detachment will take on a concave shape (will follow the shape of the globe) and demonstrate a hyper-reflective spike on the A-scan (Fig. 55.3).

55.8 Etiology

Under normal physiologic conditions, the suprachoroidal space is a potential space without fluid. This equilibrium state is maintained between the intravascular blood pressure and intraocular pressure and the colloid osmotic pressure gradient of the choriocapillaris. Albumin, the most abundant protein in the choroidal capillaries, is primarily responsible for maintaining this colloid osmotic pressure. Changes in vascular permeability, scleral composition, and intraocular pressure disrupt this balance and result in accumulation of protein and fluid in the suprachoroidal space. As discussed previously, the major causes of imbalance are abnormal scleral composition, alterations in hydrodynamic factors, inflammation, and neoplastic conditions.

55.9 Workup/Testing

Low-lying serous detachments can be seen easily with indirect ophthalmoscopy. B-scan can be used to differentiate between hemorrhagic and serous detachments. Additional testing is typically not required.

55.10 Prognosis and Management

Serous choroidal detachments, if located in the periphery, can be observed and have a good prognosis. It is important to identify and resolve the inciting cause.

Appositional or hemorrhagic choroidal detachments, however, have a poorer prognosis and require intervention.

An appositional choroidal detachment requires careful B-scan echography to determine involvement of the macula. If the macula is involved, then surgical drainage is indicated urgently. The underlying cause, typically hypotony after glaucoma surgery, should also be corrected at the same time. If treatment is initiated early, patients can do very well.

A hemorrhagic choroidal detachment carries a poor prognosis, with visual acuity often decreasing to count fingers or worse. Early surgical intervention is not advised as it is difficult to achieve satisfactory drainage of the clotted hemorrhage. Waiting at least 1 week, and often longer, allows for adequate liquefaction. This can be seen on B-scan as multiple layers of hyper- and hypo-intensity.

Treatment of serous choroidal detachments is primarily aimed at resolving the underlying condition. If the choroidal detachments are not large, then they should resolve without sequelae as long as the underlying etiology is addressed.

In cases of appositional and hemorrhagic choroidal detachments, drainage via surgical intervention is required. This consists of creating one-half to two-thirds thickness sclerotomies in each quadrant, centered 1–2 mm anterior to the equator and placed outside the meridian of each vortex vein. A sclerostomy can be created in the center of each sclerotomy to facilitate drainage of the fluid. In patients that are at high risk of developing choroidal detachments (nanophthalmic eyes undergoing glaucoma surgery), preplacement of the flaps can be considered.

55.11 Follow-Up

Patients with low-lying choroidal detachments do not necessarily need to be followed closely. However, the underlying condition does need to be addressed as long-standing effusions can result in more severe complications.

Appositional choroidal detachments require strict follow-up. Surgical intervention should be considered urgently, unless the underlying condition can be resolved and the resolution of the choroidal detachment documented.

Patients with hemorrhagic choroidal detachments also require close follow-up to address any complications that arise. As discussed previously, adequate time is required to allow for liquefaction of the hemorrhage before surgical drainage.

References and Suggested Reading

1. Gass JD. Uveal effusion syndrome. A new hypothesis concerning pathogenesis and technique of surgical treatment. Retina. 1983;3:159–63.
2. Reddy AC, Salim S. Ophthalmic Pearls: Diagnosis and management of choroidal effusions. EyeNet. 2012;47–49.
3. Ryan S, et al. Retina. 5th ed. Philadelphia: Saunders; 2013.
4. Besirli CG, Johnson MW. Uveal Effusion Syndrome and Hypotony Maculopathy. In Ryan S, et al. Retina. 5th ed. Philadelphia: Saunders. 2013;1306–17.
5. Spalton D, et al. Atlas of clinical ophthalmology. 3rd ed. Philadelphia: Elsevier Saunders. 2012; 772–834.
6. Kapuata M, et al. Choroidal hemorrhage. In Yanoff M, Duker J, et al. Ophthalmology. 4th ed. Philadelphia: Elsevier Saunders; 2014;660–4.
7. Yanoff M, Duker J, et al. Ophthalmology. 4th ed. Philadelphia: Elsevier Saunders; 2014.

Chapter 56
Optic Nerve Pit

Gregory D. Lee and Roger A. Goldberg

56.1 Definitions

OCT – optical coherence tomography
PVD – posterior vitreous detachment

56.2 Symptoms

Generally asymptomatic unless there is associated macular schisis or a serous retinal detachment, which can cause decreased vision, metamorphopsia, or a blind spot.

56.3 Signs

Grayish round depression typically seen at the optic nerve rim on clinical exam. May have associated serous retinal detachment.

56.4 Predisposing Conditions

- No known risk factors.

G.D. Lee, MD
Department of Ophthalmology, University of Kentucky/Retina Associates of Kentucky, Lexington, KY, USA

R.A. Goldberg (✉)
Bay Area Retina Associates, 122 La Casa Via #223, Walnut Creek, CA 94549, USA
e-mail: Rgoldberg.eyemd@gmail.com

C.A. Medina et al. (eds.), *Manual of Retinal Diseases: A Guide to Diagnosis and Management*, DOI 10.1007/978-3-319-20460-4_56

- Prevalence of 1/10,000.
- Occurs in both genders equally and can present in children or adults.
- Ten to 15 % of patients have bilateral optic nerve pits.

56.5 Differential Diagnosis

Optic nerve coloboma, tilted disc appearance, circumpapillary staphyloma, hypoplastic disc, and glaucomatous optic neuropathy. For a serous detachment of the macula, central serous chorioretinopathy or idiopathic choroidal neovascular membrane should be considered.

56.6 Etiology

Incomplete closure of the superior edge of the embryonic fissure. The source of the fluid causing serous retinal detachment and inner retinal schisis is unclear, with liquefied vitreous or cerebrospinal fluid being hypothesized sources. Posterior vitreous traction has been suspected to be a contributing factor based on resolution of detachments after PVD or vitrectomy.

56.7 Workup/Testing

Dilated fundus examination should be performed to monitor the patient, and disc photos may be helpful if there is any doubt to the diagnosis (Fig. 56.1a). In cases of symptomatic optic pits with serous retinal detachments, OCT imaging is recommended to detect inner retinal schisis and/or a serous retinal detachment (Fig. 56.1b). If treatment is being considered, pre- and post-treatment OCT is the preferred imaging modality. Fluorescein angiography may be useful in differentiating from central serous chorioretinopathy and choroidal neovascularization or polypoidal choroidal vasculopathy in cases with associated serous detachment.

56.8 Prognosis and Management

Prognosis is generally very good in cases of optic pit as long as there is no associated schisis or serous retinal detachments. In cases with serous macular detachment, there is no consensus about the best treatment due to the rare prevalence. Most reported studies are small, retrospective, and nonrandomized. The natural history of untreated eyes of optic pit with serous macular detachment was shown by

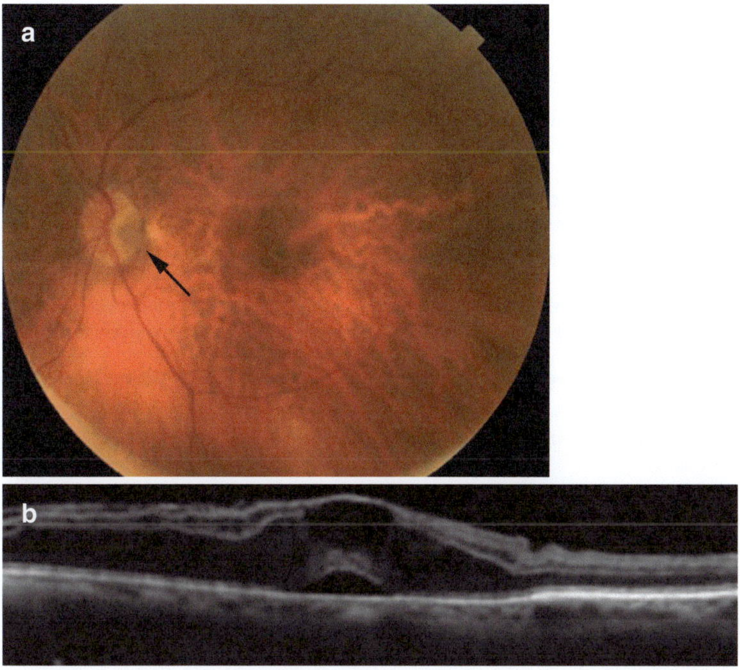

Fig. 56.1 Optic disc pit (**a**, *arrow*) with corresponding OCT scan through the macula showing retinal schisis and serous retinal detachment (**b**)

Sobol et al. to result in severely decreased vision within the first 6 months of observation for 15 patients. Surgical management has been reported as pars plana vitrectomy with and without internal limiting membrane peeling and with and without gas tamponade. Laser photocoagulation at the temporal peripapillary edge is recommended to close the communication channel for fluid between the optic pit and the macula. However focal laser without vitrectomy has been reported to be unsuccessful. More recently, some surgeons have reported success with partial thickness retinal cuts with a bent 25-gauge needle or 27-gauge cannula with limited vitrectomy and no gas tamponade to allow for passive egress of the intraretinal and subretinal fluid.

56.9 Follow-Up

Annual follow-up for asymptomatic optic pit without associated serous retinal detachment. Surgical management within the first 6 months for optic pit with associated serous macular detachment. For asymptomatic optic pits with associated schisis and no serous detachment, 3 months or sooner initially with longer intervals if findings are stable.

References and Suggested Reading

1. García-Arumí J, Guraya BC, Espax AB, Castillo VM, Ramsay LS, Motta RM. Optical coherence tomography in optic pit maculopathy managed with vitrectomy-laser-gas. Graefes Arch Clin Exp Ophthalmol. 2004;242:819–26.
2. Hirakata A, Okada AA, Hida T. Long-term results of vitrectomy without laser treatment for macular detachment associated with an optic disc pit. Ophthalmology. 2005;112:1430–5.
3. Patton N, Aslam SA, Aylward GW. Visual improvement after long-standing central serous macular detachment associated with an optic disc pit. Graefes Arch Clin Exp Ophthalmol. 2008;246:1083–5.
4. Postel EA, Pulido JS, McNamara JA, Johnson MW. The etiology and treatment of macular detachment associated with optic nerve pits and related anomalies. Trans Am Ophthalmol Soc. 1998;96:73–88; discussion 88–93.
5. Sadun A. Optic disc pits and associated macular detachment. In: Ryan SJ, editor. Retina, vol. 2. 4th ed. Philadelphia: Elsevier Mosby; 2006. p. 1883–9.
6. Schaal KB, Wrede J, Dithmar S. Internal drainage in optic pit maculopathy. Br J Ophthalmol. 2007;91:1093.
7. Sobol WM, Blodi CF, Folk JC, Weingeist TA. Long-term visual outcome in patients with optic nerve pit and serous retinal detachment of the macula. Ophthalmology. 1990;97:1539–42.
8. Spaide RF, Fisher Y, Ober M, Stoller G. Surgical hypothesis: inner retinal fenestration as a treatment for optic disc pit maculopathy. Retina. 2006;26:89–91.
9. Vedantham V, Ramasamy K. Spontaneous improvement of serous maculopathy associated with congenital optic disc pit: an OCT study. Eye (Lond). 2005;19:596–9.

Section VIII
Diabetic Retinopathy

John E. Legarreta

Chapter 57
Diabetic Retinopathy Clinical Trials

John E. Legarreta

57.1 Clinical Trials: Medical Management

Wisconsin Epidemiological Study of Diabetic Retinopathy (WESDR) Population-based epidemiologic study which determined estimates of the prevalence and incidence of diabetic retinopathy.

Diabetes Control and Complications Trial (DCCT) Assessed the effect of glycemic control in patients with Type I insulin-dependent diabetes mellitus. The study concluded that intensive glycemic control compared to conventional control delayed the onset of diabetic retinopathy (by 76 %) as well as slowed the progression of retinopathy (by 54 %).

United Kingdom Prospective Diabetes Study (UKPDS) Assessed the effect of glycemic control and blood pressure control in patients with Type 2 diabetes mellitus. The study concluded that intensive glycemic control compared to conventional control slowed the progression of retinopathy, and tight blood pressure control reduced the risk of diabetes-related complications.

57.2 Clinical Trials: Laser Therapy

Diabetic Retinopathy Study (DRS) The purpose of the study was to see if photocoagulation provided any benefit in preventing vision loss in patients with severe nonproliferative diabetic retinopathy or proliferative diabetic retinopathy. The study

J.E. Legarreta, MD
Department of Ophthalmology, Bascom Palmer Eye Institute, University of Miami,
900 NW 17th St., Miami, FL 33136, USA
e-mail: legarretaje@icloud.com

C.A. Medina et al. (eds.), *Manual of Retinal Diseases: A Guide to Diagnosis and Management*, DOI 10.1007/978-3-319-20460-4_57

found that photocoagulation reduced the risk of severe vision loss by 50 % in patients with severe nonproliferative diabetic retinopathy and proliferative diabetic retinopathy. The study also defined high-risk proliferative diabetic retinopathy.

Early Treatment Diabetic Retinopathy Study (ETDRS) The study set out to assess three questions including when to initiate panretinal photocoagulation in patients with diabetic retinopathy, the efficacy of focal photocoagulation in diabetic macular edema, and the utility of aspirin use in affecting the disease progression of diabetic retinopathy. The study found that panretinal photocoagulation should be performed in patients demonstrating high-risk proliferative diabetic retinopathy. Panretinal photocoagulation was beneficial in patients with severe nonproliferative diabetic retinopathy and early proliferative diabetic retinopathy, and laser therapy should be considered in this group of patients. For patients with mild to moderate nonproliferative diabetic retinopathy, panretinal photocoagulation should not be performed. Finally, aspirin use was not found to effect the progression of diabetic retinopathy.

57.3 Diabetic Retinopathy Clinical Research Network (DRCR.net)

Protocol A: Pilot Study of Laser Photocoagulation for Diabetic Macular Edema The purpose of the study was to compare the modified ETDRS focal photocoagulation technique to a mild macular grid technique. The study found that the mild macular grid technique was less effective and reducing retinal thickening than the modified ETDRS focal photocoagulation technique.

Protocol B: Randomized Trial Comparing Intravitreal Triamcinolone Acetonide (IVTA) and Laser Photocoagulation for Diabetic Macular Edema The purpose of this study was to assess the efficacy and safety of IVTA (1 and 4 mg doses) compared to focal/grid laser photocoagulation. The study found that at 3 years, focal/grid laser photocoagulation was more effective than IVTA (1 and 4 mg doses) for treating DME. Additionally, there were fewer side effects with focal/grid laser photocoagulation compared to the IVTA groups.

Protocol F: Observational Study of the Development of Diabetic Macular Edema Following Scatter Laser Photocoagulation The purpose of the study was to evaluate a single, complete panretinal photocoagulation session vs a four-quarter panretinal photocoagulation sessions on the development/progression of diabetic macular edema in patients with severe nonproliferative diabetic retinopathy or early proliferative diabetic retinopathy. The results showed no significant, clinically meaningful difference in vision or OCT thickness between the two groups.

57.4 Clinical Trials: Pharmacotherapy

Protocol I: Laser-Ranibizumab-Triamcinolone Study for DME The purpose of the study was to evaluate the efficacy of intravitreal ranibizumab (0.5 mg) or triamcinolone (4 mg) combined with focal/grid laser vs focal/grid laser for treatment of diabetic macular edema. The study concluded that intravitreal ranibizumab with focal/grid laser (prompt or deferred) was more efficacious in treating center-involving diabetic macular edema at 2 years compared to focal/grid laser (prompt) alone.

A Study of Ranibizumab Injection in Subjects with Clinically Significant Macular Edema with Center Involvement Secondary to Diabetes Mellitus (RISE and RIDE) The purpose of the study was to evaluate the safety and efficacy of intravitreal ranibizumab for the treatment of diabetic macular edema. Both studies found that intravitreal ranibizumab improved diabetic macular edema, improved vision, and reduced the further risk of vision loss and improved the underlying diabetic retinopathy.

A Prospective Randomized Trial of Intravitreal Bevacizumab or Laser Therapy in the Management of Diabetic Macular Edema (BOLT) The purpose of the study was to evaluate the efficacy of intravitreal bevacizumab compared to modified Early Treatment of Diabetic Retinopathy Study laser therapy in the treatment of diabetic macular edema. The study found that intravitreal bevacizumab improved vision and reduced diabetic macular edema at both 1 and 2 years.

DME and VEGF Trap Eye Investigation of Clinical Impact (DA VINCI): The purpose of this study was to evaluate different doses of intravitreal VEGF trap eye in patients with diabetic macular edema and compare this with macula laser photocoagulation only. The study found that intravitreal VEGF trap eye improved vision, and this was statistically significant when compared with macula laser photocoagulation only.

Protocol T: A Comparative Effectiveness Study of Intravitreal Aflibercept, Bevacizumab, and Ranibizumab for Diabetic Macular Edema The purpose of the study was the compare the efficacy of intravitreal aflibercept vs intravitreal bevacizumab vs intravitreal ranibizumab for the treatment of diabetic macular edema. The study concluded that intravitreal aflibercept, intravitreal bevacizumab and intravitreal ranibizumab improved vision in patients with diabetic macular edema. Furthermore, in patients with better baseline visual acuity, there were no significant differences in efficacy among the three agents. However, when the baseline vision was 20/50 or worse, aflibercept was superior to bevacizumab after 2 years. The superiority of aflibercept over ranibizumab noted at year 1 was not seen after 2 years. The study noted an increase in Anti-Platelet Trialists' Collaboration event rates with ranibizumab compared to the other agents.

References and Suggested Reading

1. Diabetic Retinopathy Clinical Research Network, Wells JA, Glassman AR, Ayala AR, Jampol LM, Aiello LP, Antoszyk AN, Arnold-Bush B, Baker CW, Bressler NM, Browning DJ, Elman MJ, Ferris FL, Friedman SM, Melia M, Pieramici DJ, Sun JK, Beck RW. Aflibercept, bevacizumab, or ranibizumab for diabetic macular edema. N Engl J Med. 2015;372(13)):1193–203.
2. Gupta AK, Aggarwal VK, Goel N. Handbook of clinical trials in ophthalmology. Wolters Kluwer Health, Inc.: Jp Medical Ltd.; 2014.

Chapter 58
Nonproliferative Diabetic Retinopathy

Colin J. Prensky and John E. Legarreta

58.1 Definitions

Nonproliferative diabetic retinopathy (NPDR)
Proliferative diabetic retinopathy (PDR)
Intraretinal microvascular anomalies (IRMA)
Clinically significant macular edema (CSME)

58.2 Symptoms

Often asymptomatic unless coexisting macular edema or macular ischemia is present. This may lead to decreased vision or metamorphopsia.

58.3 Signs

Early: Dot/blot hemorrhages, flame-shaped hemorrhages, microaneurysms (MA), hard exudates (HE), cotton wool spots (CWS) (Fig. 58.1)
Late: In addition to the above, venous beading, venous loops, IRMA (Fig. 58.2)

C.J. Prensky, MD
Department of Ophthalmology, UPMC Eye Center, 200 Lothrop Street, Pittsburgh, PA 15213, USA

J.E. Legarreta, MD (✉)
Department of Ophthalmology, Bascom Palmer Eye Institute, University of Miami, 900 NW 17th St., Miami, FL 33136, USA
e-mail: legarretaje@icloud.com

C.A. Medina et al. (eds.), *Manual of Retinal Diseases: A Guide to Diagnosis and Management*, DOI 10.1007/978-3-319-20460-4_58

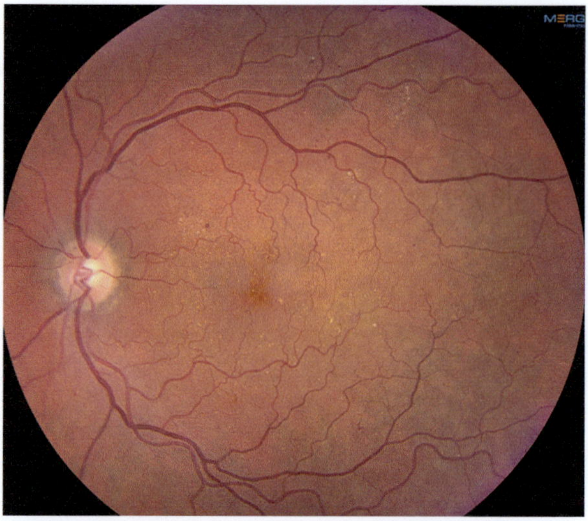

Fig. 58.1 Fundus photo showing microaneurysms and dot/blot hemorrhages along with several small hard exudates

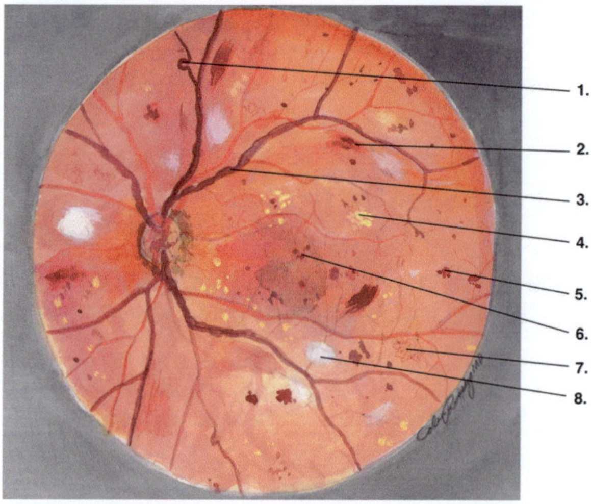

Fig. 58.2 Funduscopic findings seen in severe NPDR. (1) Venous loops, (2) flame hemorrhages, (3) venous beading, (4) hard exudates, (5) dot/blot hemorrhages, (6) microaneurysms, (7) IRMA, (8) cotton wool spots

58.4 Epidemiology

58.4.1 Predisposing Conditions

The major risk factor for development of diabetic retinopathy is duration of diabetes as well as poor control of blood glucose and systemic hypertension.

58.5 Differential Diagnosis

Hypertensive retinopathy, branch or central retinal vein occlusion, radiation retinopathy, ocular ischemic syndrome, carotid artery disease, HIV retinopathy, vasculitic disease

58.6 Etiology

As with other late complications of diabetes, diabetic retinopathy results from microvasculopathy believed to be related to the accumulation of advanced glycation end products. The findings in NPDR are related to a combination of microvascular occlusion and increased vascular permeability. Histopathology demonstrates loss of pericytes as well as thickened endothelial basement membrane. Microvascular occlusive disease includes focal ischemia, infarcts (CWS), and increase in VEG-F levels. Increased microvascular permeability leads to retinal edema, exudates, and hemorrhages.

58.7 Workup/Testing

Patients with DM type I should have comprehensive eye exam at age 20. Patients with DM type II should be examined at time of diagnosis with diabetes.

Initial workup should include:

1. Careful slit lamp exam with attention paid to excluding neovascularization of the iris (NVI).
2. Gonioscopy to exclude neovascularization of the angle (NVA).
3. Dilated exam of the macula and peripheral fundus. A slit lamp with handheld 60–90 diopter lens or contact lens is effective to examine for maculopathy and diabetic macular edema (DME). Indirect ophthalmoscopy should be used to inspect the periphery.
4. Bloodwork including fasting blood glucose, hemoglobin A1c, lipid panel (if exuberant, exudate is a feature).
5. Fluorescein angiography (FA) may be helpful to delineate areas of non-perfusion, enlarged foveolar avascular zone, macular ischemia, and subtle neovascularization that may be missed on clinical exam. FA will also highlight DME, if present.
6. OCT can be used to detect and evaluate DME.

58.8 Prognosis and Management

Prognosis and management depend largely on severity of NPDR discussed below. The International Clinical Diabetic Retinopathy Disease Severity Scale is based on funduscopic findings.

1. No retinopathy: No abnormalities
2. Mild NPDR: Microaneurysms only
3. Moderate NPDR: More than mild but less than severe NPDR
4. Severe NPDR (4:2:1 rule): Any of the following without proliferative retinopathy:
   (a) More than 20 intraretinal hemorrhages in each of four quadrants
   (b) Venous beading in two or more quadrants
   (c) Prominent IRMA in one or more quadrants
5. Very severe NPDR: Any two of the above features

Treatment focuses on strict control of blood glucose, hypertension, and lipids. Further lifestyle modifications including diet, exercise, and smoking cessation should be encouraged.

Classically, NPDR may be observed without specific ocular intervention unless high-risk PDR develops. The Early Treatment of Diabetic Retinopathy Study (ETDRS) demonstrated that risk of progression to high-risk PDR within 1 year was 15 % in patients with severe NPDR and 45 % in patients with very severe NPDR. For these patients, early panretinal photocoagulation may be considered. Some recommendations simplify the severity scale and do not distinguish between severe and very severe NPDR.

58.9 Follow-Up

Frequency of follow-up depends on severity of retinopathy (Table 58.1). According to the AAO Preferred Practice Guidelines, patients without retinopathy should be evaluated with dilated fundus exam every 12 months. For mild to moderate NPDR without CSME, 6–12 month follow-up is recommended. Severe NPDR without CSME may be seen as often as every 2–4 months to ensure that the patient is not developing PDR.

Table 58.1 Management recommendations by severity of disease

Severity	Findings	Recommendations
No retinopathy	No clinical findings	Dilated exam every 12 months
Mild NPDR	Microaneurysms only	Dilated exam every 6–12 months
Moderate NPDR	Microaneurysms, intraretinal hemorrhages, exudates, cotton wool spots, venous beading, does not meet 4:2:1 rule	Dilated exam every 6–12 months
Severe NPDR	One or more of the following (4:2:1 rule): >20 hemorrhages in four quadrants Venous beading in two quadrants Prominent IRMA in one quadrant	Dilated exam every 2–4 months May consider early PRP
Very severe NPDR	Two or more of above criteria	Dilated exam every 2–4 months Strongly consider early PRP
CSME (may exist at any stage of NPDR)	Macular thickening and exudates meeting ETDRS criteria	Follow-up at least every 2–4 months. Treat with anti-VegF or macular laser

References and Suggested Reading

1. American Academy of Ophthalmology Retina/Vitreous Panel. Preferred practice pattern guidelines. Diabetic retinopathy. San Francisco: American Academy of Ophthalmology; 2008. www.aao.org/ppp.
2. Early photocoagulation for diabetic retinopathy. ETDRS report number 9. Early Treatment Diabetic Retinopathy Study Research Group. Ophthalmology. 1991;98(5 Suppl):766–85.
3. Hammes H-P, et al. Pericytes and the pathogenesis of diabetic retinopathy. Diabetes. 2002;51(10):3107–12. doi:10.2337/diabetes.51.10.3107.
4. Wilkinson CP, et al. Proposed International clinical diabetic retinopathy and diabetic macular edema disease severity scales. Ophthalmology. 2003;110:1677–82.

Chapter 59
Diabetic Macular Edema

Aman Sharma and John E. Legarreta

59.1 Definitions

Diabetic macular edema is characterized by retinal thickening in the macula and the ETDRS defined clinically significant macular edema (CSME) as the following:

1. Thickening of the retina at or within 500 μm of the center of macula
2. Hard exudates at or within 500 μm of the center of macula
3. Retinal thickening of one disk area or larger

CSME is further defined as focal, diffuse, or both based on fluorescein angiogram leakage patterns. In focal leakage, there are points of retinal hyperfluorescence correlating with leaking microaneurysms, while in diffuse areas, there is leakage from dilated retinal capillaries and intraretinal microvascular abnormalities.

DME categories have been established using OCT as follows:

1. Diffuse DME (DRT)
2. Cystoid macular edema (DME)
3. Serous sensory retinal detachment (SRD)
4. Vitreomacular tractions (VMIA)

A. Sharma, MD • J.E. Legarreta, MD (✉)
Bascom Palmer Eye Institute, University of Miami,
900 NW 17th St., Miami, FL 33136, USA
e-mail: jel60@med.miami.edu

C.A. Medina et al. (eds.), *Manual of Retinal Diseases: A Guide to Diagnosis and Management*, DOI 10.1007/978-3-319-20460-4_59

59.2 Symptoms

Decreased vision, blurred vision, distorted vision

59.3 Signs

Exudates with retinal thickening on slit-lamp exam, cystoid maculopathy on OCT b-scans and thickening on retinal thickness map.

59.4 Epidemiology

It is estimated that in 2013, 382 million people were impacted by diabetes worldwide with diabetic retinopathy being the leading cause of visual impairment in working-age adults. DME is a common cause of vision loss related to diabetes. The incidence of DME over a 10-year period in one study was reported to be 20.1 % in those diagnosed before age 30 and 39.3 % for those diagnosed after 30.

59.5 Predisposing Conditions

Many factors have been studied for their association with DME, but only elevated diastolic blood pressure and lipid levels have shown to increase risk of developing DME.

59.6 Inheritance

Complex genetic and environmental factors play a role in individual susceptible for DME. Polymorphisms in eNOs, TGF-B1/B2, obesity-related genes, and VEGF-B gene along with SNP2543887 and rs476141 all have been proposed as playing a role in the development of macular edema.

59.7 Differential Diagnosis

Irvine-Gass syndrome, CRVO/BRVO, Uveitis, Retinitis pigmentosa, AMD, Retinal telangiectasias, Topical medical toxicity, Retinal vasculitis, Epiretinal membrane, Intraocular tumors

59.8 Etiology

The pathogenesis of DME is multifactorial involving many pathways which ultimately lead to a disruption of the blood retinal barrier, resulting in fluid accumulation in the intraretinal layers.

59.9 Workup/Testing

The American Diabetes Association recommends blood glucose, lipid, blood pressure control, and annual ophthalmic examination for diabetes. It is important to screen for sight-threatening DME early and intervene with timely management. In addition, a detailed history should be taken with questions about recent surgery, medications, history of uveitis, and night blindness along with a complete ocular examination.

Fundus stereo photography and slit-lamp microscopy play a role in workup and testing (Fig. 59.1); however, several additional ocular imaging platforms are available. Fluorescein angiography is a standard method to detect fluid leakage and identify leaking lesions and ischemic areas. OCT provides a noninvasive and high-resolution imaging for objective evaluation of DME and response to intervention (Fig. 59.2).

59.10 Prognosis and Management

DME is a common cause of central vision loss in setting of diabetic retinopathy. The Wisconsin Epidemiologic Study of diabetic retinopathy reported that 10-year incidence of macular edema was 20.1 % among type 1 diabetics and 25.4 % among type

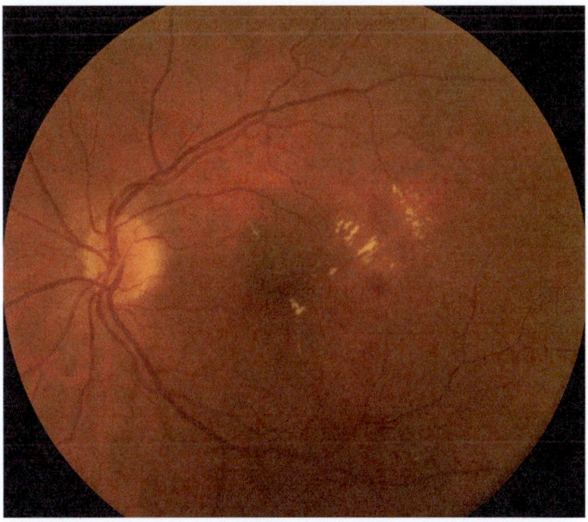

Fig. 59.1 Fundus photo showing exudates, intraretinal hemorrhages, and retinal thickening

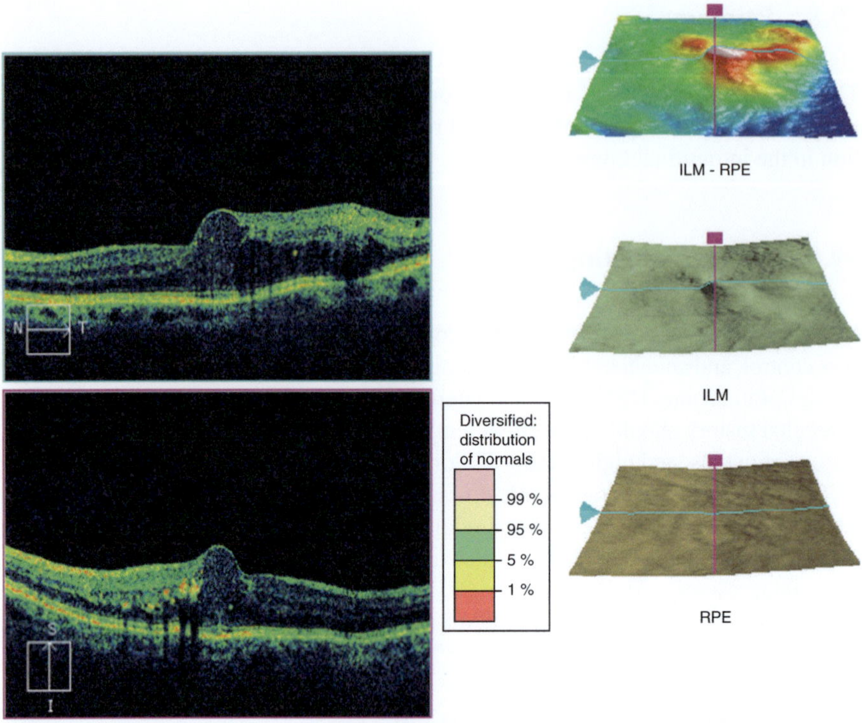

Fig. 59.2 OCT showing cystoid maculopathy and retinal thickening on retinal thickness map

2 diabetics. Strict glycemic and blood pressure control is the cornerstone of DME prevention and treatment. For CSME, the ETDRS reported that focal laser photocoagulation had a 50 % reduction in risk of moderate visual loss compared to controls making it the traditional therapy. In recent years, the treatment of DME has rapidly evolved with the development of anti-VEGF agents, glucocorticoid therapy, vitrectomy, and micropulse diode laser as additional treatment options.

59.11 Follow-Up

Based on clinical judgment and patient clinical course, other forms of CME however may require urgent workup and treatment.

References and Suggested Reading

1. Arevalo JF. Diabetic macular edema: changing treatment paradigms. Curr Opin Ophthalmol. 2014;25(6):502–7.

2. Bhagat N, Grigorian RA, Tutela A, Zarbin MA. Diabetic macular edema: pathogenesis and treatment. Surv Ophthalmol. 2009;54(1):1–32.
3. Kiire CA, Porta M, Chong V. Medical management for the prevention and treatment of diabetic macular edema. Surv Ophthalmol. 2013;58(5):459–65.
4. Shamsi HN, Masaud JS, Ghazi NG. Diabetic macular edema: new promising therapies. World J Diabetes. 2013;4(6):324–38.
5. Zhang X, Zeng H, Bao S, Wang N, Gillies MC. Diabetic macular edema: new concepts in patho-physiology and treatment. Cell Biosci. 2014;4:27. doi:10.1186/2045-3701-4-27.

Chapter 60
Proliferative Diabetic Retinopathy

Shilpa Kodati and John E. Legarreta

60.1 Definitions

Proliferative diabetic retinopathy (PDR)
Neovascularization (NV)

60.2 Symptoms

Decreased vision, floaters

60.3 Signs

Vitreous hemorrhage, preretinal hemorrhage, tractional retinal detachment (TRD)
NV is characterized by location: neovascularization of the disk (NVD) or neovascularization elsewhere (NVE). Patients with neovascularization of the iris (NVI) or angle (NVA) are at high risk of developing neovascular glaucoma (NVG).

S. Kodati, MD
Department of Ophthalmology, UPMC Eye Center, 200 Lothrop Street, Pittsburgh, PA 15213, USA

J.E. Legarreta, MD (✉)
Department of Ophthalmology, Bascom Palmer Eye Institute, University of Miami, 900 NW 17th St., Miami, FL 33136, USA
e-mail: legarretaje@icloud.com

C.A. Medina et al. (eds.), *Manual of Retinal Diseases: A Guide to Diagnosis and Management*, DOI 10.1007/978-3-319-20460-4_60

60.4 Epidemiology

The prevalence of PDR in the United States has been reported as 1.5 % in diabetics over the age of 40 years. Type I diabetics have a higher prevalence of PDR. The Wisconsin Epidemiologic Study of Diabetic Retinopathy reported a 25-year progression to PDR of 42 % in type 1 diabetics.

60.5 Risk Factors

- Hyperglycemia
- Duration since diagnosis of diabetes
- Pregnancy (PDR typically progresses more rapidly in pregnancy)
- Smoking
- Cardiovascular risk factors
- Renal disease

60.6 Differential Diagnosis

The patient's history and features of NPDR on exam will help distinguish PDR from other causes of proliferative retinopathy (Table 60.1).

60.7 Etiology

VEGF and other angiogenic factors are produced by ischemic retina, resulting in new vessel formation. The new vessels are initially intraretinal (intraretinal microvascular abnormalities) and subsequently penetrate through the ILM. The new vessels will proliferate and may be associated with fibrous tissue. The fine and delicate

Table 60.1 Differential diagnosis of proliferative retinopathy

Neovascularization secondary to CRAO, CRVO, or BRVO
Ocular ischemic syndrome
Sickle cell retinopathy
Occlusive retinal vascular disease (e.g., Eales disease, Behcet's disease)
Other inflammatory eye diseases (e.g., sarcoid, systemic lupus erythematous, pars planitis)
Radiation retinopathy
Hypercoagulability

new vessels are prone to rupture with either contraction of fibrovascular tissue or posterior vitreous detachment, resulting in vitreous or preretinal hemorrhage.

60.8 Workup/Testing

- Anterior segment slit examination and gonioscopy are recommended prior to dilation for evaluation of NVI and NVA.
- Dilated fundus exam with careful attention to the disk and posterior pole, which are the most common sites for NV (Fig. 60.1).
- Fluorescein angiography (FA) may be used to evaluate areas of retinal ischemia and NV. FA combined with wide field imaging is especially beneficial in the assessment of peripheral NV.
- Consider performing an OCT to determine the presence of coexistent cystoid macular edema (CME), as well as to detect changes in the vitreo-macula interface (such as VMT or VMA).
- If dense vitreous hemorrhage is present, B-scan ultrasound is necessary to rule out a TRD.
- Check most recent glycated hemoglobin (a1c).

60.9 Prognosis and Management

Panretinal photocoagulation (PRP) is indicated if any of the high-risk features of PDR are present (Table 60.2). However, some specialists will perform PRP for any degree of PDR, especially in poorly compliant patients or type 1 diabetics,

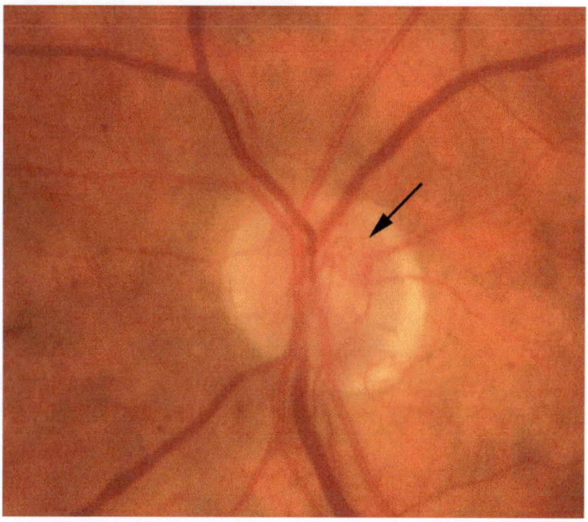

Fig. 60.1 Neovascularization of the disk

Table 60.2 Diagnostic features of high-risk PDR (*as defined by the Diabetic Retinopathy Study*)

1 of the following:
Preretinal hemorrhage or vitreous hemorrhage and NVE >0.5DD
Preretinal hemorrhage or vitreous hemorrhage and NVD
NVD >0.25DD

Table 60.3 Laser parameters for PRP

Laser: Argon green. Kryton red or diode laser can be used in media opacity
Widefield lens ~ ×2.0 magnification
Spot size – 500 μm
Separation – half a spot size
Duration – 0.05–0.2 s
Power – 130 mW, titrate until white-gray burn
1200 spots or more
Location: burns should extend from the arcades to the equator. Start nasally >500 μm from optic disk. Start temporally >2.5DD from fovea

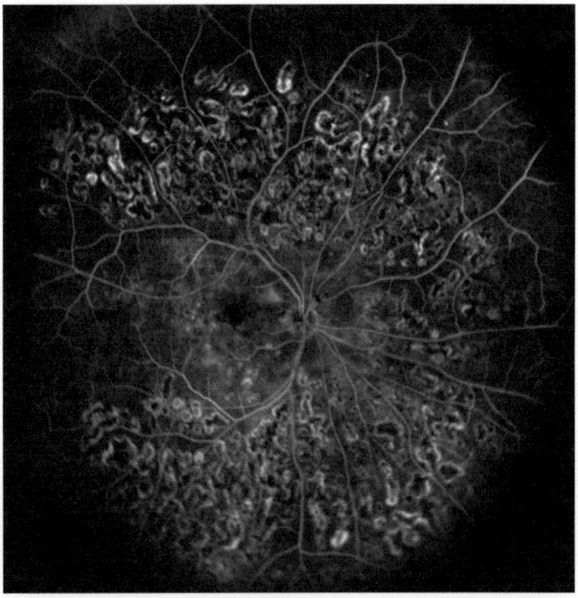

Fig. 60.2 Late-phase fluorescein angiography showing staining of PRP scars

who usually progress more rapidly. PRP induces regression of NV and reduces further neovascular tissue formation (Table 60.3). Peripheral ischemic retina is destroyed, thereby lowering the VEGF drive from ischemic retina. Furthermore, decreased oxygen consumption and increased choroidal perfusion of oxygen in areas of PRP scars both serve to increase the overall oxygen tension of the retina (Figs. 60.2 and 60.3).

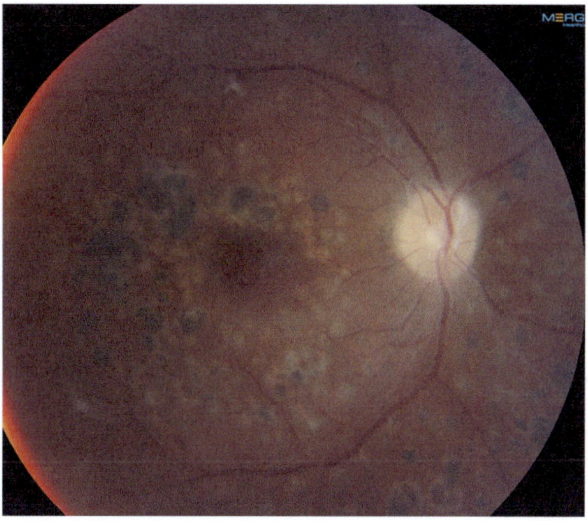

Fig. 60.3 Fundus photo showing regressed NVD and dense PRP laser scars in the periphery and dense focal laser scars in the macula

Table 60.4 Indications for vitrectomy in PDR

Dense non-clearing vitreous hemorrhage or dense pre-macula hemorrhage
Macula involving TRD
Tractional-rhegmatogenous RD
Severe fibrovascular proliferation refractory to PRP
Diabetic CME refractory to treatment or CME associated with significant traction of the posterior hyaloid
Ghost cell glaucoma
NVI or NVA with vitreous hemorrhage precluding PRP

Complications from resultant fibrovascular tissue contraction include vitreous hemorrhage, TRD, and combined tractional-rhegmatogenous detachment. Involvement of the long ciliary nerves can disrupt accommodation and pupillary function and impair corneal sensation. Other adverse effects from PRP include decreased visual acuity, reduced peripheral vision, nyctalopia, worsening macula edema, decreased color vision, reduced contrast sensitivity, choroidal detachment, and serous retinal detachment.

Anti-VEGF drugs may be used as a temporizing measure to decrease vessel leakage and induce regression of NV (both anterior segment and retinal). Due to its short-term effect, anti-VEGF therapy is beneficial as an adjunct to laser photocoagulation, either to cause regression of vessels prior to vitrectomy (Table 60.4), in treatment refractory PDR, or to expedite resolution of NVA. However, anti-VEGF in this setting carries the risk of retinal tears and combined tractional-rhegmatogenous retinal detachment from sudden fibrovascular tissue contraction, as well as potentially worsening macula ischemia. Non-clearing vitreous hemorrhage or TRD requires vitrectomy (Table 60.4).

60.10 Follow-Up

Dilated fundus exam is recommended every 2–3 months for PDR not classified as high risk. More frequent follow-up is needed for high-risk PDR. Pregnant women with PDR should have dilated exams monthly.

References and Suggested Reading

1. Klein R, Klein BE, Moss SE, et al. The Wisconsin Epidemiologic Study of Diabetic Retinopathy: XVII. The 14-year incidence and progression of diabetic retinopathy and associated risk factors in type 1 diabetes. Ophthalmology. 1998;105:1801–15.
2. Photocoagulation treatment of proliferative diabetic retinopathy: the second report of diabetic retinopathy study findings. Ophthalmology. 1978;85:82–106.
3. Zhang X, Saaddine JB, Chou CF, et al. Prevalence of diabetic retinopathy in the United States, 2005–2008. JAMA. 2010;304:649–56.

Section IX
Retinal Vascular Diseases

Amir Mohsenin

Chapter 61
Retinal Vascular Occlusions: Review of Clinical Trials

Andrew S. Camp

61.1 Natural History and Laser

CVOS (Central Vein Occlusion Study): Patients with good vision (≥20/40) or poor vision (<20/200) at presentation are likely to maintain good and poor vision, respectively. Conversion to ischemic CRVO is most likely in the first 4 months. Eyes with ischemic CRVO and early NV respond well to PRP; prophylactic PRP is not indicated.

BVOS (Branch Vein Occlusion Study): Patients with BRVO ≥3 months, macular edema, and vision ≤20/40 benefit from macula grid laser. Patients with BRVO that receive sectoral PRP have a lower risk of neovascularization; however, prophylactic sectoral PRP is not recommended. Patients with BRVO and neovascularization that receive sectoral PRP are less likely to develop vitreous hemorrhage.

61.2 Corticosteroid Therapy

SCORE (Standard care vs. corticosteroid for retinal vein occlusion):

BRVO: Compared intravitreal triamcinolone 1 or 4 mg with grid laser photocoagulation. There was no difference in visual acuity gain between the three groups. Grid laser photocoagulation remains standard of care compared to intravitreal triamcinolone.

CRVO: Compared intravitreal triamcinolone 1 or 4 mg with observation. One milligram and 4 mg groups both had significant improvements in vision compared

A.S. Camp, MD
Bascom Palmer Eye Institute, University of Miami,
900 NW 17th St., Miami, FL 33136, USA
e-mail: ascamp@med.miami.edu

C.A. Medina et al. (eds.), *Manual of Retinal Diseases: A Guide to Diagnosis and Management*, DOI 10.1007/978-3-319-20460-4_61

to observation, but 4 mg group had higher rates of elevated intraocular pressure and cataract. Therefore, 1 mg intravitreal triamcinolone is recommended.

GENEVA (Global evaluation of implantable dexamethasone in retinal vein occlusion with macular edema):

BRVO/CRVO: Compared intravitreal dexamethasone 0.35 and 0.7 mg implants to sham injections in pooled BRVO and CRVO patients with macular edema. BRVO patients responded better to therapy than CRVO patients. Vision improved significantly faster in both implant groups compared to sham with no statistically significant difference between 0.35 and 0.7 mg implants. Response peaked at day 60, but by day 180, there was no difference in improvement from sham, although more sham patients had a decrease in vision.

61.3 Anti-VEGF Therapy (Ranibizumab)

BRAVO (Ranibizumab for the treatment of macular edema following branch retinal vein occlusion study: Compared monthly intravitreal ranibizumab 0.3 or 0.5 mg to sham injections. Patients receiving ranibizumab had improved visual acuity compared to sham.
CRUISE: (Ranibizumab for the treatment of macular edema after central retinal vein occlusion study: Compared monthly intravitreal ranibizumab 0.3 or 0.5 mg to sham injections. Patients receiving ranibizumab had improved visual acuity. Although both groups had similar gains at 12 months, 0.5 mg ranibizumab is currently the recommended dose.
HORIZON: Extension study to evaluate the safety and tolerability of ranibizumab in subjects with macular edema secondary to retinal vein occlusion. Patients from BRAVO and CRUISE were followed for an additional year at reduced intervals (at least every 3 months). BRVO: Vision remained stable in BRVO patients with reduced follow-ups and injections. CRVO: Patients with reduced follow-up and injections had a decline in vision. Based on these results, CRVO follow-up should be individualized, and patients will likely require injections more frequently than every 3 months.
RETAIN: Extended follow-up of patients with macular edema due to retinal vein occlusion. Patients from HORIZON were followed for a mean 49 months with continued PRN dosing of intravitreal ranibizumab 0.5 mg. Patients requiring injections on 2 consecutive visits were treated with ranibizumab plus scatter photocoagulation.
BRVO: 80 % of patients retained good vision, but half required continued injections.
CRVO: Less than half the patients had good visual outcomes; the rest of the patients lost significant vision and required frequent injections. The long-term prognosis of patients with CRVO is guarded.

SHORE: Study evaluating dosing regimens for treatment with intravitreal ranibizumab injections in subjects with macular edema following retinal vein occlusion (BRVO and

CRVO). Compared PRN versus monthly intravitreal ranibizumab 0.5 mg in patients that already had 7 consecutive months of intravitreal ranibizumab 0.5 mg. There was no significant difference in vision between patients receiving PRN or monthly intravitreal ranibizumab. Both BRVO and CRVO patients responded well to PRN dosing.

61.4 Anti-VEGF Therapy (Bevacizumab)

Russo et al. (2009) [BRVO]: Compared intravitreal bevacizumab 1.25 mg to grid laser in patients with BRVO. Patients receiving intravitreal bevacizumab had greater vision gains compared to those receiving grid laser.
Donati et al. (2012) [BRVO]: Compared intravitreal bevacizumab 1.25 mg to intravitreal bevacizumab 1.25 mg together with grid laser in patients with BRVO. Patients receiving intravitreal bevacizumab and grid laser together had greater vision gains compared to those receiving bevacizumab alone.
Epstein et al. (2012) [CRVO]: Compared intravitreal bevacizumab 1.25 mg to sham injections in patients with CRVO. Patients treated with bevacizumab 1.25 mg every 6 weeks had a significant gain in vision compared to those treated with sham.

61.5 Anti-VEGF Therapy (Aflibercept)

Evaluation of Repeated Intravitreal Administration of VEGF Trap-Eye in Central Retinal Vein Occlusion (*COPERNICUS*) [CRVO]: Compared intravitreal aflibercept 2 mg to sham injection. Patients in the aflibercept group had improved visual acuity compared to sham. An extension of the study showed that patients maintained visual acuity when converted to PRN dosing.
Intravitreal Aflibercept Injection for Macular Edema Resulting from Central Retinal Vein Occlusion (*GALILEO*) [CRVO]: Compared intravitreal aflibercept 2 mg to sham injection. Patients in the aflibercept group had improved visual acuity which was maintained when converted to PRN dosing after 6 months.
Complications: Major complications (not including increased intraocular pressure or cataract formation) for all above trials include uveitis (11), retinal tear (6), endophthalmitis (4), retinal detachment (3), and traumatic lens damage (0).

61.6 Retinal Artery Occlusions

EAGLE: European Assessment Group for Lysis in the Eye study. Randomized patients with CRAO for <20 h to conservative standard treatment or local intra-arterial fibrinolysis using tPA. There was no significant difference in outcomes between the two groups. Given the higher rate of adverse reactions in the tPA group, conservative management is recommended.

Chen et al. (2011): Randomized patients with CRAO for <24 h to intravenous saline or local intra-arterial fibrinolysis using tPA. Patients receiving tPA within 6 h of symptoms had improvement in vision, but greater complication rates and the improvement were not sustained at 6 months.

References and Suggested Reading

1. Argon laser scatter photocoagulation for prevention of neovascularization and vitreous hemorrhage in branch vein occlusion. A randomized clinical trial. Branch Vein Occlusion Study Group. Arch Ophthalmol. 1986;104(1):34–41.
2. Gupta AK, Aggarwal VK, Goel N. Handbook of clinical trials in ophthalmology. New Delhi: Jay Pee Medical Ltd.; 2014.
3. Haller JA, Bandello F, Belfort Jr R, Blumenkranz MS, Gillies M, Heier J, Loewenstein A, Yoon YH, Jacques ML, Jiao J, Li XY, Whitcup SM, OZURDEX GENEVA Study Group. Randomized, sham-controlled trial of dexamethasone intravitreal implant in patients with macular edema due to retinal vein occlusion. Ophthalmology. 2010;117(6):1134–46.e3.
4. Ip MS, Scott IU, VanVeldhuisen PC, Oden NL, Blodi BA, Fisher M, Singerman LJ, Tolentino M, Chan CK, Gonzalez VH, SCORE Study Research Group. A randomized trial comparing the efficacy and safety of intravitreal triamcinolone with observation to treat vision loss associated with macular edema secondary to central retinal vein occlusion: the Standard Care vs Corticosteroid for Retinal Vein Occlusion (SCORE) study report 5. Arch Ophthalmol. 2009;127(9):1101–14.
5. Natural history and clinical management of central retinal vein occlusion. The Central Vein Occlusion Study Group. Arch Ophthalmol. 1997;115(4):486–91.
6. Ogura Y, Roider J, Korobelnik JF, Holz FG, Simader C, Schmidt-Erfurth U, Vitti R, Berliner AJ, Hiemeyer F, Stemper B, Zeitz O, Sandbrink R, GALILEO Study Group. Intravitreal aflibercept for macular edema secondary to central retinal vein occlusion: 18-month results of the phase 3 GALILEO study. Am J Ophthalmol. 2014;158(5):1032–8.
7. Rofagha S, Bhisitkul RB, Boyer DS, Sadda SR, Zhang K, SEVEN-UP Study Group. Seven-year outcomes in ranibizumab-treated patients in ANCHOR, MARINA, and HORIZON: a multicenter cohort study (SEVEN-UP). Ophthalmology. 2013;120(11):2292–9.
8. Schumacher M, Schmidt D, Jurklies B, Gall C, Wanke I, Schmoor C, Maier-Lenz H, Solymosi L, Brueckmann H, Neubauer AS, Wolf A, Feltgen N, EAGLE-Study Group. Central retinal artery occlusion: local intra-arterial fibrinolysis versus conservative treatment, a multicenter randomized trial. Ophthalmology. 2010;117(7):1367–75.e1.
9. Scott IU, Vanveldhuisen PC, Oden NL, Ip MS, Domalpally A, Doft BH, Elman MJ, Blodi BA, SCORE Study Investigator Group. Baseline characteristics and response to treatment of participants with hemiretinal compared with branch retinal or central retinal vein occlusion in the standard care vs corticosteroid for retinal vein occlusion (SCORE) study: SCORE study report 14. Arch Ophthalmol. 2012;130(12):1517–24.
10. Thach AB, Yau L, Hoang C, Tuomi L. Time to clinically significant visual acuity gains after ranibizumab treatment for retinal vein occlusion: BRAVO and CRUISE trials. Ophthalmology. 2014;121(5):1059–66.

Chapter 62
Branch Retinal Artery Occlusion

Daniel Gologorsky and Amir Mohsenin

62.1 Definitions

- BRAO: Branch retinal artery occlusion
- CVA: Cerebrovascular accident
- TIA: Transient ischemic attack

62.2 Symptoms

- Sudden, unilateral, and painless loss of a visual field segment.
- Central acuity is preserved in 50 % of patients.
- Patients may have a prior history of amaurosis fugax (in up to 25 % of cases), TIA, or CVA.

62.3 Signs

- Superficial retinal whitening and edema along the distribution of ischemic branch of the retinal artery
- Visible retinal emboli
- Arteriolar constriction
- Segmentation of arterial blood flow (boxcarring)
- May have a RAPD

D. Gologorsky, MD, MBA • A. Mohsenin, MD, PhD (✉)
Bascom Palmer Eye Institute, University of Miami, 900 NW 17th St., Miami, FL 33136, USA
e-mail: dangologorsky@med.miami.edu; amohsenin@gmail.com

C.A. Medina et al. (eds.), *Manual of Retinal Diseases: A Guide to Diagnosis and Management*, DOI 10.1007/978-3-319-20460-4_62

62.4 Epidemiology

- Typically occurs in older patients, mean age 60–65.
- Men: Women = 2:1.
- BRAO occurs in OD 60 % versus OS 40 %. Likely reflecting the tendency of cardiac emboli to enter the right carotid.

62.5 Predisposing Conditions

- Hypertension, diabetes, carotid atherosclerotic disease, and cardiac valve disease.
- Cigarette smoking and oral contraceptives are known risk factors for younger women.

62.6 Differential Diagnosis

- Commotio retinae
- Central retinal artery obstruction
- Cilioretinal artery obstruction
- Inflammatory/infectious retinitis
- Cotton wool spot

62.7 Etiology

- Most cases of BRAO are secondary to emboli ($\frac{2}{3}$ of all cases).
- Emboli are often visible on examination, most often as bright reflective crystals at vascular bifurcation points.
- Emboli types:
  - Cholesterol (Hollenhorst plaque) from carotid artery atheromas
  - Calcium (cardiac valves)
  - Platelet fibrin (carotid atheromas)
  - Fat (long bone fractures)
- Hypercoagulable disorders
- Other causes: thrombus, temporal arteritis rarely, trauma, syphilis, sickle cell disease, mitral valve prolapse, and IV drug abuse

62.8 Workup/Testing

- Ophthalmic history and exam
  - Macular OCT
  - FA: abrupt diminution in fluorescence at the site and distal to the obstruction. Leakage from the embolus site may occur.
  - If desired, a visual field can be obtained to document the extent of field loss.
- Blood pressure, fasting blood glucose, CBC, glycosylated hemoglobin, and PT/PTT.
- Cardiovascular workup: EKG, echocardiogram, and duplex carotid Doppler ultrasound.
- In younger patients: protein C/S, RF, ANA, antiphospholipid antibody, lipid panel, FTA-ABS, antithrombin III, homocysteine, and serum protein electrophoresis.
- GCA is an exceedingly rare cause of BRAO, so ESR, CRP, and platelets are not routinely measured in most cases unless the review of systems is positive.

62.9 Treatment

- No treatment has been proven effective for BRAO.
- Similar interventions to those described in the CRAO chapter have been employed with variable success.
- Optimization of systemic medical conditions in conjunction with the patient's primary care doctor is recommended.

62.10 Prognosis and Management

Most patients remain with a fixed visual field defect and intact central acuity. 80 % of patients recover to vision better than 20/40. Pallor fades and retinal circulation is restored within several weeks. Neovascularization is rare after BRAO.

62.11 Follow-Up

- Medical management.
- Reevaluate every 3–6 months.

References and Suggested Reading

1. Arruga J, Sanders MD. Ophthalmologic findings in 70 patients with evidence of retinal embolism. Ophthalmology. 1982;89(12):1336–47.
2. Margolis R, Singh RP, Kaiser PK. Branch retinal vein occlusion: clinical findings, natural history, and management. Compr Ophthalmol Update. 2006;7(6):265–76.
3. Sharma S, Brown GC, Pater JL, Cruess AF. Does a visible retinal embolus increase the likelihood of hemodynamically significant carotid artery stenosis in patients with acute retinal arterial occlusion? Arch Ophthalmol. 1998;116:1602.

Chapter 63
Central Retinal Artery Occlusion

Daniel Gologorsky and Amir Mohsenin

63.1 Definitions

- CRAO: Central retinal artery occlusion
- CVA: Cerebrovascular vascular attack
- TIA: Transient ischemic attack

63.2 Symptoms

- Sudden, unilateral, and painless profound loss of vision to counting fingers (CF) or light perception (LP).
- Patients may describe past history of amaurosis fugax (in up to 10 % of cases), TIA, or CVA.

63.3 Signs

- RAPD
- Diffuse superficial retinal whitening
- Cherry-red spot in macula (Fig. 63.1)
- Arteriolar constriction

D. Gologorsky, MD, MBA • A. Mohsenin, MD, PhD (✉)
Bascom Palmer Eye Institute, University of Miami,
900 NW 17th St., Miami, FL 33136, USA
e-mail: dangologorsky@med.miami.edu; amohsenin@gmail.com

C.A. Medina et al. (eds.), *Manual of Retinal Diseases: A Guide to Diagnosis and Management*, DOI 10.1007/978-3-319-20460-4_63

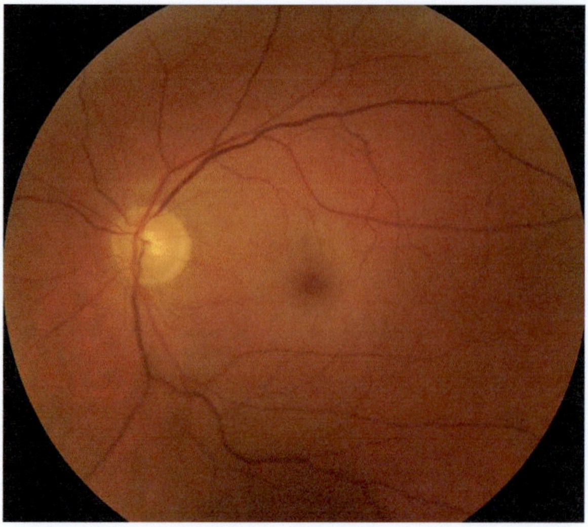

Fig. 63.1 CRAO. Cherry-red spot in macula

- Segmentation of arterial blood flow (boxcarring)
- Visible retinal arterial emboli

63.4 Epidemiology

- Typically occurs in older patients, mean age 60–65
- Men:Women = 2:1

63.5 Predisposing Conditions

- Hypertension (60 %), diabetes (25 %), carotid atherosclerotic disease, and cardiac valve disease

63.6 Differential Diagnosis

- Commotio retinae
- Ophthalmic artery occlusion
- Necrotizing retinitis
- Storage disorders: Tay-Sachs, Niemann-Pick, GM1 gangliosidosis, and mucolipidosis
  - Usually bilateral

63.7 Etiology

- Thrombus
  - Secondary to atherosclerotic disease
  - The most common etiology of CRAO
- Emboli
  - Cholesterol: Hollenhorst plaques from carotid artery atheromas
  - Calcium: cardiac valves
  - Platelet-fibrin: carotid atheromas
  - Fat: long bone fractures
- GCA
- Hypercoagulable disorders
- Other
  - Trauma, compression, vasospasm, direct vascular damage, syphilis, sickle cell disease, cardiac valvular disease, and IV drug abuse

63.8 Workup/Testing

- Ophthalmic history and exam:
  - Macular OCT: thickening of inner retinal layers in acute setting
  - FA: delayed retinal arterial filling time and arteriovenous transit time, normal choroidal filling, and extensive capillary nonperfusion
  - Electrophysiology: ERG (reduced b wave amplitude, normal a wave)
- Systemic: blood pressure, fasting blood glucose, glycosylated hemoglobin, CBC, and lipid panel.
- Cardiology referral: EKG, echocardiogram, and duplex carotid Doppler ultrasound.
- If over 50 years old: ESR, CRP, platelets.
  - Although GCA is the causative etiology in <5 % of cases, it must still be ruled out in patients over 50. In cases of GCA, bilateral involvement can occur within hours to days.
- If under 50 years old: rule out coagulation abnormalities with PT/PTT, protein C/S, antithrombin III, homocysteine, RF, ANA, antiphospholipid antibody, VDRL, FTA-ABS, serum protein electrophoresis, and hemoglobin electrophoresis.

63.9 Treatment

- No treatment has been proven effective for CRAO
- Nonevidence-based treatments exist. The goal of these treatments is to push the occlusive agent or embolus distally in order to restore proximal retinal blood flow. These interventions are best utilized within 120 min of the occlusive event:

- Manual dislodgement of embolus: digital ocular massage
- Increase retinal oxygenation: breathing carbogen (95 % oxygen, 5 % carbon dioxide)
- Increase retinal blood flow:
  - Systemic acetazolamide (500 mg IV or PO)
  - AC paracentesis
  - IOP-lowering agents
  - Hyperventilation inducing respiratory acidosis and subsequent vasodilation
  - Hyperbaric oxygen

- Revascularization: intravenous thrombolytic therapy with tPA

63.10 Prognosis and Management

CRAO often results in severe, permanent loss of vision. Retinal pallor fades as retinal circulation is restored within 4–6 weeks. The prognosis is poor as most affected patients have persistent severe visual loss with constricted retinal arterioles and optic atrophy. Must monitor for iris, optic disc, and retinal neovascularization which may require treatment with panretinal photocoagulation and/or anti-VEGF agents. Secondary iris and optic disc neovascularization occurs in 18 % and 2 % of cases, respectively. Systemic medical issues should be managed in conjunction with a primary care physician.

63.11 Follow-Up

Within 1 month for neovascularization

References and Suggested Reading

1. Brown GC, Magargal LE. Central retinal artery obstruction and visual acuity. Ophthalmology. 1982;89:14.
2. Cugati S, Varma DD, Chen CS, Lee AW. Treatment options for central retinal artery occlusion. Curr Treat Options Neurol. 2013;15(1):63–77.
3. Hayreh SS, Podhajsky PA, Zimmerman MB. Retinal artery occlusion: associated systemic and ophthalmic abnormalities. Ophthalmology. 2009;116:1928.
4. Hayreh SS, Zimmerman MB. Central retinal artery occlusion: visual outcome. Am J Ophthalmol. 2005;140(3):376–91.
5. Rudkin AK, Lee AW, Chen CS. Vascular risk factors for central retinal artery occlusion. Eye (Lond). 2010;24:678.
6. Varma DD, Cugati S, Lee AW, Chen CS. A review of central retinal artery occlusion: clinical presentation and management. Eye (Lond). 2013;27(6):688–97.

Chapter 64
Cilioretinal Artery Occlusion

Daniel Gologorsky and Amir Mohsenin

64.1 Definitions

- CLRAO: cilioretinal artery occlusion
- CRAO: central retinal artery occlusion
- CRVO: central retinal vein occlusion
- GCA: giant cell arteritis

64.2 Symptoms

- Loss of central visual acuity with preservation of peripheral field

64.3 Signs

- Macular whitening and/or edema
- Cherry-red spot

D. Gologorsky, MD, MBA • A. Mohsenin, MD, PhD (✉)
Bascom Palmer Eye Institute, University of Miami,
900 NW 17th St., Miami, FL 33136, USA
e-mail: dangologorsky@med.miami.edu; amohsenin@gmail.com

C.A. Medina et al. (eds.), *Manual of Retinal Diseases: A Guide to Diagnosis and Management*, DOI 10.1007/978-3-319-20460-4_64

64.4 Epidemiology

Typically occurs in older patients (50–80 years of age)

64.5 Predisposing Conditions

Hypertension, carotid occlusive disease, diabetes, cardiac valvular disease, and collagen vascular disorders.

64.6 Differential Diagnosis

- Commotio retinae
- CRAO

64.7 Etiology

CLRAO occurs in three groups:

- Isolated CLRAO
  - Often in younger patients with collagen vascular disorders
- CLRAO in conjunction with CRVO
  - Most common form (40 %)
  - May occur secondary to CRVO associated increased hydrostatic pressure that reduces flow to the cilioretinal artery to the point of infarction
- CLRAO in conjunction with anterior ischemic optic neuropathy
  - Older patients in association with GCA

64.8 Workup/Testing

Ophthalmic history and exam

- Macular OCT
- FA

- If over 50 years old, rule out GCA with ESR, CRP, and platelets.
- If under 50 years old, rule out coagulation abnormalities with PT/PTT, protein C/S, antithrombin III, homocysteine, RF, ANA, antiphospholipid antibody, VDRL, FTA-ABS, serum protein electrophoresis, and hemoglobin electrophoresis.
- Cardiovascular workup: EKG, echocardiogram, and duplex carotid Doppler ultrasound.

64.9 Treatment

Treatment is aimed at the underlying etiology.

64.10 Prognosis and Management

- Young patients with CLRAO secondary to collagen vascular disorders carry a favorable prognosis, with 90 % of eyes achieving 20/40 or better vision.
- CLRAO in the context of CRVO carries a positive prognosis, although the central scotoma from the occlusion is often permanent.
- CLRAO in the context of GCA typically portends a poor visual prognosis.

64.11 Follow-Up

Depends on underlying etiology

References and Suggested Reading

1. Galasso JM, Jay WM. An occult case of giant cell arteritis presenting with combined anterior ischemic optic neuropathy and cilioretinal artery occlusion. Semin Ophthalmol. 2004;19(3–4):75–7.
2. Hayreh SS, Fraterrigo L, Jonas J. Central retinal vein occlusion associated with cilioretinal artery occlusion. Retina. 2008;28(4):581–94.
3. Schatz H, Fong AC, McDonald HR, et al. Cilioretinal artery occlusion in young adults with central retinal vein occlusion. Ophthalmology. 1991;98(5):594–601.

Chapter 65
Branch Retinal Vein Occlusion

Andrew S. Camp and Amir Mohsenin

65.1 Definitions

- BRVO: branch retinal vein occlusion
- CRVO: central retinal vein occlusion
- FA: fluorescein angiography
- IOP: intraocular pressure
- NVA: neovascularization of the angle
- NVI: neovascularization of the iris
- OCT: optical coherence tomography
- VEGF: vascular endothelial growth factor

65.2 Symptoms

- Sudden, unilateral, painless decreased vision or loss of vision
- May complain of a visual field defect

A.S. Camp, MD • A. Mohsenin, MD, PhD (✉)
Bascom Palmer Eye Institute, University of Miami,
900 NW 17th St., Miami, FL 33136, USA
e-mail: ascamp@med.miami.edu; amohsenin@gmail.com

C.A. Medina et al. (eds.), *Manual of Retinal Diseases: A Guide to Diagnosis and Management*, DOI 10.1007/978-3-319-20460-4_65

65.3 Signs

- Sectoral retinal hemorrhages with associated venous dilation/tortuosity
- May see cotton wool spots and retinal edema

65.4 Epidemiology

- Retinal vein occlusion is the second most common retinal vascular disease (after diabetic retinopathy).
- Prevalence: 4.42 per 1000, increasing risk with age.

65.5 Predisposing Conditions

Age >65 years old, hypertension, and diabetes mellitus

65.6 Differential Diagnosis

- Diabetic retinopathy
- Hypertensive retinopathy

65.7 Classification

- Perfused: <5 disk areas of non-perfusion on FA
- Ischemic: >5 disk areas of non-perfusion on FA

65.8 Etiology

- Thrombotic occlusion of a branch retinal vein
- Usually at an arteriovenous crossing

65.9 Workup/Testing

- History:
  - Past medical history of hypertension or diabetes
  - Past ocular history of vein occlusion

- Ophthalmic:
  - Careful examination of the iris, angle, and fundus for evidence of neovascularization
- Imaging:
  - Macular OCT
  - FA to evaluate perfusion status if visualization not too obscured by hemorrhage
- Systemic:
  - Primary care workup for hypertension and diabetes.
  - In younger patients, consider hypercoagulable workup.
    - CBC, PT/PTT, protein C/S, antiphospholipid antibody, factor V Leiden mutation, serum homocysteine, antinuclear antibodies, and lupus anticoagulant.
  - In suspected cases, consider infectious disease workup for Lyme disease, syphilis, or human immunodeficiency virus.

65.10 Prognosis

- 50–60 % of eyes have a final vision of 20/40 or better without treatment.
- Retinal neovascularization develops in 25 % of eyes.
- Persistent macular edema develops in 60 % of eyes.

65.11 Management

- Medical management and treatment of underlying etiology in conjunction with primary care physician
- Macular edema:
  - Intravitreal anti-VEGF therapy is first-line, safe, and effective.
  - Intravitreal corticosteroids are inexpensive and effective but have a higher side effect profile (IOP elevation, cataract).
  - Grid laser photocoagulation improves vision in eyes with BRVO ≥3 months and vision ≤20/40 but is unlikely to benefit eyes with BRVO >1 year duration or vision <20/200 (Fig. 65.1).
- Neovascularization:
  - Sectoral laser photocoagulation is recommended.

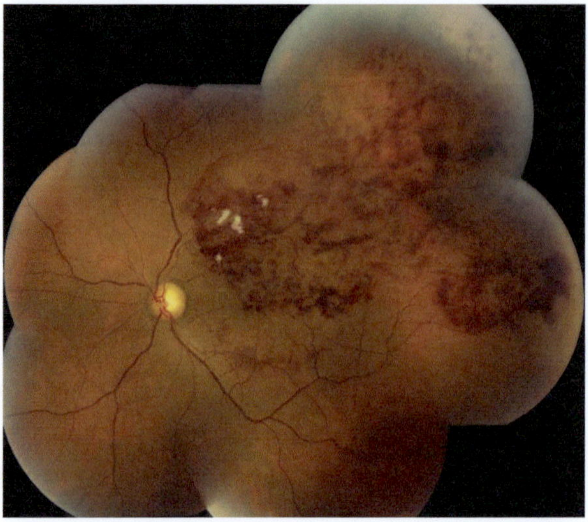

Fig. 65.1 Montage fundus photo of a patient with BRVO demonstrating intraretinal hemorrhages in the vascular distribution of the occluded vessel

65.12 Follow-Up

- No macular edema:
  - Every 1–2 months for 4 months, then extend based on stability.
- Macular edema:
  - Every month for 4 months, then consider extension depending on response to treatment.

References and Suggested Reading

1. McIntosh RL, Mohamed Q, Saw SM, et al. Interventions for branch retinal vein occlusion: an evidence-based systematic review. Ophthalmology. 2007;114(5):835–54.
2. Newman-Casey PA, Stem M, Talwar N, et al. Risk factors associated with developing branch retinal vein occlusion among enrollees in a United States managed care plan. Ophthalmology. 2014;121(10):1939–48.

Chapter 66
Central Retinal Vein Occlusion

Andrew S. Camp and Amir Mohsenin

66.1 Definitions

CRVO: central retinal vein occlusion
FA: fluorescein angiography
IOP: intraocular pressure
NVA: neovascularization of the angle
NVI: neovascularization of the iris
OCT: optical coherence tomography
VEGF: vascular endothelial growth factor

66.2 Symptoms

Sudden, unilateral, painless vision loss

66.3 Signs

- Diffuse retinal hemorrhages (blood and thunder) (Fig. 66.1).
- Tortuous retinal venous vasculature.

A.S. Camp, MD • A. Mohsenin, MD, PhD (✉)
Bascom Palmer Eye Institute, University of Miami,
900 NW 17th St., Miami, FL 33136, USA
e-mail: ascamp@med.miami.edu; amohsenin@gmail.com

C.A. Medina et al. (eds.), *Manual of Retinal Diseases: A Guide to Diagnosis and Management*, DOI 10.1007/978-3-319-20460-4_66

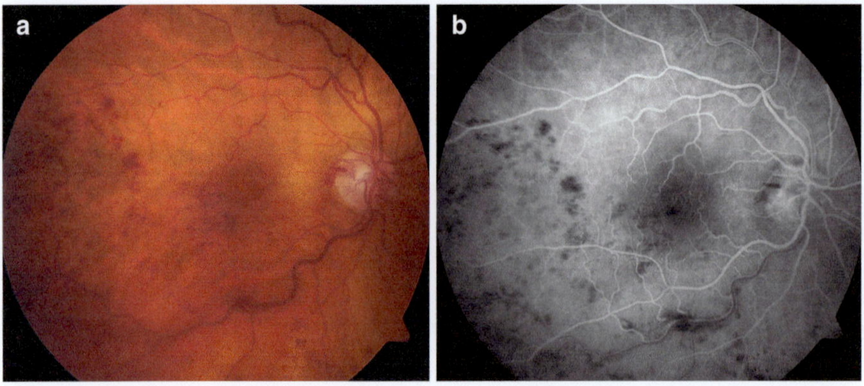

Fig. 66.1 Color fundus photograph of the right eye with an inferior hemiretinal vein occlusion. Dilated veins and intraretinal hemorrhages in a classic "blood and thunder" distribution are observed inferiorly. Collateral vessels are observed along the inferonasal aspect of the optic nerve (**a**). Fluorescein angiography shows delayed filling of the inferotemporal veins compared to the superior where laminar flow is already observed (**b**)

- May see optic nerve edema, cotton wool spots, and macular edema to varying degrees.
- Neovascularization of the iris, angle, optic disc, and retina can be present in non-acute cases.
- Afferent pupillary defect may be present.

66.4 Epidemiology

- Prevalence less than 0.5 %
- Increasing risk with age

66.5 Predisposing Conditions

Age >65 years old; hypertension, diabetes mellitus, vascular disease, optic disc edema, optic disc drusen, hypercoagulable state, and glaucoma.

66.6 Etiology

Not fully understood. Thrombotic occlusion of the central retinal vein has been demonstrated in enucleated specimens. Atherosclerotic changes in the central retinal artery compress the central retinal vein near the lamina cribrosa resulting in turbulent flow and thrombus formation.

66.7 Differential Diagnosis

- Proliferative diabetic retinopathy
- Hypertensive retinopathy
- Ocular ischemic syndrome
- Impending CRVO
- Valsalva retinopathy

66.8 Classification

- Perfused: <10 disk areas of non-perfusion on FA
- Ischemic: >10 disk areas of non-perfusion on FA, 20 % of CRVO cases

66.9 Workup/Testing

- History:
  - Past medical history of hypertension, diabetes, stroke, peripheral artery disease, or hypercoagulable state
  - Past ocular history of vein occlusion or glaucoma
  - Review of medications including oral contraceptives
- Ophthalmic:
  - Complete ocular examination with gonioscopy paying close attention to the iris, angle, and fundus for evidence of neovascularization
- Imaging:
  - Macular OCT
  - FA to evaluate perfusion status if visualization not too obscured by hemorrhage
- Systemic:
  - Primary care workup for hypertension, diabetes, and vascular disease.
  - Medication review:
  - In patients less than 60 years of age, consider laboratory workup:

    CBC, PT/PTT, protein C/S, antithrombin III, antiphospholipid antibody, factor V Leiden mutation

  - In atypical cases and if indicated, consider FTA-ABS, serum protein electrophoresis, and hemoglobin electrophoresis.

66.10 Prognosis

- Presenting visual acuity correlates with final visual acuity.
- Patients presenting with vision ≥20/40 are likely to maintain good vision.
- Patients with vision ≤20/200 at first visit are less likely to experience significant gains.
- Risk of vascular occlusion in fellow eye is 1 % per year.

66.11 Management

- Treatment of underlying etiology with cessation of inciting medications if applicable.
- Macular edema:
  - Intravitreal anti-VEGF therapy is first-line and effective.
  - Intravitreal corticosteroids are inexpensive and effective but have a higher side effect profile (IOP elevation, cataract).
  - Focal laser can be considered if persistent and unresponsive macular edema is present.
- Neovascularization: PRP is recommended if neovascularization is present.
- Prophylactic PRP is not indicated.

66.12 Follow-Up

- Vision ≥20/40: Every 1–2 months for 6 months, then taper to annually once stabilized
- Vision 20/50–20/200: Initially every 1–2 months, decrease interval if vision or exam worsening
- Vision <20/200: Every month for 6 months, then reassess
- For all patients, monitoring of IOP, pupillary border for NVI, and gonioscopy for NVA at every exam

References and Suggested Reading

1. Natural history and clinical management of central retinal vein occlusion. Arch Ophthalmol. 1997;115(4):486–91.
2. Rogers S, McIntosh RL, Cheun N, et al. The prevalence of retinal vein occlusion: pooled data from population studies from the United States, Europe, Asia, and Australia. Ophthalmology. 2010;117:313–9.

3. Stem MS, Talwar N, Comer GM, et al. A longitudinal analysis of risk factors associated with central retinal vein occlusion. Ophthalmology. 2013;120(2):362–70.
4. Yeh S, Kim SJ, Ho AC, et al. Therapies for macular edema associated with central retinal vein occlusion: a report by the American Academy of Ophthalmology. Ophthalmology. 2015;122(4):769–78.

Chapter 67
Idiopathic Juxtafoveal Telangiectasis

Daniel Gologorsky and Amir Mohsenin

67.1 Definitions

- IJT = idiopathic juxtafoveal telangiectasis
- PDT=photodynamic therapy

67.2 Background

Idiopathic juxtafoveal telangiectasis (IJT) refers to a heterogeneous group of rare clinical conditions that entail telangiectatic changes of the juxtafoveal or parafoveal capillary network in one or both eyes.

67.3 Group 1: Unilateral Parafoveal Telangiectasia, Congenital or Acquired

67.3.1 Symptoms

Mild to moderate blurring of vision in one eye

D. Gologorsky, MD, MBA • A. Mohsenin, MD, PhD (✉)
Bascom Palmer Eye Institute, University of Miami, 900 NW 17th St., Miami, FL 33136, USA
e-mail: dangologorsky@med.miami.edu; amohsenin@gmail.com

C.A. Medina et al. (eds.), *Manual of Retinal Diseases: A Guide to Diagnosis and Management*, DOI 10.1007/978-3-319-20460-4_67

67.3.2 Signs

- >1 disk diameter (DD) telangiectasia located temporal to the fovea
- Frequently associated with macular edema and hard exudates

67.3.3 Epidemiology

- Men > women
- Mean age 40

67.3.4 Differential Diagnosis

- Must exclude other secondary causes of telangiectasia
- Diabetic retinopathy
- Retinal venous occlusions
- Radiation retinopathy
- Sickle cell maculopathy
- Ocular ischemic syndrome
- Hypertensive retinopathy
- Other conditions: polycythemia vera retinopathy and macular capillary hemangioma

67.3.5 Diagnosis

- Macular OCT (cystic or non-cystic macular edema)
- FA (capillary dilatation with late-phase leakage)

67.3.6 Prognosis

Macular edema and exudation are the main cause of visual loss. Many patients do well without any treatment. However, if progressive visual loss occurs, treatment with laser photocoagulation may be effective in reducing the exudation and stabilizing vision. Other treatment modalities include intravitreal injections of steroids or anti-VEGF agents.

67.4 Group 2: Bilateral Parafoveal Telangiectasia

67.4.1 Symptoms

- Slowly progressive disruption of central vision. These visual changes can be mild to severe in nature, and patients may note asymmetric vision changes with respect to both eyes.
- Symptoms may include blurred vision, metamorphopsia, or paracentral positive scotoma.

67.4.2 Signs

- <1 DD of telangiectasia involving the parafoveal retina bilaterally without hard exudates. Perifoveal changes are most noticeable temporally and include thickening, RPE hyperplasia, loss of transparency with a grayish foveal appearance, or a cystic foveal appearance.
- Superficial crystalline deposits, including stellate intraretinal pigment epithelial plaques and refractile retinal crystals, are a common finding in this condition.
- Proliferative disease with CNVM manifestation may develop.

67.4.3 Epidemiology

- Both genders affected equally.
- Typically affects middle-aged patients.
- Mean age 56.
- This is an acquired, non-congenital form of IJT.

67.4.4 Diagnosis

- FA: dilation and telangiectasis of the perifoveal capillary network with late intraretinal staining (Fig. 67.1a), possible CNVM
- Macular OCT: may demonstrate foveal cyst, RPE hyperplasia, foveal atrophy, and absence of edema (Fig. 67.1b)

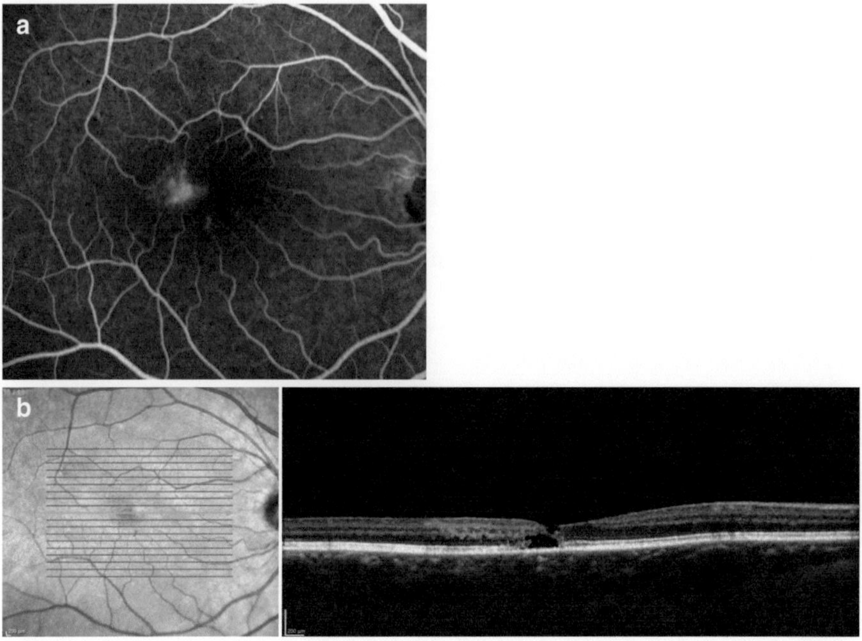

Fig. 67.1 Bilateral parafoveal telangiectasia (*Group 2*): FA demonstrating telangiectatic vessels temporal to the fovea with leakage (**a**). OCT with foveal cyst that is more prominent temporally. Retinal pigment epithelium hyperplasia, atrophy, and absence of edema are also noted (**b**)

67.4.5 Prognosis

As opposed to Group 1 IJT, vision loss in Group 2 IJT is due to retinal atrophy and subretinal neovascularization (rather than edema and exudation). About $\frac{1}{3}$ of patients demonstrate impaired glucose tolerance on testing.

- Depends on the type of Group 2 IJT.
- *Nonproliferative*: Guarded prognosis. Laser photocoagulation is of limited utility. PDT and anti-VEGF intravitreal injections have been reported in the literature.
- *Proliferative*: Poor prognosis. Intravitreal anti-VEGF injections and PDT have been used in cases of CNVM formation.

67.5 Group 3: Bilateral Parafoveal Telangiectasia and Retinal Capillary Obliteration

67.5.1 Symptoms

Gradual and progressive loss of central vision

67.5.2 Signs

Terminal capillaries with aneurysmal dilatation and progressive occlusion of parafoveal capillaries. May note optic atrophy on exam as well

67.5.3 Epidemiology

- Typically affects female > male.
- Most patients are in their 50s.

67.5.4 Diagnosis

- Macular OCT
- FA: capillary occlusion, widening of FAZ without leakage.

67.5.5 Prognosis

Typically poor. Type 3 is the most rare and severe. It represents progressive obliteration of the perifoveal capillary network, often in association with a systemic medical or neurologic condition.

References and Suggested Reading

1. Charbel Issa P, Helb HM, Holz FG, Scholl HP, MacTel Study Group. Correlation of macular function with retinal thickness in nonproliferative type 2 idiopathic macular telangiectasia. Am J Ophthalmol. 2008;145:169–75.
2. Gass JD, Blodi BA. Idiopathic juxtafoveolar retinal telangiectasis. Update of classification and follow-up study. Ophthalmology. 1993;100:1536–46.
3. Yannuzzi LA, Bardal AM, Freund KB, Chen KJ, Eandi CM, Blodi B. Idiopathic macular telangiectasia. Arch Ophthalmol. 2006;124:450–60.

Chapter 68
Radiation Retinopathy

Nikisha Kothari and Amir Mohsenin

68.1 Definitions

- VEGF = Vascular endothelial growth factor
- Gy = Gray

68.2 Symptoms

- Asymptomatic or decreased vision

68.3 Signs

- Microaneurysms
- Cotton-wool spots
- Intraretinal hemorrhages
- Retinal edema
- Can also see exudates, perivascular sheathing, disc edema, neovascularization, and optic atrophy.

N. Kothari, MD • A. Mohsenin, MD, PhD (✉)
Bascom Palmer Eye Institute, University of Miami,
900 NW 17th St., Miami, FL 33136, USA
e-mail: nkothari@med.miami.edu; amohsenin@gmail.com

C.A. Medina et al. (eds.), *Manual of Retinal Diseases: A Guide to Diagnosis and Management*, DOI 10.1007/978-3-319-20460-4_68

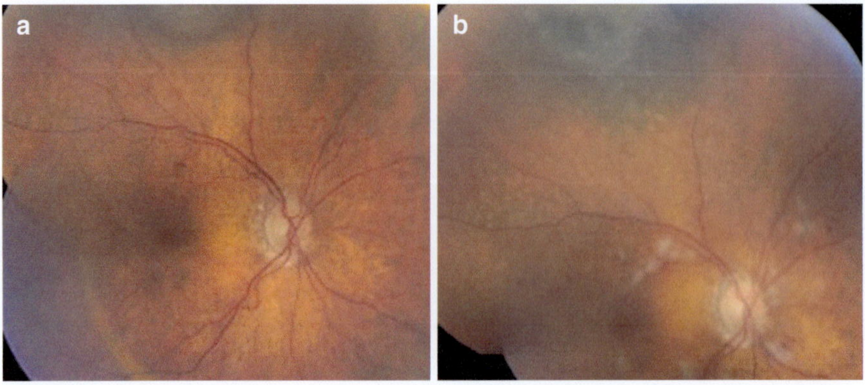

Fig. 68.1 Uveal melanoma superiorly prior to plaque therapy (a) Development of radiation retinopathy after plaque brachytherapy. (b)

68.4 Predisposing Conditions

- External beam radiation
- Local plaque brachytherapy (Fig. 68.1)
- Gamma knife therapy

68.5 Differential Diagnosis

- Diabetic retinopathy
- Hypertensive retinopathy
- Retinal vein occlusions
- Bone marrow transplant retinopathy

68.6 Etiology

Radiation results in DNA damage and the production of free radicals. Injury to the retinal vascular endothelial cells is at the core of the resulting vision-threatening complications. The loss of capillary integrity leads to microaneurysms, capillary closure, retinal edema, exudation, and ischemia. Retinal nonperfusion can lead to increased VEGF levels and proliferative disease.

68.7 Workup/Testing

- History with attention to radiation modality, radiation dose, date of treatment, and reason for treatment.
- Complete ophthalmic examination with dilation.

  - Careful attention to the presence or absence of neovascularization in the anterior and posterior segments should be made.

- OCT to assess for macular edema.
- If warranted, fluorescein angiography can be performed to assess for leakage, proliferative disease, and capillary nonperfusion.

68.8 Prognosis and Management

Radiation retinopathy is nearly indistinguishable from diabetic retinopathy. The higher the radiation dose received, the more radiation retinopathy is to be expected. The latency between radiation treatment and the onset of radiation retinopathy is highly variable ranging from weeks to years.

- Treatment is similar to the management of diabetic retinopathy.
- If macular edema is present:
  - Intravitreal anti-VEGF therapy is typically a first-line treatment.
  - Focal laser and intravitreal steroids can also be employed.
- If neovascularization is present, anti-VEGF agents and panretinal photocoagulation have been shown to be effective.

68.9 Follow-Up

- If macular edema or neovascularization is present, then monthly follow-up is warranted.
- Follow-up intervals can be extended once edema and neovascularization have regressed.

References and Suggested Reading

1. Horgan N, Shields CL, Mashayekhi A, Shields JA. Classification and treatment of radiation maculopathy. Curr Opin Ophthalmol. 2010;21(3):233–8.
2. Reichstein D. Current treatments and preventive strategies for radiation retinopathy. Curr Opin Ophthalmol. 2015;26(3):157–66.

Chapter 69
Sickle Cell Retinopathy

Nikisha Kothari and Amir Mohsenin

69.1 Definitions

- HbAS = sickle cell trait
- HbSS = sickle cell disease, hemoglobin SS
- HbSC = sickle cell disease, hemoglobin SC
- HbS-Thal = sickle cell beta-thalassemia
- ILM = internal limiting membrane

69.2 Symptoms

Asymptomatic or decreased vision

69.3 Signs

- Nonproliferative retinopathy:
  - Salmon patch hemorrhages: Hemorrhage between the retina and ILM

N. Kothari, MD • A. Mohsenin, MD, PhD (✉)
Bascom Palmer Eye Institute, University of Miami,
900 NW 17th St., Miami, FL 33136, USA
e-mail: nkothari@med.miami.edu; amohsenin@gmail.com

C.A. Medina et al. (eds.), *Manual of Retinal Diseases: A Guide to Diagnosis and Management*, DOI 10.1007/978-3-319-20460-4_69

Table 69.1 Goldberg's classification of sickle cell retinopathy

Stage 1: Peripheral arteriolar occlusions
Stage 2: Peripheral arteriovenular anastomoses
Stage 3: Neovascularization
Stage 4: Vitreous hemorrhage
Stage 5: Retinal detachment

  - Iridescent spots: Schisis cavity at a site of previous hemorrhage containing hemosiderin-laden macrophages
  - Black sunburst lesions: Oval or round hyperpigmented spots. Histopathologically, these show focal hypertrophy of the retinal pigment epithelium.
  - Angioid streaks

- Proliferative retinopathy (Table 69.1): Sea fan-shaped neovascularization

- Other ocular signs:

  - Conjunctiva: comma-shaped blood vessels.
  - Iris: sectoral iris atrophy and pupillary irregularities.
  - Optic disc: dilated capillaries that may look like small dark dots. Neovascularization of the disk can be present but is rare.
  - Choroid: choroidal infarction.

69.4 Epidemiology

Predilection for African American, Hispanic, and Mediterranean populations

69.5 Inheritance

- Autosomal recessive.
- One allele is HbS and the other is HbS, C, or Thal.

69.6 Differential Diagnosis

- Diabetic retinopathy
- Retinal vein occlusion

- Retinal artery occlusion
- Retinopathy of prematurity
- Familial exudative vitreoretinopathy

69.7 Etiology

Mutations in the β-globin gene result in erythrocytes that undergo sickling in response to hypoxic, acidotic, and hyperosmolar conditions. Sickled erythrocytes are not pliable thereby resulting in mechanical occlusion of arterioles. Arteriolar occlusion is at the core of sickle cell retinopathy as it causes both nonproliferative and proliferative disease.

69.8 Workup/Testing

- Complete medical, family, and ocular history.
- Complete ophthalmic examination with dilation.
- Wide-field fluorescein angiography to assess for ischemia and neovascular disease (Fig. 69.1).
- SD-OCT can be obtained to evaluate for subclinical thinning in the macula.
- Laboratory testing:
  - Screening test: sickle cell preparation. False negatives and positives may occur in patients with severe anemia or with recent history of blood transfusion.
  - Definitive testing: hemoglobin electrophoresis

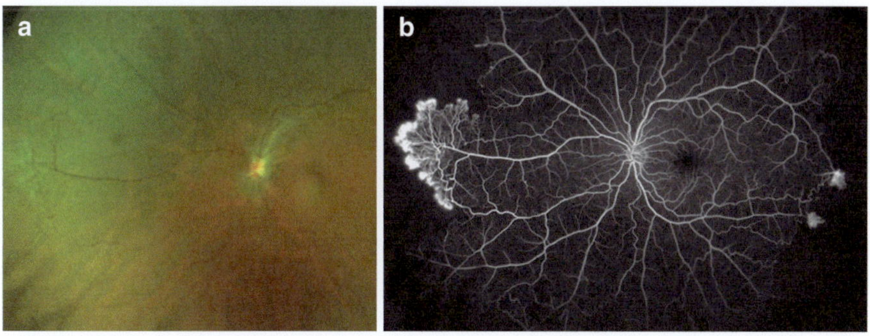

Fig. 69.1 Sea fan-shaped neovascularization demonstrated in periphery on (**a**) Optos fundus photos and (**b**) fluorescein angiography

69.9 Prognosis and Management

- HbSC and HbS-Thal have a higher incidence of retinopathy than HbSS.
- Vision loss is variable and based on severity of disease.
- Proliferative sickle cell lesions frequently undergo autoinfarction frequently making observation a good initial treatment choice.
- Observation is appropriate for asymptomatic peripheral lesions.
- Treatment can be instituted if there is significant vision loss or if the fellow eye has poor vision.
- Treatment options include:
  - Peripheral scatter photocoagulation in areas of ischemia.
  - Anti-VEGF agents have been successfully used for proliferative disease but should be used with caution as data is limited.
  - Pars plana vitrectomy for non-clearing vitreous hemorrhage and/or retinal detachment.
- Of note, sickle cell patients with hyphema have an increased risk of complications including a difficult-to-control intraocular pressure. In these patients, carbonic anhydrase inhibitors should be avoided as they cause acidosis and precipitate sickling.

69.10 Follow-Up

Frequency of screening is not established, though patients with HbSC should be monitoring more carefully for the development of retinopathy.

References and Suggested Reading

1. Chen RW, Flynn Jr HW, Lee WH, Parke DW, Isom RF, Davis JL, Smiddy WE. Vitreoretinal management and surgical outcomes in proliferative sickle retinopathy: a case series. Am J Ophthalmol. 2014;157(4):870–5.
2. Downes SM, Hambleton I, Chuang E, Lois N, Serjeant G, Bird A. Incidence and natural history of proliferative sickle cell retinopathy. Ophthalmology. 2011;112(11):1869–75.
3. Lim J. Ophthalmic manifestations of sickle cell disease: update of latest findings. Curr Opin Ophthalmol. 2012;23(6):533–6.

Chapter 70
Ocular Ischemic Syndrome

Daniel Gologorsky and Amir Mohsenin

70.1 Definitions

- NVA: neovascularization of the angle
- NVE: neovascularization elsewhere
- NVI: neovascularization of the iris
- OIS: ocular ischemic syndrome

70.2 Symptoms

- Gradual loss of vision over days to weeks.
- Often accompanied by ocular or periocular pain or a significant headache.
- Prolonged recovery of vision after bright-light exposure.
- Patients will often describe a history of amaurosis fugax.

70.3 Signs

- Vision ranges from 20/20 to NLP
- 80 % of cases are unilateral; 20 % are bilateral
- Anterior segment findings

D. Gologorsky, MD, MBA • A. Mohsenin, MD, PhD (✉)
Bascom Palmer Eye Institute, University of Miami, 900 NW 17th St.,
Miami, FL 33136, USA
e-mail: dangologorsky@med.miami.edu; amohsenin@gmail.com

C.A. Medina et al. (eds.), *Manual of Retinal Diseases: A Guide to Diagnosis and Management*, DOI 10.1007/978-3-319-20460-4_70

- Mild uveitis
- Corneal edema
- NVI or NVA that may progress to neovascular glaucoma
- Posterior segment findings
- Dilated and irregular veins
- Narrowed arterioles
- Scattered mid-peripheral retinal hemorrhages, retinal microaneurysms, and cotton wool spots
- Macular edema
- NVD or NVE may occur in 1/3 of cases

70.4 Epidemiology

- Typically occurs in elderly patients, ages 50–80, mean age 65
- Men:women = 2:1

70.5 Predisposing Conditions

Hypertension (73 % of cases), carotid occlusive disease, diabetes (56 % of cases), cardiac valvular disease, stroke (25 % of cases), and peripheral vascular disease (20 % of cases)

70.6 Differential Diagnosis

- CRVO
- Diabetic retinopathy
- Aortic arch syndrome caused by atherosclerosis, Takayasu's arteritis, or giant cell arteritis

70.7 Etiology

- OIS is usually caused by occlusive carotid disease. Most often, atheromas cause stenosis at the bifurcation of the common carotid artery.
- OIS occurs with >90 % occlusion of the ipsilateral carotid artery (or rarely, ophthalmic artery). With this degree of stenosis, central retinal artery perfusion drops by 50 %.
- Note that only 5 % of internal carotid artery stenosis patients develop OIS.

70.8 Workup/Testing

- Ophthalmic exam and history
- Fluorescein angiography showing delayed filling and prolonged transit times. May see macular leakage and edema
- Duplex carotid artery ultrasound, magnetic resonance angiogram (MRA)
- Cardiology consultation

70.9 Treatment

- Multidisciplinary approach with ophthalmology, cardiology, neurology, and vascular surgery.
- Ophthalmic treatment is focused on controlling anterior segment inflammation, sequela of retinal ischemia, and neovascular glaucoma.
- Anterior segment inflammation is managed with topical steroidal agents.
- Anterior or posterior segment neovascularization is managed with panretinal photocoagulation and/or intravitreal injections.
- Neovascular glaucoma may require topical IOP-lowering drops or glaucoma surgery.
- Surgical candidates, defined as those with <99 % carotid artery occlusion, should be evaluated by vascular surgery for possible carotid endarterectomy.
- Primary care physicians must coordinate the management of hypertension, diabetes, and atherosclerotic disease.
- Smoking cessation must be emphasized for all patients.

70.10 Prognosis and Management

Whenever encountering asymmetric retinopathy, always think of carotid occlusive disease and OIS. Cardiac death is the main cause of mortality. Remember the rule of thirds: $\frac{1}{3}$ of cases improve with carotid endarterectomy, $\frac{1}{3}$ remain the same, and $\frac{1}{3}$ deteriorate. Cases of OIS carry a poor visual prognosis.

70.11 Follow-Up

- Depends on the clinical picture. Cases of neovascularization should be followed more closely for PRP and intraocular pressure control.
- Surgical candidates should be referred urgently.

References and Suggested Reading

1. Brown GC, Magargal LE. The ocular ischemic syndrome. Clinical, fluorescein angiographic and carotid angiographic features. Int Ophthalmol. 1988;11(4):239–51.
2. Chen CS, Miller NR. Ocular ischemic syndrome: review of clinical presentations, etiology, investigation, and management. Compr Ophthalmol Update. 2007;8(1):17–28.
3. Mendrinos E, Machinis TG, Pournaras CJ. Ocular ischemic syndrome. Surv Ophthalmol. 2010;55(1):2–34.
4. Mizener JB, Podhajsky P, Hayreh SS. Ocular ischemic syndrome. Ophthalmology. 1997; 104(5):859–64.

Chapter 71
Retinal Arterial Macroaneurysm

Nikisha Kothari and Amir Mohsenin

71.1 Definitions

- RAM: retinal arterial macroaneurysm
- CNVM: choroidal neovascular membrane
- RPE: retinal pigment epithelium

71.2 Symptoms

- Asymptomatic or decreased vision

71.3 Signs

- Macroaneurysm, typically temporal.
- Hemorrhage (Fig. 71.1). Sub-RPE, subretinal, intraretinal, preretinal, or break-through into the vitreous.
- Exudation.
- Hypertensive retinopathy with arteriovenous nicking.
- Retinal vein and arterial occlusions have been described in association with RAM.

N. Kothari, MD • A. Mohsenin, MD, PhD (✉)
Department of Ophthalmology, Bascom Palmer Eye Institute, University of Miami,
900 NW 17th St., Miami, FL 33136, USA
e-mail: nkothari@med.miami.edu; amohsenin@gmail.com

C.A. Medina et al. (eds.), *Manual of Retinal Diseases: A Guide to Diagnosis and Management*, DOI 10.1007/978-3-319-20460-4_71

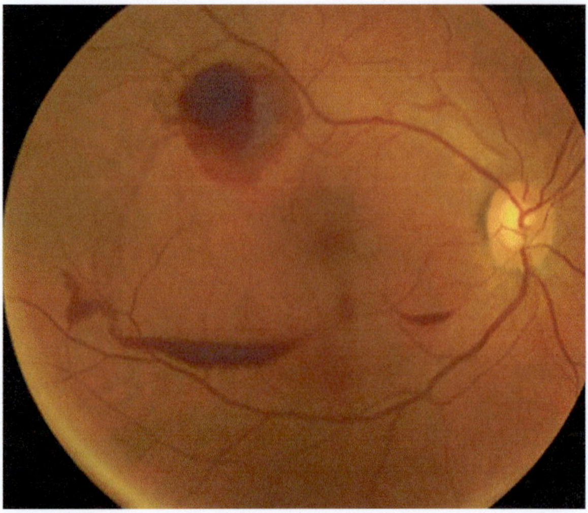

Fig. 71.1 Retinal macroaneurysm in superotemporal macula with associated subhyaloid hemorrhage

71.4 Predisposing Conditions

- Systemic hypertension (present in 90 % of patients with RAM)
- Age (typically over 60 years)
- Gender (typically female)

71.5 Differential Diagnosis

- Diabetic retinopathy
- Radiation retinopathy
- Von Hippel-Lindau with capillary hemangioblastoma
- Coats' disease
- Age-related macular degeneration with CNVM

71.6 Etiology

Systemic hypertension leads to hyaline degeneration and increased collagen in the intima resulting in decreased vessel wall elasticity. Hypertension increases transmural pressure causing outpouching of the wall within the first three orders of the arterial tree. Leakage may occur from the aneurysm or from the surrounding capillaries. If the aneurysm ruptures, then hemorrhage at all levels is possible.

71.7 Workup/Testing

- Complete ophthalmic examination with attention to vascular changes
- Fluorescein angiography
  - Demonstrates a saccular or fusiform aneurysm filling during the early arterial phase
  - Leakage if the blood-retinal barrier is disrupted
  - Blockage if hemorrhage is present
- Indocyanine green angiography
  - Can be beneficial if hemorrhage is present due to its greater penetration compared to fluorescein
- Primary care physician consultation
  - For management of hypertension and evaluation for other systemic vascular diseases

71.8 Prognosis and Management

- Good overall prognosis as these lesions tend to spontaneously resolve.
- Quiescent lesions should be monitored.
- No clear treatment method or treatment criteria have been established.
- Laser photocoagulation to the surrounding capillary bed can be considered if the lesion threatens the macula.
- Hemorrhagic macroaneurysms can be observed as they typically undergo spontaneous thrombosis.
- Vitrectomy can be considered for non-clearing vitreous hemorrhage or a large submacular hemorrhage.

71.9 Follow-Up

Examination interval based on RAM location, presence of hemorrhage, exudates, and macular status

References and Suggested Reading

1. Lavin MJ, Marsh RJ, Peart S, Rehman A. Retinal arterial macroaneurysms: a retrospective study of 40 patients. Br Ophthalmol. 1987;71(11):817–25.
2. Moosavi RA, Fong KC, Chopdar A. Retinal artery macroaneurysms: clinical and fluorescein angiographic features in 34 patients. Eye (Lond). 2006;20(9):1011–20.

Section X
Age Related Macular Degeneration

John E. Legarreta

Chapter 72
Clinical Trials in Age-Related Macular Degeneration

John E. Legarreta

Age-related macular degeneration (AMD) is a leading cause of blindness in elderly adults in the United States and other developed countries across the world. Exudative or "wet" AMD remains the leading cause of AMD-related blindness.

The last 15 years have seen radical changes in the treatment of wet AMD from focal laser photocoagulation and photodynamic therapy to the recent development of anti-vascular endothelial growth factor (anti-VEGF) intravitreal injections, which are now the gold standard for treatment of wet AMD. Several clinical trials are underway as the treatment modalities continue to evolve. Below is a summary of important clinical trials over the last couple of decades.

72.1 Age-Related Eye Disease Study (AREDS)

The purpose of this study was to evaluate the effects of antioxidants and zinc on the progression of AMD. The study concluded that eyes with intermediate AMD or advanced AMD and vision loss in one eye could reduce their risk of developing advanced AMD by 25 % by taking antioxidants and zinc.

72.2 Age-Related Eye Disease Study 2 (AREDS2)

The purpose of this study was to evaluate the effects of lutein, zeaxanthin, docosahexaenoic acid, and eicosapentaenoic acid on the progression of AMD. The study concluded that the addition of lutein, zeaxanthin, docosahexaenoic acid, and

J.E. Legarreta, MD
Bascom Palmer Eye Institute, University of Miami,
900 NW 17th St., Miami, FL 33136, USA
e-mail: legarretaje@icloud.com

C.A. Medina et al. (eds.), *Manual of Retinal Diseases: A Guide to Diagnosis and Management*, DOI 10.1007/978-3-319-20460-4_72

eicosapentaenoic acid to the original AREDS formulation did not further reduce risk of progression to advanced AMD. Additionally, due to concerns for increased incidence of lung cancer in former smokers, lutein and zeaxanthin were determined to be an equivalent carotenoid substitute in the AREDS2 formulation.

72.3 Treatment of Age-Related Macular Degeneration with Photodynamic Therapy (TAP)

The purpose of this study was to evaluate the use of verteporfin in photodynamic therapy (PDT) in patients with wet AMD and classic subfoveal choroidal neovascularization. The primary outcome measure for this study was less than 15 letters of vision loss at 2 years. The results of the study showed a statistically significant benefit in the PDT-treated eyes compared to placebo; however, this was only true for eyes that had predominantly classic CNV. There was no statistically significant benefit in eyes with only minimally classic CNV.

72.4 Verteporfin in Photodynamic Therapy (VIP)

The purpose of this study was to evaluate the use of verteporfin in photodynamic therapy (PDT) in patients with subfoveal CNV due to myopia as well as occult subfoveal CNV due to AMD. The results of the study found a benefit for PDT-treated eyes with CNV due to myopia. The study also found a treatment benefit in PDT-treated eyes that had occult lesions that were less than four disk areas and eyes with vision worse than 20/50.

72.5 VEGF Inhibition Study in Ocular Neovascularization (VISION)

The purpose of this study was to evaluate the benefit of pegaptanib sodium (Macugen) in patients with wet AMD. The primary outcome measure for this study was less than 15 letters of vision loss at 1 year. The study found a benefit in patients treated with pegaptanib sodium compared with placebo.

72.6 Anti-VEGF Antibody for the Treatment of Predominantly Classic Choroidal Neovascularization in AMD (ANCHOR)

The purpose of this study was to evaluate the use of ranibizumab (Lucentis) in patients with predominantly classic CNV in AMD and compare it to verteporfin in photodynamic therapy (PDT). The primary outcome measures were the number of eyes losing less than 15 letters and the numbers of eyes gaining more than 15 letters. The results of the study concluded that ranibizumab was superior to PDT at 2 years.

72.7 Minimally Classic/Occult Trial of Anti-VEGF Antibody Ranibizumab in the Treatment of Neovascular ARMD (MARINA)

The purpose of this study was to evaluate the use of ranibizumab (Lucentis) in patients with minimally classic/occult CNV in AMD. The primary outcome measure was the number of eyes losing less than 15 letters and the numbers of eyes gaining more than 15 letters. The results of the study concluded that ranibizumab showed a statistically significant difference in reducing and improving vision compared to sham injections in this patient population.

72.8 Comparison of Age-Related Macular Degeneration Treatment Trials (CATT)

The purpose of the study was to compare ranibizumab and bevacizumab for the treatment of wet AMD and evaluate monthly versus as-needed treatment for 2 years. The primary outcome measure was the change in vision at 1 year. The results of the study showed that ranibizumab and bevacizumab have similar vision acuity effects at 1 year. Monthly bevacizumab was similar to monthly ranibizumab on visual acuity outcomes, and as-needed bevacizumab was similar to as-needed ranibizumab on visual acuity outcomes.

72.9 VEGF Trap-Eye: Investigation of Efficacy and Safety in Wet AMD (VIEW 1 and 2)

The purpose of these studies was to compare monthly and every-2-month VEGF Trap-Eye (aflibercept or Eylea) with monthly ranibizumab. The results of the studies show that VEGF Trap-Eye was similar in efficacy at monthly and every-2-month dosing when compared to monthly ranibizumab.

References and Suggested Reading

1. Ciulla TA, Rosenfeld PJ. Anti-vascular endothelial growth factor therapy for neovascular age-related macular degeneration. Curr Opin Ophthalmol. 2009;20:158–65.
2. Gupta AK, Aggarwal VK, Goel N. Handbook of clinical trials in ophthalmology. Wolters Kluwer Health, Inc.: Jp Medical Ltd.; 2014.

Chapter 73
Nonexudative Age-Related Macular Degeneration

Andrew D. Legarreta and John E. Legarreta

73.1 Definitions

- Age-related macular degeneration (AMD)
- Geographic atrophy (GA)
- Reticular pseudodrusen (RPD)

73.2 Symptoms

Gradual vision loss (central vision), distorted vision, or blurred vision

73.3 Signs

- Early: Appearance of few drusen and/or RPD, disruption of retinal pigment epithelium (Fig. 73.1a)
- Intermediate: Appearance of numerous drusen and/or RPD, GA not involving the central macula
- Late: Appearance of numerous drusen and/or RPD, GA in the central macula

A.D. Legarreta, BA
Research Associate, Department of Ophthalmology,
Bascom Palmer Eye Institute, University of Miami,
900 NW 17th St., Miami, FL 33136, USA

J.E. Legarreta, MD (✉)
Bascom Palmer Eye Institute, University of Miami,
900 NW 17th St., Miami, FL 33136, USA
e-mail: jel60@med.miami.edu

C.A. Medina et al. (eds.), *Manual of Retinal Diseases: A Guide to Diagnosis and Management*, DOI 10.1007/978-3-319-20460-4_73

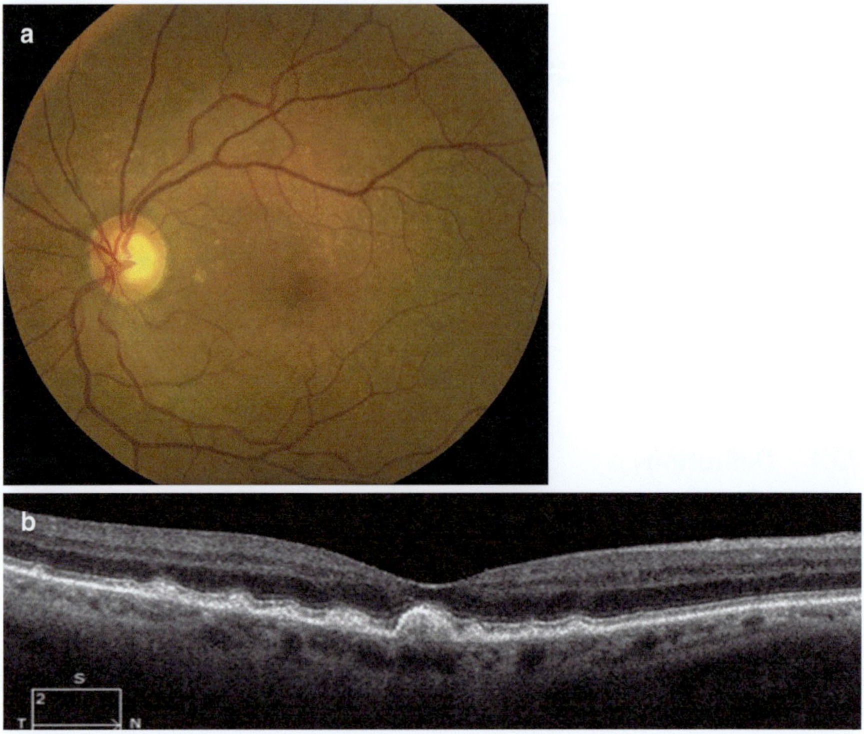

Fig. 73.1 Fundus photo showing multiple drusen in the macula along with mild mottling of the RPE (**a**). OCT showing drusen with absence of macular fluid (**b**)

73.4 Epidemiology

- Nonexudative AMD is believed to account for 80–90 % of all AMD cases.
- In Caucasian people over 40, the prevalence of early AMD is estimated at 6.8 %; late AMD is at 1.5 %.
- Occurrence of AMD is nine to ten times more common in a white population compared to a black population.

73.5 Predisposing Conditions

- Advanced age
- History of smoking
- Genetic inheritance
- White race
- Obesity
- Hypertension
- Hypercholesterolemia

73.6 Inheritance

AMD involves the inheritance of multiple heterogeneous phenotypes. It has been reported that polymorphisms in complement factor H, complement factor B, and C2 genes may be responsible for 75 % of cases of AMD. Twin studies and familial analyses have provided clear evidence of the heritability of AMD, but further research is required to elucidate the genetic roots of the disease.

73.7 Differential Diagnosis

Drusen, Central serous retinopathy, Myopic degeneration, Stargardt disease, Pattern dystrophy, Inherited retinal dystrophy

73.8 Workup/Testing

- Complete ocular examination with Amsler grid testing documentation and dilated fundus examination
- Optical coherence tomography (Fig. 73.1b)
- Color fundus photography
- Fundus autofluorescence
- Fluorescein angiography (consider when exam/testing concerning for exudative process)

73.9 Prognosis and Management

Individuals with intermediate dry AMD or advanced dry AMD or wet AMD in the other eye should have dietary supplementation with AREDS vitamins, which have been shown to provide some benefit in slowing the progression to advanced AMD in about 25 % of patients. Additionally, several clinical trials are underway targeting various pathways for the treatment/prevention of dry AMD.

73.10 Follow-Up

Recommended follow-up is every 6–12 months. Patient should be instructed to check their Amsler grid daily in each eye and report any changes immediately.

References and Suggested Reading

1. Age-Related Eye Disease Study 2 Research Group. Lutein + zeaxanthin and omega-3 fatty acids for age-related macular degeneration: the Age-Related Eye Disease Study 2 (AREDS2) randomized clinical trial. JAMA. 2013;309(19):2005–15.
2. Jager RD, et al. Age-related macular degeneration. N Engl J Med. 2008;358(24):2606–17.
3. Lim LS, et al. Age-related macular degeneration. Lancet. 2012;379(9827):1728–38.

Chapter 74
Exudative Age-Related Macular Degeneration

Andrew D. Legarreta and John E. Legarreta

74.1 Definitions

- Vascular endothelial growth factor (VEGF)
- Neovascular age-related macular degeneration (NVAMD)

74.2 Symptoms

Sudden vision loss, metamorphopsia, and scotoma

74.3 Signs

Drusen, pigmentary changes, RPE mottling, subretinal fluid, intraretinal fluid, retinal pigment epithelium detachment, fibrotic scar, hemorrhage, and hard exudates (Fig. 74.1).

A.D. Legarreta, BA
Research Associate, Department of Ophthalmology,
Bascom Palmer Eye Institute, University of Miami,
900 NW 17th St., Miami, FL 33136, USA

J.E. Legarreta, MD (✉)
Bascom Palmer Eye Institute, University of Miami,
900 NW 17th St., Miami, FL 33136, USA
e-mail: jel60@med.miami.edu

C.A. Medina et al. (eds.), *Manual of Retinal Diseases: A Guide to Diagnosis and Management*, DOI 10.1007/978-3-319-20460-4_74

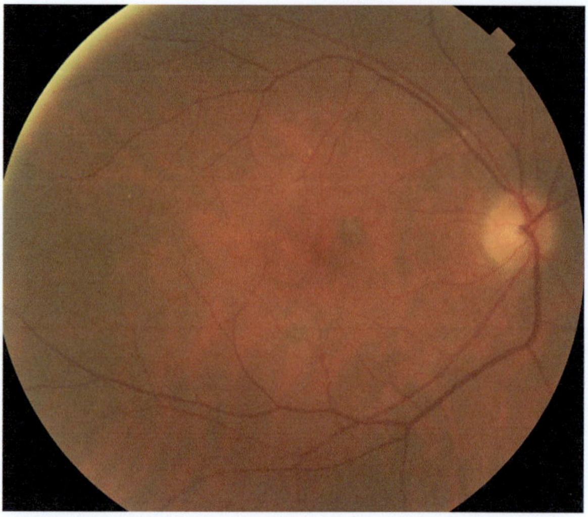

Fig. 74.1 Fundus photo showing drusen, RPE mottling, and choroidal neovascular membrane superior and nasal to fovea

74.4 Epidemiology

- In white people over 40 years of age, the prevalence of early AMD is estimated at 6.8 % and late AMD 1.5 %.
- Occurrence of AMD is nine to ten times more common in a white population compared to a black population.
- Polypoidal choroidal vasculopathy (PCV), a variant of choroidal neovascularization, is more common in Asians. Roughly 50 % of NVAMD cases occur as PCV in Asians but only 8–13 % in whites [1].

74.5 Predisposing Conditions

- Advanced age
- History of smoking
- Genetic inheritance
- White race
- Obesity

74.6 Inheritance

AMD involves the inheritance of multiple heterogeneous phenotypes. It has been reported that polymorphisms in complement factor H, complement factor B, and C2 genes may be responsible for 75 % of cases of AMD. Twin studies and familial analyses have provided clear evidence of the heritability of AMD, but further research is required to elucidate all genetic roots of the disease.

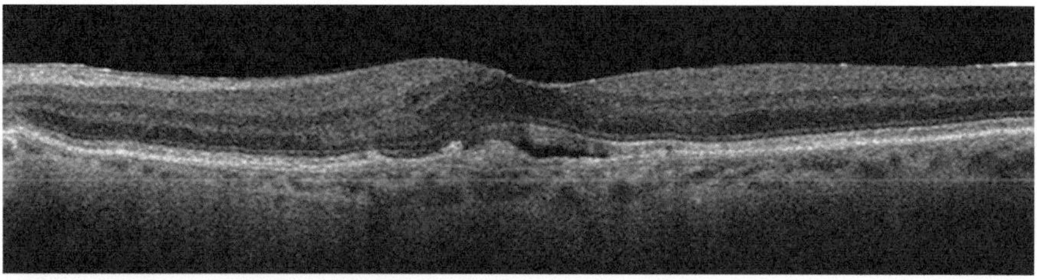

Fig. 74.2 OCT B-scan showing PED with associated SRF

74.7 Differential Diagnosis

Central serous chorioretinopathy, macular telangiectasia, vitelliform dystrophy, myopic degeneration, idiopathic polypoidal choroidal vasculopathy (IPCV), and CNV from other etiologies.

74.8 Etiology

Vascular endothelial growth factor (VEGF) pathway has been strongly implicated in the formation of NVAMD. VEGF is most closely linked to the development of choroidal neovascularization (CNV) and retinal angiomatous proliferation (RAP) lesions. Polypoidal choroidal vasculopathy (PCV) is believed to have a weaker association with the VEGF pathway.

74.9 Workup/Testing

- Complete ocular examination with dilated fundus examination
- Optical coherence tomography (Fig. 74.2)
- Color fundus photography
- Fundus autofluorescence (Fig. 74.3)
- Fluorescein angiography
- Indocyanine green angiography

74.10 Prognosis and Management

Intravitreal antiangiogenic therapy is the first choice of treatment. Bevacizumab, ranibizumab, or aflibercept can be injected intravitreously. Three treatment strategies are commonly used:

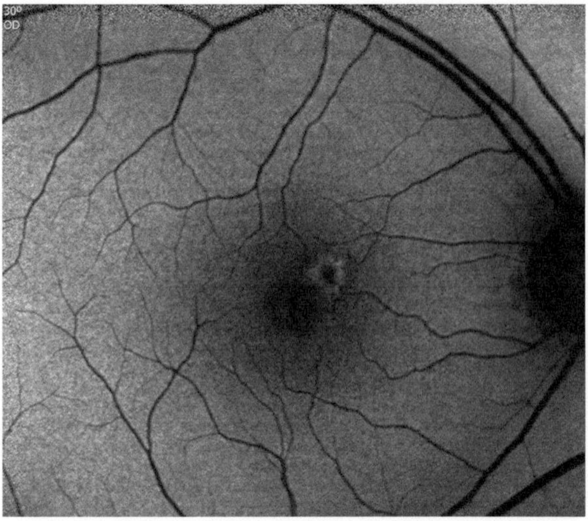

Fig. 74.3 Fundus autofluorescence showing area of increased autofluorescence superior and nasal to fovea corresponding to a choroidal neovascular membrane

1. Monthly – An anti-VEGF agent is injected every 4 weeks.
2. Pro re nata or "as needed" – An anti-VEGF agent is injected every time fluid or blood is present.
3. Treat and extend – An anti-VEGF agent is injected when fluid or blood is present, and the patient is brought back at a set interval. If there is no blood or fluid on the follow-up exam, the patient is injected, and the interval between visits is increased. If there is blood or fluid on the follow-up exam, the patient is injected, and the interval between visits decreases. The goal is to extend a patient to the maximum interval of visits before blood or fluid reappears.

74.11 Caveat

Not all fluid in the retina is caused by VEGF and therefore will not respond to intravitreal injection of anti VEGF agents. Consider a "VEGF challenge" when it is unclear if the fluid is caused by VEGF. The following strategies are used:

1. Inject an anti-VEGF agent and assess response to therapy 1–2 weeks later. Maximal response to an anti-VEGF agent is apparent 1–2 weeks following the injection. Improved outcome indicates the process has a VEGF-mediated component.
2. Inject an anti-VEGF agent at a smaller time interval and assess for response to therapy (i.e., injection frequency changes from monthly to biweekly).
   (a) Improved outcome indicates the process has a VEGF-mediated component.
   (b) It is possible that the amount of VEGF present requires a greater treatment frequency.

3. Forego an anti-VEGF injection and examine the patient again 1–2 weeks later.
    (a) Diminished outcome indicates the process has a VEGF-mediated component.
    (b) Neutral outcome indicates the process may not be caused by VEGF.

74.12 Follow-Up

Depending on the severity of the subretinal or intraretinal fluid, follow-up can range from 1 to 4 weeks following the first injection. Subsequent follow-up frequency depends on the treatment regimen selected.

References and Suggested Reading

1. Lim LS, et al. Age-related macular degeneration. Lancet. 2012;379(9827):1728–38.
2. Jager RD, et al. Age-related macular degeneration. N Engl J Med. 2008;358(24):2606–17.

Chapter 75
AMD Masquerade Syndromes

John E. Legarreta

75.1 Definitions

Age-related macular degeneration (AMD) masquerade syndromes can mimic both dry AMD and wet AMD.

75.2 Dry AMD Masquerade Syndromes

Geographic atrophy is a common feature of dry AMD masquerade syndromes (Fig. 75.1).

75.3 Wet AMD Masquerade Syndromes

Typically diagnosed after treatment with anti-VEGF therapy.
Lack of response to anti-VEGF therapy raises suspicion.

75.4 Workup/Testing

- Dilated fundus examination
- Fundus photography (including red-free and infrared reflectance)
- Fundus autofluorescence (FAF)

J.E. Legarreta, MD
Department of Ophthalmology, Bascom Palmer Eye Institute, University of Miami, 900 NW 17th St., Miami, FL 33136, USA
e-mail: jel60@med.miami.edu

C.A. Medina et al. (eds.), *Manual of Retinal Diseases: A Guide to Diagnosis and Management*, DOI 10.1007/978-3-319-20460-4_75

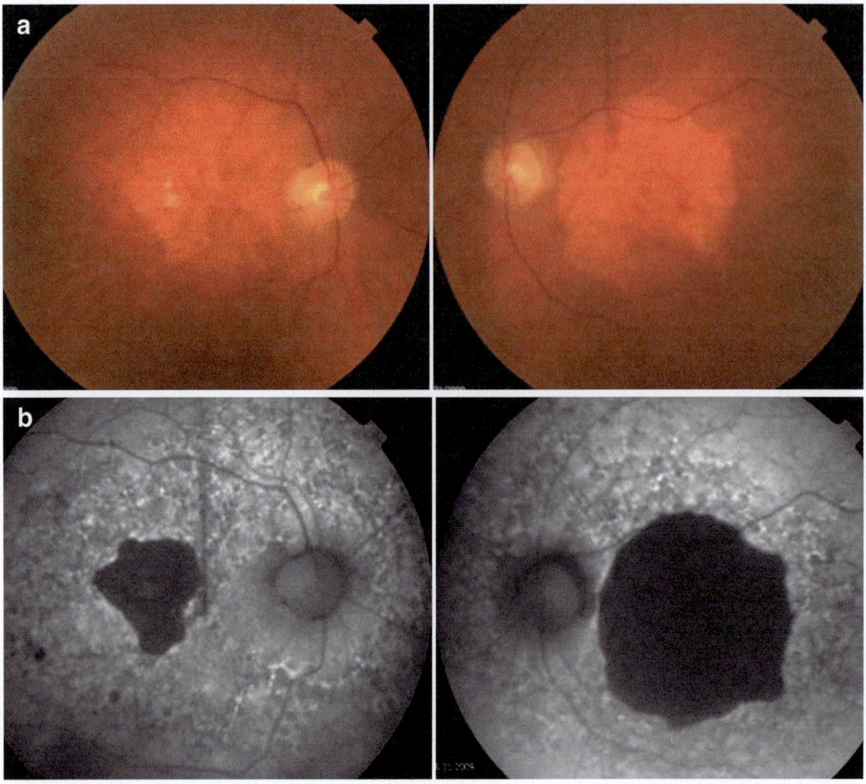

Fig. 75.1 Fundus photos (**a**) and bottom autofluorescence (**b**) reveal well-circumscribed geographic atrophy in the central macula. This case is of genetically confirmed Stargardt's disease

Table 75.1 Differential diagnosis for dry AMD masquerade syndromes with geographic atrophy

Late-onset Stargardt's disease
Advanced pathologic myopia
Advanced pattern dystrophy
Advanced vitelliform lesions
Adult onset vitelliform dystrophy/Best disease

Table 75.2 Differential diagnosis for wet AMD masquerade syndromes with a lack of response to anti-VEGF therapy

Non-vascularized PEDs
Vitelliform lesions (Fig. 75.2)
Polypoidal choroidal vasculopathy
Central serous chorioretinopathy (Fig. 75.3)
Choroidal nevus with subretinal fluid (Fig. 75.4)
Retinal tubulation
Vitreomacular traction
Macular telangiectasia type II (Fig. 75.5)

Myopic CNV and idiopathic CNV respond to anti-VEGF therapy

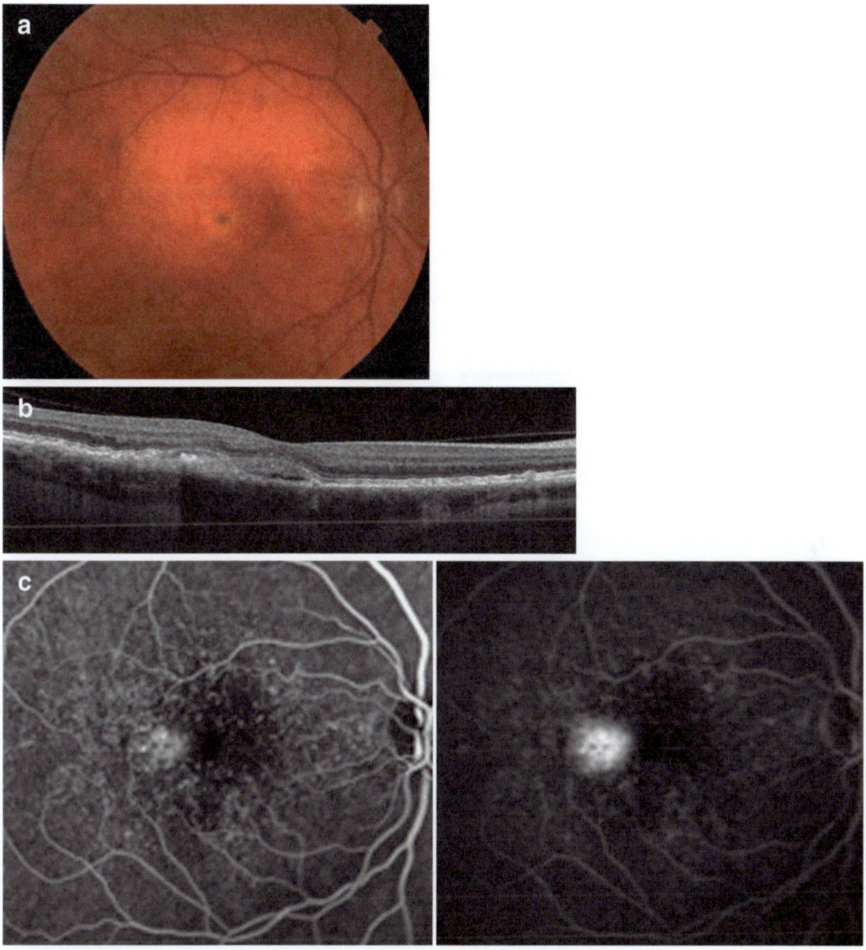

Fig. 75.2 Vitelliform lesion non-responsive to anti-VEGF therapy. Fundus photo showing RPE and pigmentary changes (**a**) and OCT showing PED with small amount of SRF (**b**). FA showing increasing hyperfluorescence consistent with leakage (**c**)

- Optical coherence tomography (OCT)
- Enhanced depth imaging OCT (EDI-OCT)
- Fluorescein angiography (FA)
- Indocyanine green angiography (ICGA)

75.5 Prognosis and Management

Management depends on determining the exact etiology. If a diagnosis is not ascertained with careful examination and multimodal imaging, close observation may be warranted. Alternatively performing an anti-VEGF challenge may be helpful in

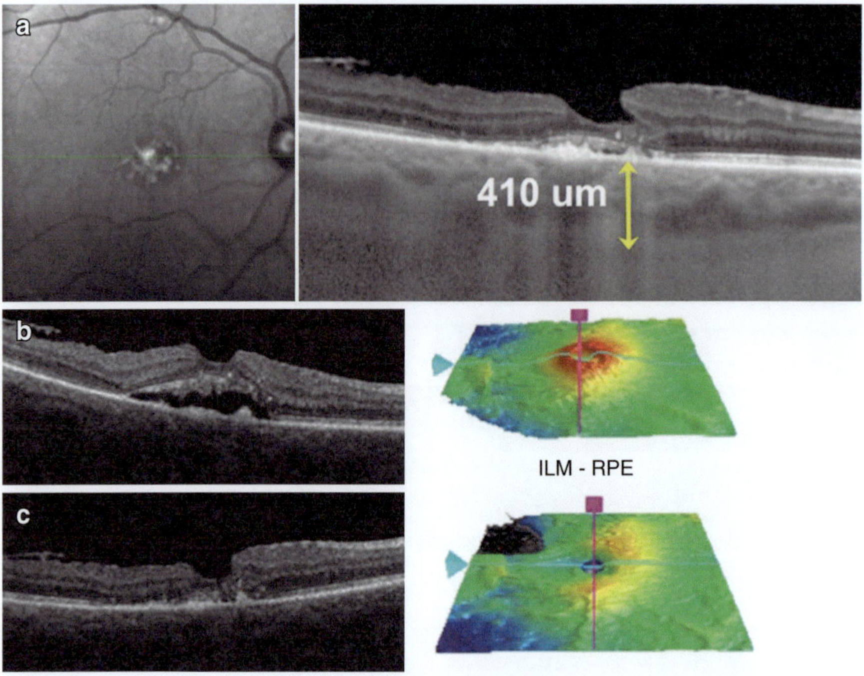

Fig. 75.3 Chronic CSR. OCT with EDI showing thickened choroid (**a**), OCT showing chronic SRF prior to therapy (**b**), resolved SRF after reduced fluence PDT (**c**)

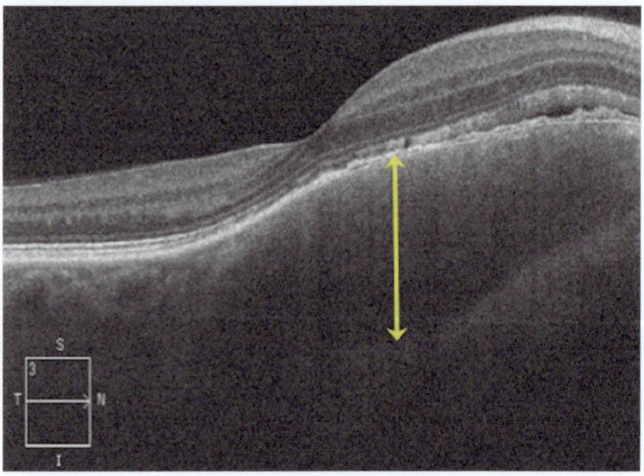

Fig. 75.4 OCT showing choroidal nevus with associated SRF

elucidating whether or not the process is mediated by VEGF. This can be done by administering an anti-VEGF agent and having the patient return in 1–2 weeks to assess for response to therapy on OCT. If no response is seen on OCT (improvement or resolution of macular fluid), then a masquerade syndrome should be considered. Specific prognoses depend on the underlying pathology.

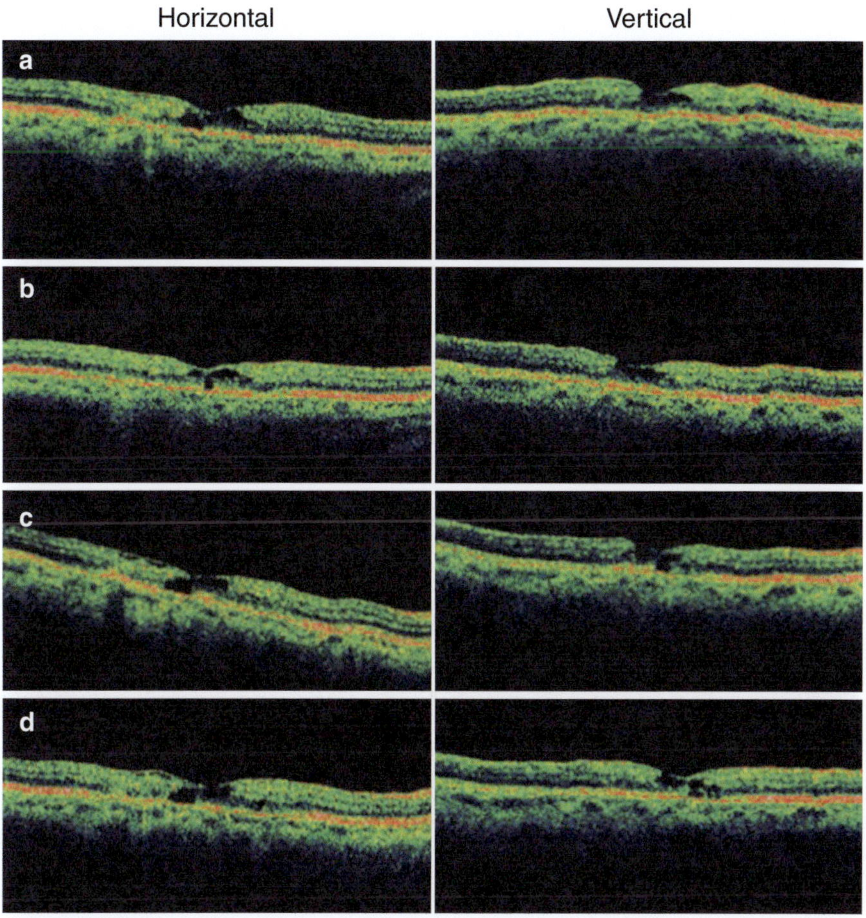

Fig. 75.5 MacTel2. OCT showing cystic cavitations. Anti-VEGF agent given (**a**). One month after anti-VEGF agent showing no significant changes in cystoid maculopathy (**b**). Two months (**c**) and 3 months (**d**) after anti-VEGF agent showing stable cystoid maculopathy

75.6 Follow-Up

Variable depending on the underlying etiology.

References and Suggested Reading

1. Karmel M. Wet AMD Look-alikes. Eyenet. Dec 2014. http://www.aao.org/eyenet/article/wet-amd-lookalikes?december-2014.
2. Kovach JL, Rosenfeld PJ. Bevacizumab (avastin) therapy for idiopathic macular telangiectasia type II. Retina. 2009;29(1):27–32.

3. Schulze S, Hoerle S, Mennel S, Kroll P. Vitreomacular traction and exudative age-related macular degeneration. Acta Ophthalmol. 2008;86(5):470–81.
4. Sikorski BL, Bukowska D, Kaluzny JJ, Szkulmowski M, Kowalczyk A, Wojtkowski M. Drusen with accompanying fluid underneath the sensory retina. Ophthalmology. 2011;118(1):82–92.

Section XI
Macular Diseases

Royce W.S. Chen

Chapter 76
Myopic Degeneration

Elona Dhrami-Gavazi and Royce W.S. Chen

76.1 Definitions

Degenerative or pathological myopia: characterized by a high myopic refractive error (usually > –6.00 D or, in countries like Japan, > –8.00 D), which typically is due to progressive increase of the axial length in excess of 26 mm; associated with degenerative changes.

76.2 Signs

A study of 308 eyes by Grossniklaus and Green described the histopathological findings in pathological myopia. They include:

- An insidiously progressive thinning and atrophy of the retinal pigment epithelium (RPE) and choriocapillaris that leads to the typical appearance of the *tessellated* or *tigroid* fundus and ultimately *geographic atrophy* formation and *bare sclera* (Figs. 76.1, 76.2, and 76.3)

E. Dhrami-Gavazi, MD
Department of Ophthalmology, Edward S. Harkness Eye Institute, Columbia University College of Physicians and Surgeons, 635 W. 165th Street, Box 104, New York, NY 10032, USA

Vitreous-Retina-Macula Consultants of New York, The LuEsther T. Mertz Retinal Research Center, Manhattan Eye, Ear and Throat Hospital, New York, NY, USA

R.W.S. Chen, MD (✉)
Department of Ophthalmology, Edward S. Harkness Eye Institute, Columbia University College of Physicians and Surgeons, 635 W. 165th Street, Box 104, New York, NY 10032, USA
e-mail: rc2631@cumc.columbia.edu

C.A. Medina et al. (eds.), *Manual of Retinal Diseases: A Guide to Diagnosis and Management*, DOI 10.1007/978-3-319-20460-4_76

- Breaks in Bruch's membrane that appear as fine, yellowish-white linear lesions overlaid by an intact neuroretina, known as *lacquer cracks* (Fig. 76.3). They may be organized concentrically to the optic disk or in a fashion that is dictated by the configuration of the posterior staphyloma. Lacquer cracks could be heralded by subretinal hemorrhages in the absence of neovascularization, could be complicated by neovascularization, and could be iatrogenically extended by attempted laser photocoagulation, or they could spontaneously heal by retinal gliosis that fills the defect and hyperplasia of the RPE that extends into the choroid and is noted clinically as a pigmentary change.
- A hallmark of degenerative myopia, the ectatic *posterior staphylomatous* changes are in essence outpouchings of all the layers of the posterior eye wall in the terrain of an abnormal sclera. Posterior staphyloma may be overlooked on clinical exam.

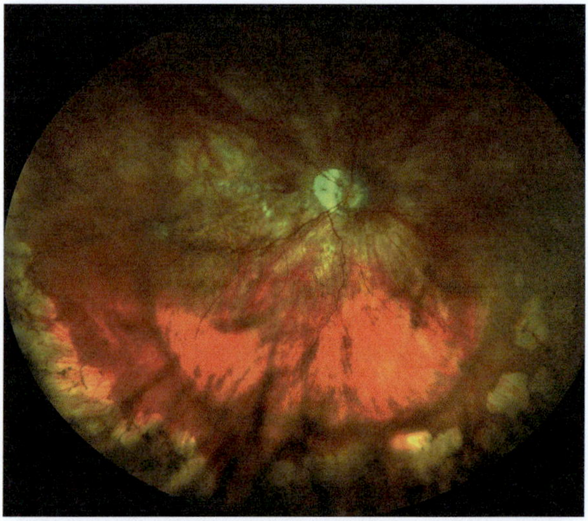

Fig. 76.1 Staphyloma, peripapillary atrophy, cobblestone degeneration

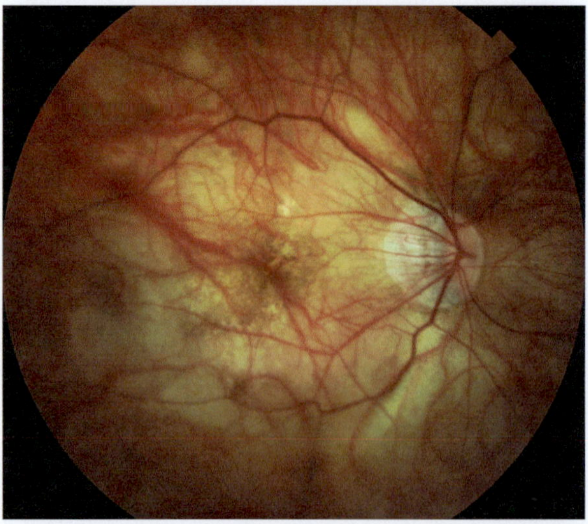

Fig. 76.2 Staphyloma, peripapillary atrophy

- *Subretinal hemorrhages* with or without *neovascularization* (known as *the Fuchs spot in its later stage*). The neovascularization is a type 2 lesion (subretinal), it may develop at a discernible lacquer crack, and it is typically smaller both in the size of the "dirty gray" membrane and the leakage extent when compared to the neovascular age-related macular degeneration lesions. The scar and atrophy caused by myopic neovascularization can extend significantly, exhibiting the phenomenon known as "atrophic creep" (Fig. 76.3).
- *The peripapillary changes and the myopic arrangement of the optic disk* which appears tilted, associated by an area of depigmentation temporally (infrequently nasally or circumferential) which is called the *temporal crescent* or *myopic conus* (Figs. 76.1, 76.2, and 76.3). There is a higher prevalence of normal tension glaucoma in myopic patients, and the configuration of the myopic disk makes its evaluation challenging both clinically and on retinal nerve fiber layer analysis by optical coherence tomography (OCT).
- *Degenerative changes of the vitreous* (early syneresis) and *vitreoretinal interface, compounded by a staphylomatous configuration in an elongated eye*, contribute to the formation of the *myopic foveoschisis, macular and retinal holes and detachment* (Figs. 76.4 and 76.5).
- *Lattice* and *cobblestone degeneration*.

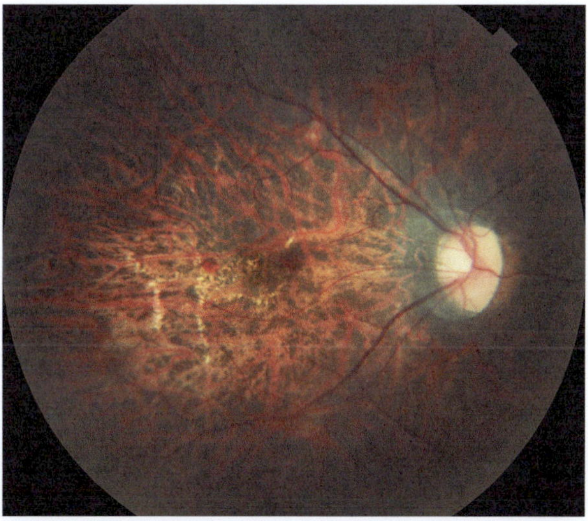

Fig. 76.3 Tilted optic disk, tigroid fundus, lacquer cracks, subretinal hemorrhages

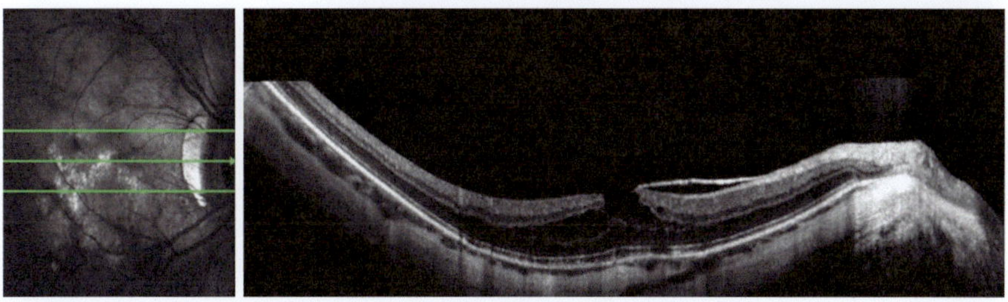

Fig. 76.4 Enhanced depth imaging optical coherence tomography showing a very thin choroid and retinoschisis of the macular region with lamellar macular hole formation

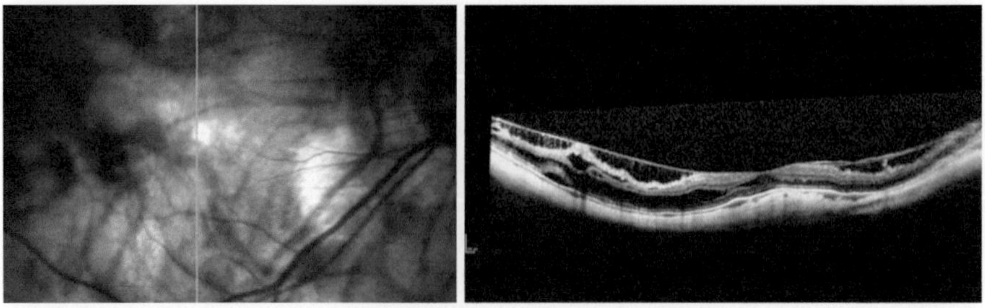

Fig. 76.5 Enhanced depth imaging optical coherence tomography showing a very thin choroid, vitreoretinal interface abnormalities, and foveoschisis

76.3 Symptoms

Depending on the type of degenerative change present, patients might complain of slow or rapid onset decline in acuity, metamorphopsia, central scotoma, flashes, and floaters, or they might be asymptomatic.

76.4 Epidemiology and Predisposing Factors

Myopia is a leading cause of visual impairment in developed countries. As a complex multifactorial trait, the development of degenerative myopia is governed by both genetic and environmental factors. Myopia is encountered much more commonly than glaucoma, cataract, and diabetic retinopathy in East Asian populations. The rapid global increase (1–3 % of the general population) in the prevalence of visual impairment caused by high myopia could be due to the increase in the time spent with activities that require near vision. In addition, urbanization seems to be of greatest importance, which is the highest among Taiwanese, Japanese, and Singaporeans. Outdoor time appears to be the most important modifiable factor in the prevention of high myopia.

76.5 Inheritance

Since the middle of the past century, studies have demonstrated the heritability of myopia. Genome-wide association studies (GWAS) have been performed in both population-based and case–control cohorts. MYP2-3 loci, respectively, 18p11.31 and 12q21-23, were the first to be associated with high myopia.

76.6 Differential Diagnosis

The myopic etiology of type 2 neovascularization (subretinal) should be kept in mind in young patients that develop an "idiopathic" lesion. Anecdotal experience in young, myopic women shows that these lesions are a unifocal manifestation of multifocal choroiditis (MFC)/punctate inner choroidopathy (PIC) that will eventually develop additional findings within the MFC/PIC spectrum.

76.7 Workup/Testing

- Spectral domain OCT (SD-OCT) yields fast and accurate invaluable information on the configuration of foveoschisis, macular holes, and neovascular tissue.
- Enhanced depth imaging (EDI-OCT) evaluates the degree of choroidal thinning.
- Enhanced vitreous imaging (EVI-OCT) evaluates vitreoretinal degeneration.
- Fundus autofluorescence (FAF) evaluates the RPE–choriocapillaris loss.
- Angiogram with fluorescein or indocyanine green when neovascularization is suspected has been largely replaced by the high-resolution, noninvasive modality of SD-OCT.
- Ultrasound B-scan is valuable in the preoperative localization of staphyloma.
- Magnetic resonance imaging yields accurate information on the staphyloma.

76.8 Prognosis and Management

Degenerative myopia can have a guarded prognosis and can result in permanent, severe visual impairment despite attempts to surgically treat the vitreoretinal interface changes via pars plana vitrectomy and repeated surgical procedures. Neovascularization is typically treated with anti-angiogenic regimens.

76.9 Follow-Up

Asymptomatic patients with degenerative myopia should be followed at least twice a year, and patients with active lesions should be examined every 4–6 weeks with dilated funduscopy and imaging (SD-OCT, color photos).

References and Suggested Reading

1. Curtin BJ. The posterior staphyloma of pathologic myopia. Trans Am Ophthalmol Soc. 1977;75:67–86.
2. Curtin BJ. Physiologic vs pathologic myopia: genetics vs environment. Ophthalmology. 1979;86(5):681–91.
3. Grossniklaus HE, Green WR. Pathologic findings in pathologic myopia. Retina. 1992; 12(2):127–33.
4. Ohno-Matsui K, Akiba M, Moriyama M, Ishibashi T, Hirakata A, Tokoro T. Intrachoroidal cavitation in macular area of eyes with pathologic myopia. Am J Ophthalmol. 2012;154(2): 382–93.
5. Ohno-Matsui K, Ikuno Y, Yasuda M, Murata T, Sakamoto T, Ishibashi T. Section 3. Chapter 68: Myopic macular degeneration. In: Ryan S, editor. Retina. 5th ed. China: Saunders Elsevier; 2014. p. 1256–66.
6. Spaide R, Ohno-Matsui K, Yannuzzi LA, editors. Pathologic myopia. New York, Heidelberg, Dordrecht, London: Springer; 2014. p. 1–360.
7. Yannuzzi LA. The retinal atlas. China: Saunders Elsevier; 2010. p. 526–43.

Chapter 77
Angioid Streaks

Stacy Scofield and Royce W.S. Chen

77.1 Definitions

Angioid streak: discontinuity or break in an abnormally calcified Bruch's membrane

77.2 Symptoms

- Often asymptomatic
- Decreased vision in the setting of choroidal neovascularization

77.3 Signs

- Dark reddish-brown or gray irregular lines of varying width present deep within the retina radiating from the optic nerve in a concentric pattern; they taper and fade a few millimeters from the optic disk (Fig. 77.1).

S. Scofield, MD
Department of Ophthalmology, Edward S. Harkness Eye Institute, Columbia University College of Physicians and Surgeons, New York, NY, USA

R.W.S. Chen, MD (✉)
Department of Ophthalmology, Edward S. Harkness Eye Institute, Columbia University College of Physicians and Surgeons, New York, NY, USA

Edward S. Harkness Eye Institute, Columbia University Medical Center, 635 W. 165th Street, Box 104, New York, NY 10032, USA
e-mail: rc2631@cumc.columbia.edu

C.A. Medina et al. (eds.), *Manual of Retinal Diseases: A Guide to Diagnosis and Management*, DOI 10.1007/978-3-319-20460-4_77

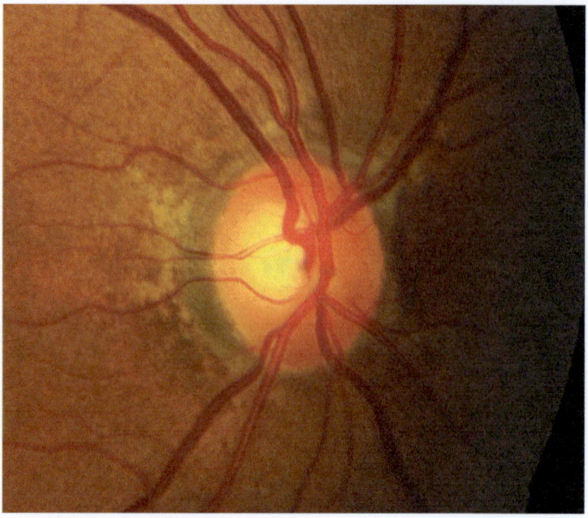

Fig. 77.1 Fundus photograph of right eye showing angioid streaks: deep, *yellow-gray* irregular lines radiating from the optic disk in a concentric fashion

- Choroidal neovascularization with secondary serous or hemorrhagic retinal detachment.
- Retinal hemorrhages.
- Optic disk drusen.
- Focal peripheral chorioretinal scars (salmon spots).
- Peau d'orange mottling of RPE (often temporal to macula).
- Crystalline bodies: mid-peripheral multiple, small, round subretinal lesions that can cause atrophy of the RPE.

77.4 Epidemiology

Not thought to be present at birth. Develops between the second and fifth decade.

77.5 Predisposing Conditions

- Pseudoxanthoma elasticum (PXE): autosomal recessive disorder with mutation in ABCC6
  - Most common associated disorder.
  - 85 % develop angioid streaks.
  - Other findings: loose skin folds in the neck, axillae, and flexor surface of joints, increased risk of gastrointestinal bleeding, and cardiovascular complications.

- Ehlers-Danlos syndrome:
  - Increased elasticity of skin and loose joints
- Paget disease of the bone:
  - 10–15 % have angioid streaks.
  - Enlarged skull, bone fractures, hearing loss, high-output cardiac failure, and hyperparathyroidism.
  - Elevated urine calcium and serum alkaline phosphatase.
  - Visual loss can occur from enlarged bone compressing optic nerve.
- Sickle cell disease:
  - 1.5 % have angioid streaks.
  - Recurrent infections and painful sickle cell crises.
- Others: acromegaly, senile elastosis, lead poisoning, and Marfan syndrome

77.6 Differential Diagnosis

- Choroidal rupture: yellow-white subretinal streaks concentric to the optic disk
- Lacquer cracks: seen in myopic degeneration
- Age-related macular degeneration

77.7 Etiology

Half of cases are associated with an underlying systemic disease, while the rest are idiopathic.

77.8 Workup/Testing

- Complete history (including systemic disorders, ocular trauma) along with ocular examination for choroidal neovascularization and physical examination for systemic diseases
- Fluorescein angiography: hyperfluorescence (window defect) in early phase due to RPE atrophy in region of streak, important for identification of CNV
- ICG: hyperfluorescent lines that are larger and more numerous than those seen on FA and can be used to evaluate for choroidal neovascularization
- Serum alkaline phosphatase and urine calcium if Paget disease of the bone suspected
- Sickle cell preparation and hemoglobin electrophoresis if sickle cell suspected
- Skin biopsy if PXE suspected

77.9 Prognosis and Management

- No treatment is known to prevent the development of angioid streaks.
- Manage underlying systemic disease if present.
- Choroidal neovascularization occurs in up to 80 % of patients and if left untreated can lead to scarring with visual acuity worse than 20/200.
- Treatment of choroidal neovascularization is with anti-VEGF therapy.
- The use of laser photocoagulation, transpupillary thermotherapy, photodynamic therapy, and feeder vessel occlusion has poor visual outcomes with a high recurrence rate; these have limited utility.
- These eyes are susceptible to choroidal rupture and subretinal hemorrhage even after minor blunt injury, so the use of polycarbonate glasses is important in prevention of these complications.

77.10 Follow-Up

- Every 4–8 weeks if actively treating with anti-angiogenic therapy, otherwise biannually to monitor for choroidal neovascularization.
- Encourage use of an Amsler grid at home with PRN visits if newly symptomatic.

References and Suggested Reading

1. Abdelkader E, Scott NW, Lois N. Epidemiology of angioid streak-associated choroidal neovascular membranes in the United Kingdom. Cureus. 2013;5(9):e138.
2. Clarkson JG, Altman RD. Angioid streaks. Surv Ophthalmol. 1982;26(5):235–46.
3. Gliem M, Finger RP, Fimmers R, Brinkmann CK, Holz FG, Issa PC. Treatment of choroidal neovascularization due to angioid streaks: a comprehensive review. Retina. 2013;33:1300–14.
4. Lim JI, Bressler NM, Marsh MJ, Bressler SB. Laser treatment of choroidal neovascularization in patients with angioid streaks. Am J Ophthalmol. 1993;116(4):414–23.

Chapter 78
Polypoidal Choroidal Vasculopathy

Frank Siringo

78.1 Definitions

PCV was first described in 1990 by Yannuzzi and colleagues, as a diagnosis distinct from exudative age-related macular degeneration (AMD) characterized as a bilateral exudative age-related macular disease characterized by orange-red subretinal nodules, with associated subretinal pigment epithelium (RPE) and/or subretinal serous fluid or hemorrhage.

78.2 Symptoms

Decreased visual acuity (VA), metamorphopsia

78.3 Signs

- Bilateral involvement, though often asymmetric.
- Orange-red subretinal nodules.
- Serous and/or hemorrhagic detachment of the RPE and neurosensory retina.
- The funduscopic signs are accompanied by angiographic evidence of hyperfluorescent polyp- or grape-like choroidal vascular lesions, often with lacy interconnected inner choroidal vasculature, seen within the first 6 min of indocyanine green angiography (ICG-A).

F. Siringo, MD, OD
Department of Ophthalmology, University of Colorado School of Medicine,
1675 Aurora Court, Stop F731, Aurora, CO 80045, USA
e-mail: frank.siringo@ucdenver.edu

C.A. Medina et al. (eds.), *Manual of Retinal Diseases: A Guide to Diagnosis and Management*, DOI 10.1007/978-3-319-20460-4_78

78.4 Epidemiology

- Age (typically diagnosed between 50 and 65)
- More common in nonwhite races
- Females more likely affected than males

78.5 Predisposing Conditions

- Hypertension, arteriosclerosis
- Smoking
- Genetic risk factors include polymorphisms in the following genes:
  - ARMS2 (Age-related maculopathy susceptibility 2)
  - CFH (complement factor H)
  - HTRA2 (high temperature requirement A2)
  - C2 (complement component 2)

78.6 Differential Diagnosis

Consider PCV in nonwhite patients younger than 65 who have an exudative or hemorrhagic maculopathy with orange-red subretinal nodules and/or in those initially diagnosed with exudative AMD who do not respond favorably to anti-VEGF therapy. ICG-A is needed to differentiate from exudative AMD and central serous chorioretinopathy (CSR).

78.7 Etiology

Largely unknown. Not a typical choroidal neovascular membrane as is seen in exudative age-related macular degeneration. In pathologic studies, choroidal vascular lesions demonstrate hyalinization similar to arteriosclerosis.

78.8 Workup/Testing

- ICG-A is required to make the diagnosis.
- Fluorescein angiography (FA).
- Optical coherence tomography (OCT); high/narrow PEDs are more characteristic of PCV than exudative AMD/CRS.

78.9 Prognosis and Management

PCV can have a stable or recurrent course. Poor initial visual acuity and recurrent subretinal or sub-RPE hemorrhage are associated with a worse prognosis (Fig. 78.1). Disease activity is graded by loss of five or more ETDRS letters and presence of subretinal or sub-RPE fluid or hemorrhage. PCV generally exhibits a less robust response to anti-VEGF therapy compared to EAMD (Fig. 78.2). Photodynamic therapy (PDT) has been studied in PCV as well; similar visual acuity outcomes at 2 years were found when comparing ranibizumab monotherapy (loading followed by PRN dosing) to PDT. The combination of PDT with anti-VEGF treatment has been shown to be more effective in closing polyps and improving visual acuity than anti-VEGF alone. Less frequently, thermal laser can be considered for extramacular lesions.

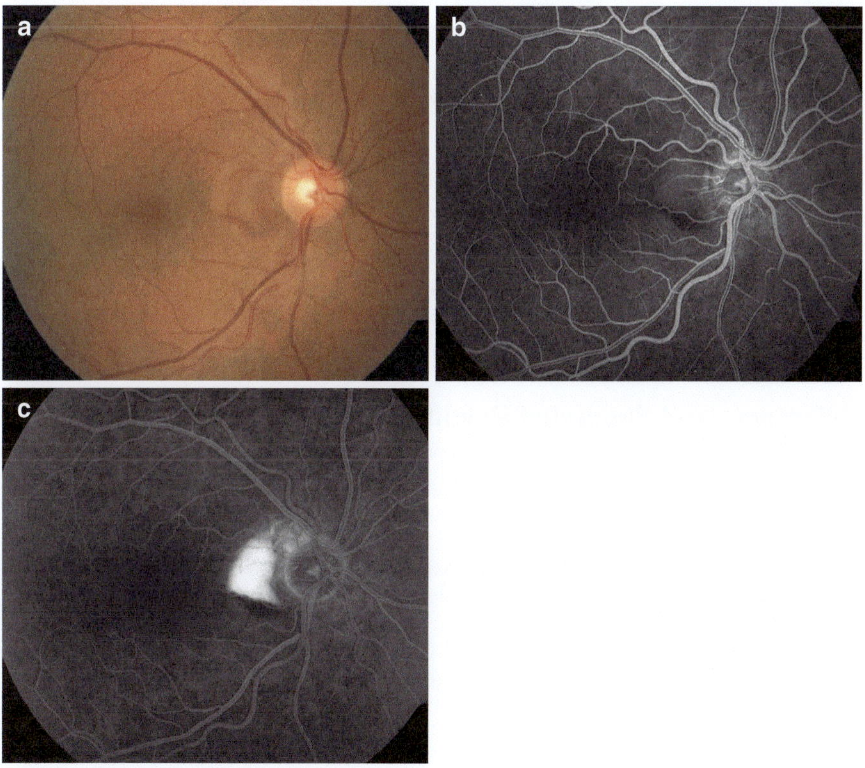

Fig. 78.1 Color fundus photo and fluorescein angiographic images of a 67-year-old Mediterranean man demonstrating orange-red sub-RPE nodule with subretinal hemorrhage (**a**), blocking hypofluorescence from subretinal hemorrhage (**b**) and late pooling into the sub-RPE lesion (**c**)

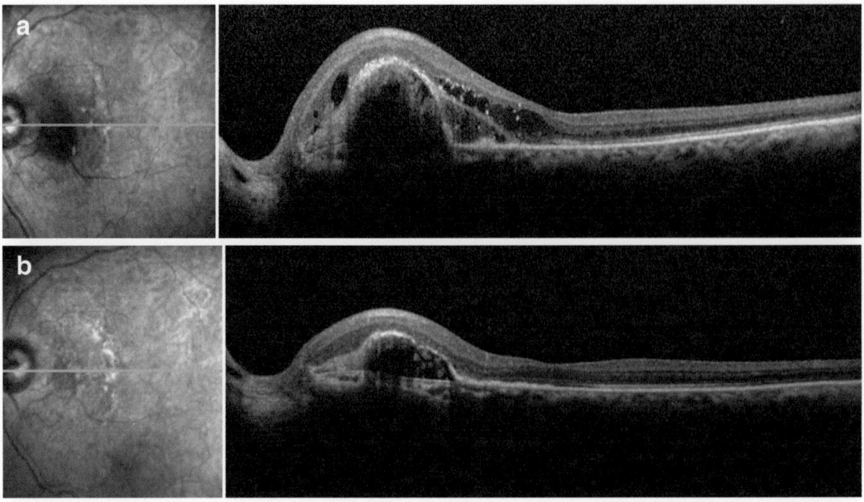

Fig. 78.2 Spectral domain OCT (SD-OCT) images of an 87-year-old South Asian woman with PCV at date of diagnosis (**a**). After 9 months of treatment with intravitreal bevacizumab, while the intra- and subretinal fluid has resolved, the hemorrhagic pigment epithelial detachment has decreased in size but persists (**b**)

78.10 Follow-Up

Every 4–8 weeks if actively treating with anti-VEGF therapy, otherwise biannually with PRN visits if newly symptomatic

References and Suggested Reading

1. Chen H, Liu K, Chen LJ, Hou P, Chen W, Pang CP. Genetic associations in polypoidal choroidal vasculopathy: a systematic review and meta-analysis. Mol Vis. 2012;18:816–29.
2. Koh AH, Expert PCV Panel, Chen LJ, Chen SJ, Chen Y, Giridhar A, Iida T, Kim H, Yuk Yau Lai T, Lee WK, Li X, Han Lim T, Ruamviboonsuk P, Sharma T, Tang S, Yuzawa M. Polypoidal choroidal vasculopathy: evidence-based guidelines for clinical diagnosis and treatment. Retina. 2013;33(4):686–716.
3. Koh E, Lee WK, Chen LJ, et al. EVEREST study: efficacy and safety of verteporfin photodynamic therapy in combination with ranibizumab or alone versus ranibizumab monotherapy in patients with symptomatic macular polypoidal choroidal vasculopathy. Retina. 2012;32: 1453–64.
4. Ohishi A, Miyamoto N, Honda M, et al. LAPTOP study: a 24-month trial of vertiporfin versus ranibizumab for polypoidal choroidal vasculopathy. Ophthalmology. 2014;121:1151–2.
5. Yannuzzi LA, Sorenson J, Spaide RF, Lipson B. Idiopathic polypoidal choroidal vasculopathy (IPCV). Retina. 1990;10:1–8.
6. Yuan D, Yuan D, Yuan S, Liu Q. The age-related maculopathy susceptibility 2 polymorphism and polypoidal choroidal vasculopathy in Asian populations: a meta-analysis. Ophthalmology. 2013;120(10):2051–7.

Chapter 79
Macular Retinoschisis

Stacy Scofield and Royce W.S. Chen

79.1 Definitions

Retinoschisis: splitting of the neurosensory retina

79.2 Symptoms

- Infants: squint, nystagmus, and strabismus
- Children (school aged): bilateral poor vision and difficulty reading

79.3 Signs

- Mild to severe central visual loss (often 20/60–20/120).
- Foveal schisis: Often bilateral spoke wheel or petaloid pattern of folds radiating outward from the foveola that contain small cystoid spaces (seen in 98–100 %).

S. Scofield, MD
Department of Ophthalmology, Edward S. Harkness Eye Institute,
Columbia University College of Physicians and Surgeons, New York, NY, USA

R.W.S. Chen, MD (✉)
Department of Ophthalmology, Edward S. Harkness Eye Institute,
Columbia University College of Physicians and Surgeons, New York, NY, USA

Edward S. Harkness Eye Institute, Columbia University Medical Center,
635 W. 165th Street Box 104, New York, NY, USA
e-mail: rc2631@cumc.columbia.edu

C.A. Medina et al. (eds.), *Manual of Retinal Diseases: A Guide to Diagnosis and Management*, DOI 10.1007/978-3-319-20460-4_79

  - With age, microcystic spaces coalesce leading to flattening of the schisis cavity and the petaloid pattern can disappear.
- Peripheral retinoschisis: Predominantly inferotemporally, seen in 50 %.
  - Infants can have large cavities that typically undergo spontaneous regression, but they often leave pigment lines.
  - Vessels crossing walls of the schisis cavity are at risk for rupture leading to vitreous hemorrhage.
  - Breaks can occur within the inner layer of the cavity. These can range from small holes to large tears with subsequent retinal detachment.
  - Vitreous veils: elevation of the surface layer of the retina into the vitreous.
- Can develop pigmentary deposits in regions of peripheral retinal damage.
- Hyperopia is common.

79.4 Epidemiology

Prevalence is 1 in 15,000 to 1 in 30,000.

79.5 Inheritance

- X-linked mutation in RS1 gene, which encodes an adhesion protein called retinoschisin. This protein is essential for Müller cell health with mutations leading to Müller cell degeneration.
- Female carriers are often asymptomatic, but can have minor retinal abnormalities.

79.6 Differential Diagnosis (Table 79.1)

Table 79.1 Differential diagnosis of juvenile X-linked retinoschisis

Differential diagnosis	
Degenerative retinoschisis	Usually older patients Two types: (1) typical, splitting at outer plexiform layer; (2) reticular, splitting at inner retinal layer Foveal retinoschisis is very uncommon
Retinal detachment	Unilateral, pigmented cells in the vitreous
Cystoid macular edema	FA with late hyperfluorescence in petaloid pattern
Retinitis Pigmentosa	Peripheral RPE atrophy, bone spicules, nyctalopia Reduced or extinguished ERG
Goldmann-Favre syndrome	Central and peripheral schisis present Nyctalopia, pigmentary clumping, extinguished ERG
Norrie disease	X-linked disorder with bilateral retinal detachments at birth or in infancy Associated with sensorineural deafness and mental retardation

79.7 Workup/Testing

- Obtain family history.
- Dilated fundus examination to rule out retinal break or tear (Fig. 79.1).
- OCT: major diagnostic technique; although histopathological studies initially reported splitting of the nerve fiber layer, OCT studies show splitting of the retina typically in the inner nuclear layer, outer plexiform layer, and outer nuclear layer; less commonly, cysts are present in nerve fiber layer and ganglion cell layer (Fig. 79.2).
- FA: often normal without staining or leakage; older individuals may have atrophic RPE changes; patients with peripheral schisis may demonstrate leakage of dye within areas of schisis.
- ERG: electronegative ERG with reduced b-wave amplitude (indicates inner retinal abnormality; seen in only 50 %), but some have normal ERGs. With the advent of OCT, this is no longer the primary diagnostic tool.

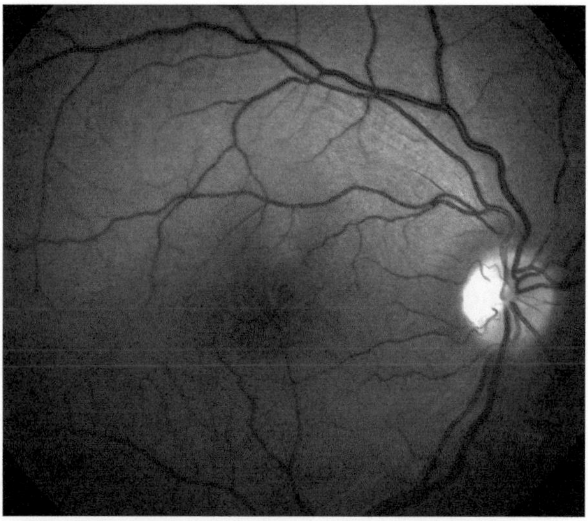

Fig. 79.1 Red-free fundus photograph showing petaloid pattern of schisis within the macula

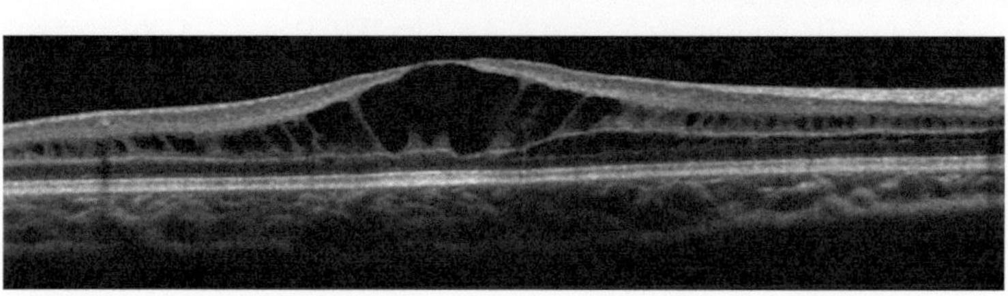

Fig. 79.2 Spectral-domain OCT image showing cystic spaces within the macula. Schisis cavities are present predominantly in the inner nuclear layer and outer plexiform layer

79.8 Prognosis and Management

The goal should be diagnosis and management of secondary complications including retinal detachment and vitreous hemorrhage.

There is no treatment for the foveal or peripheral retinoschisis, and prophylactic laser therapy is not recommended due to the increased risk of retinal detachment. Visual function varies depending on the development of vitreous hemorrhage or retinal detachment, which can lead to severe visual loss. Apart from these complications, vision typically remains stable or slowly deteriorates until the fifth to sixth decade life. In children with vitreous hemorrhage, earlier intervention with vitrectomy may be necessary for amblyopia treatment. There is some evidence that carbonic anhydrase inhibitors may decrease foveal thickening and cystic spaces. All patients should be offered low vision aids. To reduce the risk of retinal detachment and vitreous hemorrhage, there should be avoidance of head trauma or contact sports.

Families should also undergo genetic counseling given the X-linked recessive inheritance.

79.9 Follow-Up

Patients should be monitored annually with closer follow-up for those with new symptoms such as changes in vision indicative of secondary complication such as retinal detachment or vitreous hemorrhage.

References and Suggested Reading

1. Gregori NZ, Berrocal AM, Gregori G, Murray TG, Knighton RW, Flynn Jr HW, Dubovy S, Puliafito CA, Rosenfeld PJ. Macular spectral-domain optical coherence tomography in patients with X linked retinoschisis. Br J Ophthalmol. 2009;93(3):373–8. doi:10.1136/bjo.2007.136127. Epub 2008 Nov 19.
2. Molday RS, Kellner U, Weber BHF. X-linked juvenile retinoschisis: clinical diagnosis, genetic analysis and molecular mechanisms. Prog Retin Eye Res. 2012;31(3):195–212.
3. Sikkink SK, Biswas S, Parry NRA, Stanga PE, Trump D. X-linked retinoschisis: an update. J Med Genet. 2007;44:225–32.
4. Tantri A, Vrabec TR, Cu-Unjieng A, Frost A, Annesley WH, Donoso LA. X-linked retinoschisis: a clinical and molecular genetic review. Surv Ophthalmol. 2004;49(2):214–30.

Chapter 80
Macular Hole

Stacy Scofield and Royce W.S. Chen

80.1 Definitions

Macular hole: full-thickness retinal defect in the foveal neurosensory retina

80.2 Symptoms

Decreased visual acuity, metamorphopsia, loss of central vision, and central scotoma

80.3 Signs

Initially can have yellow spot or ring with loss of the normal foveal depression. In later stages, a round, red spot develops in the center of the macula with or without surrounding subretinal fluid. Operculum can be present.

S. Scofield, MD
Department of Ophthalmology, Edward S. Harkness Eye Institute,
Columbia University College of Physicians and Surgeons, New York, NY, USA

R.W.S. Chen, MD (✉)
Department of Ophthalmology, Edward S. Harkness Eye Institute,
Columbia University College of Physicians and Surgeons, New York, NY, USA

Edward S. Harkness Eye Institute, Columbia University Medical Center,
635 W. 165th Street Box 104, New York, NY 10032, USA
e-mail: rc2631@cumc.columbia.edu

C.A. Medina et al. (eds.), *Manual of Retinal Diseases: A Guide to Diagnosis and Management*, DOI 10.1007/978-3-319-20460-4_80

80.4 Epidemiology

- Women are affected 3 times more than men.
- Unilateral in 80 %.
- Most common in sixth to eighth decade of life.
- Prevalence is 0.3 % of the population.

80.5 Predisposing Conditions

Myopia and ocular trauma

80.6 Differential Diagnosis

- Macular pucker with pseudohole
- Lamellar hole
- Vitreomacular traction
- Cystoid macular edema
- Subfoveal drusen
- Solar retinopathy

80.7 Etiology

Can be idiopathic or secondary to vitreomacular traction or an epiretinal membrane

80.8 Workup/Testing

- Complete history and physical examination (including history of trauma, prior surgery).
- Watzke-Allen Test: a narrow slit beam is projected across the macular hole; a positive test indicates a true macular hole and occurs when the patient reports a gap in the slit beam.
- Fluorescein angiography: early foveal hyperfluorescence at the bottom of the hole without associated leakage.
- OCT (gold standard): confirms diagnosis; used in staging and progression of disease (Fig. 80.1).

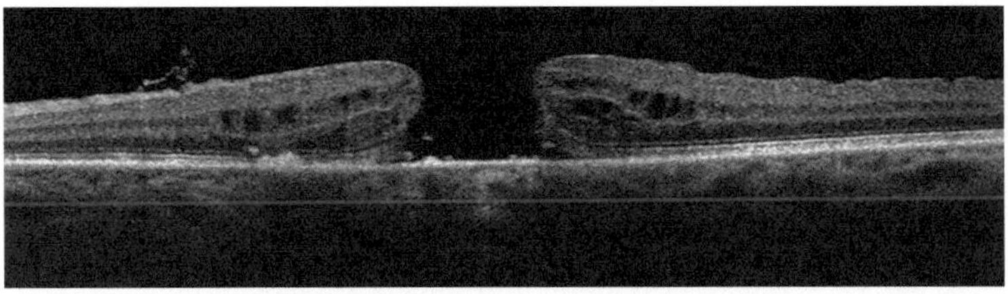

Fig. 80.1 Spectral-domain optical coherence tomography of stage 4 macular hole. A full-thickness defect is accompanied by cystic thickening of the retina. A posterior vitreous detachment is present

Table 80.1 Stages of macular hole formation

Stage	Characteristics	Prognosis
0	Premacular hole Perifoveal vitreous detachment develops Loss of foveal depression Normal visual acuity (VA)	Most do not progress to advanced stages
1	Impending macular hole Yellow spot or yellow ring Vision 20/25–20/60 Foveal pseudocyst associated with vitreous detachment from the perifoveal retina, but not from the foveal center Can have a break in the outer foveal layer	50 % regress and 40 % progress
2	Full-thickness defect <400 um in diameter Posterior vitreous is attached to foveal center VA 20/40–20/100	15 % close spontaneously and 75 % enlarge
3	Full-thickness defect >400 um in diameter Operculum often present suspended by posterior hyaloid VA 20/60–20/200	<5 % close and 50 % progress
4	Full-thickness hole with complete PVD VA 20/60–20/400	<5 % close and 20 % enlarge

80.9 Prognosis and Management

Prognosis is based on the stage of the hole (Table 80.1).

- Observation is recommended for stage 1 holes because there is a high rate of spontaneous resolution.
- Pharmocologic vitreolysis is sometimes effective in small holes with persistent areas of narrow vitreoretinal adhesion.
- Vitrectomy with removal of posterior cortical vitreous with or without internal limiting membrane (ILM) can be performed for stage 2–4 macular holes. Removal of ILM improves the rate of hole closure, especially in stage 3 and 4 holes.

- Prognosis depends on duration and size of macular hole.
- Vitrectomy has 80–90 % closure rate overall.

Risk to the fellow eye of developing macular hole:

- Presence of PVD in the fellow eye has a <2 % risk of macular hole formation.
- Presence of normal macula and attached posterior vitreous in the fellow eye: fellow eye has 15 % risk of developing full-thickness macular hole.

80.10 Follow-Up

Home Amsler grid testing of both the involved and fellow eye
Yearly follow-up examination (high myopia should have biannual examinations)

References and Suggested Reading

1. Chew EY, Sperduto RD, Hiller R, Nowroozi L, Siegel D, Yanuzzi LA, Burton TC, Seddon JM, Gragoudas ES, Haller JA, Blair NP, Farber M. Clinical course of macular holes: the eye disease case-control study. Arch Ophthalmol. 1999;117(2):242–6.
2. Duker JS, Kaiser PK, Binder S, de Smet MD, Gaudric A, Reichel E, Sadda SR, Sebag J, Spaide RF, Stalmans P. The International Vitreomacular Traction Study Group classification of vitreomacular adhesion, traction and macular hole. Ophthalmology. 2013;120:2611–9.
3. Ezra E. Idiopathic full thickness macular hole: natural history and pathogenesis. Br J Ophthalmol. 2001;85(1):102–8.
4. Gass JDM. Reappraisal of biomicroscopic classification of stages of development of a macular hole. Am J Ophthalmol. 1995;119:752–9.
5. Haouchine B, Massin P, Gaudric A. Foveal pseudocyst as the first step in macular hole formation: a prospective study by optical coherence tomography. Ophthalmology. 2001;108(1): 15–22.
6. Johnson MW, Van Newkirk MR, Meyer KA. Perifoveal vitreous detachment is the primary pathogenic event in idiopathic macular hole formation. Arch Ophthalmol. 2001;119(2): 215–22.
7. Kumagai K, Furukawa M, Ogino N, Uemura A, Demizu S, Larson E. Vitreous surgery with and without internal limiting membrane peeling for macular hole repair. Retina. 2004;24(5): 721–7.
8. Steel DHW, Lotery AJ. Idiopathic vitreomacular traction and macular hole: a comprehensive review of pathophysiology, diagnosis and treatment. Eye. 2013;27:S1–21.

Chapter 81
Epiretinal Membrane

Sergio Groman-Lupa, Richard Hwang, and Frank Siringo

81.1 Definitions

Epiretinal membrane (ERM): fibrocellular proliferation on the inner surface of the retina.

81.2 Symptoms

Frequently asymptomatic. Depending on the severity can cause decreased visual acuity and/or metamorphopsia.

81.3 Signs

The severity of retinal distortion caused by the ERM was used by Gass [1] to develop a clinical grading system to describe different stages of the disease (Table 81.1).

S. Groman-Lupa, MD (✉) • R. Hwang, MD, PhD • F. Siringo, MD
Rocky Mountain Lions Eye Institute, University of Colorado School of Medicine,
Academic Office One 1675 Aurora Ct, Aurora, CO 80045, USA
e-mail: sergio.groman-lupa@ucdenver.edu; sergiogroman@gmail.com

C.A. Medina et al. (eds.), *Manual of Retinal Diseases: A Guide to Diagnosis and Management*, DOI 10.1007/978-3-319-20460-4_81

Table 81.1 Epiretinal membrane clinical stages

Grade	Description
Grade 0 cellophane maculopathy	The ERM is translucent and is not associated with distortion of the inner retinal surface. The only clinical finding is a characteristic "cellophane" light reflex. These membranes are asymptomatic
Grade 1 crinkled cellophane maculopathy	The ERM is associated with irregular wrinkling of the inner retina producing an irregular light reflex. May remain invisible or appear as a gray-white translucent membrane with indistinct details of small underlying retinal vessels. Can cause metamorphopsia and reduced visual acuity (VA) typically no worse than 20/40
Grade 2 macular pucker	A distinct grayish membrane on the inner retinal surface is present preventing the visualization of underlying vessels and causing marked full-thickness retinal distortion. May be associated with other retinal abnormalities (retinal folds radiating from the membrane, macular edema, serous retinal detachment). VA may be less than 20/200, associated with metamorphopsia and monocular diplopia

81.4 Epidemiology

The overall prevalence of ERM in the United States is between 28.9 and 34.1 %, typically affecting people older than 50 years.

81.5 Predisposing Conditions

Increasing age, posterior vitreous detachment (PVD), retinal disease (diabetic retinopathy, retinal vein occlusion, retinal tear, retinal detachment), vitreoretinal, and cataract surgery.

81.6 Differential Diagnosis

- *Vitreomacular traction syndrome*: Incomplete separation of the posterior vitreous with persistent macular adhesion and traction.
- *Macular hole*: A spontaneous contraction of an ERM surrounding the fovea may simulate a full-thickness macular hole. Differentiate with OCT.
- *Cystoid macular edema* (CME): May appear similar to ERM; however in CME there is no distortion of the retinal microvasculature; it is always centered on the fovea and typically presents a "star" or "petaloid" pattern on fluorescein angiography.

Table 81.2 Causes of secondary epiretinal membranes

Retinal vascular occlusion (BRVO, CRVO)
Diabetic retinopathy
Vitreous hemorrhage
Telangiectasias
Macroaneurysm
Retinal angioma
Sickle cell retinopathy
Uveitis
Trauma
Retinal tear or detachment
Hamartomas
Retinitis pigmentosa
Retinal dystrophies

81.7 Etiology

- *Idiopathic*: There is no associated ocular retinopathy or ocular abnormality; splitting of the cortical vitreous lamellae during posterior vitreous detachment leaving a residual cellular membrane over the retinal surface is believed to be the trigger.
- *Secondary*: Due to a coexisting or antecedent ocular disease which influenced the development of an ERM (Table 81.2).
- *Iatrogenic*: A traumatic or surgical intervention which spurred the development of an ERM (diathermy, photocoagulation, cryopexy).

81.8 Workup/Testing

- History with emphasis on diabetes, ocular disease, and ocular surgery.
- Complete ophthalmological evaluation including an Amsler grid test and dilated fundus exam. The macula should be evaluated with slit lamp and a 60-, 90-diopter, Hruby, or fundus contact lens as well as peripheral examination to rule out a retinal break.
- OCT allows a more precise evaluation of the vitreoretinal interface and retinal morphology. The ERM appears as a highly reflective layer overlying the inner retina. Additional findings can be seen depending on the severity of the ERM including distortion of the inner retina, loss of foveal contour, retinal thickening, and irregularity of the retinal surface (Fig. 81.1). Idiopathic ERMs tend to be adherent globally, whereas secondary ERMs are more likely to be characterized by focal retinal adhesion.
- FA: Distortion of the retinal blood vessels with leakage at the macula may be found.

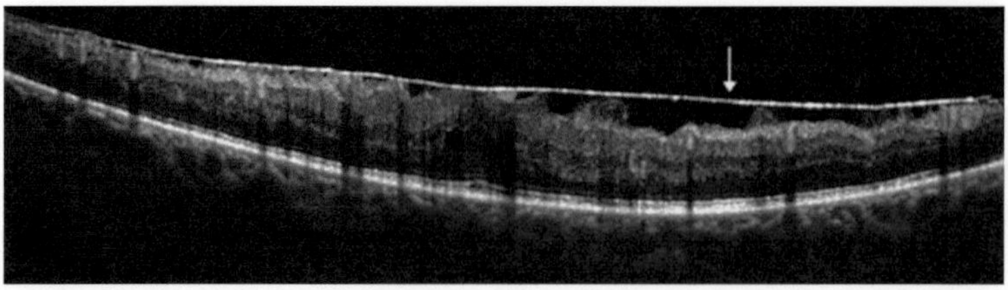

Fig. 81.1 Spectral-domain OCT image showing presence of an ERM (*arrow*), macular edema, and distortion of retinal layers

81.9 Prognosis and Management

The majority of patients who present with ERM will remain stable if observed over a period of time [6]. Surgery is indicated when there is significant or progressive vision loss, debilitating metamorphopsia, or diplopia. Although surgery is usually reserved for patients with a reduction in visual acuity to ≤20/60, it can be performed in patients with better VA if symptoms are debilitating, particularly metamorphopsia. When indicated, a standard pars plana vitrectomy with membrane peel is performed. The use of internal limiting membrane (ILM) and ERM staining ensures complete membrane removal. Commonly used dyes include triamcinolone, indocyanine green (ICG), trypan blue (TB), and brilliant blue. Most patients have improved postoperative visual acuity with a low rate of recurrence (<20 %), the rate of which is lower when the ILM is removed.

81.10 Follow-Up

This is not an emergent condition. Patients should be advised to have periodic visits and monitor their vision and symptoms for appropriate timing of surgical intervention. Rarely, membranes separate from the retina, resulting in spontaneously improved vision.

References and Suggested Reading

1. Agarwal A, Gass JDM, Gass JDM. Gass' atlas of macular diseases. 5th ed. Edinburgh: Elsevier Saunders; 2012.
2. Meuer SM, Myers CE, Klein BE, Swift MK, Huang Y, Gangaputra S, et al. The epidemiology of vitreoretinal interface abnormalities as detected by spectral-domain optical coherence tomography: the beaver dam eye study. Ophthalmology. 2014;122(4):787–95.
3. Ng CH, Cheung N, Wang JJ, Islam AF, Kawasaki R, Meuer SM, et al. Prevalence and risk factors for epiretinal membranes in a multi-ethnic United States population. Ophthalmology. 2011;118(4):694–9.

4. Mitchell P, Smith W, Chey T, Wang JJ, Chang A. Prevalence and associations of epiretinal membranes. The Blue Mountains Eye Study, Australia. Ophthalmology. 1997;104(6):1033–40.
5. Ryan SJ. Retina. 5th ed. London: Saunders/Elsevier; 2013.
6. Fraser-Bell S, Guzowski M, Rochtchina E, Wang JJ, Mitchell P. Five-year cumulative incidence and progression of epiretinal membranes: the Blue Mountains Eye Study. Ophthalmology. 2003;110(1):34–40.

Chapter 82
Vitreomacular Traction

Stacy Scofield and Royce W.S. Chen

82.1 Definitions

- Vitreomacular traction (VMT): presence of vitreous adhesion to central macula with exertion of tractional forces on the macula
- Vitreomacular adhesion (VMA): presence of vitreous adhesion to central macula without exertion of tractional forces on the macula

82.2 Symptoms

Decreased vision, photopsias, micropsias, and metamorphopsia

82.3 Signs

- Hyperreflective and thickened posterior hyaloid
- Hyperreflective adhesion to macula with distortion of foveal contour
- Subretinal or subfoveal fluid

S. Scofield, MD
Department of Ophthalmology, Edward S. Harkness Eye Institute, Columbia University College of Physicians and Surgeons, New York, NY, USA

R.W.S. Chen, MD (✉)
Department of Ophthalmology, Edward S. Harkness Eye Institute, Columbia University College of Physicians and Surgeons, New York, NY, USA

Edward S. Harkness Eye Institute, Columbia University Medical Center,
635 W. 165th Street Box 104, New York, NY 10032, USA
e-mail: rc2631@cumc.columbia.edu

C.A. Medina et al. (eds.), *Manual of Retinal Diseases: A Guide to Diagnosis and Management*, DOI 10.1007/978-3-319-20460-4_82

- Cystic changes within the macula
- Tractional macular schisis

82.4 Epidemiology

- Higher incidence in women due to a postmenopausal low estrogen state leading to premature vitreous liquefaction and earlier onset of PVD.
- Most common in sixth to eighth decade of life.
- Prevalence is 22.5 per 100,000.
- Incidence is 0.6 per 100,000.

82.5 Differential Diagnosis

- Epiretinal membrane (ERM)
- Full-thickness macular hole
- Cystoid macular edema

82.6 Etiology

Development of an incomplete or partial posterior vitreous detachment (PVD) with persistent attachment to the macula.

82.7 Workup/Testing

Complete history and physical examination. There is no correlation between clinical findings and symptoms.

- FA can show leakage from macular vessels as well as from the optic nerve.
- OCT (gold standard) reveals two categories of VMT:
  - Focal VMT: the maximal diameter of attachment is 1500 μm or less. More likely to develop full-thickness macular hole, cystoid macular edema (CME), and subfoveal detachment (Fig. 82.1).
  - Broad VMT: maximal diameter of attachment is greater than 1500 μm. More likely to develop diffuse retinal thickening with secondary ERM.

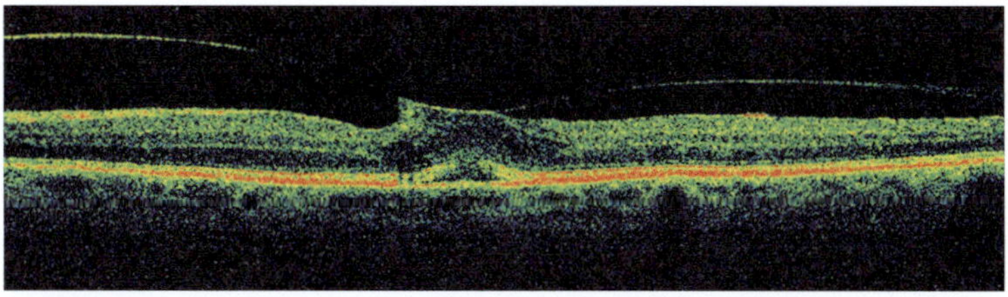

Fig. 82.1 Spectral-domain optical coherence tomography demonstrating focal VMT. Adhesion is present in the parafovea, causing tractional elevation of fovea with subretinal fluid

82.8 Prognosis and Management

- If visual acuity is preserved and metamorphopsia is mild: observation is recommended, as a significant proportion of patients may remain stable or improve in early stages.
- The traction can resolve spontaneously if a complete PVD develops.
- Vitrectomy with peeling of cortical vitreous is recommended for those with poor or worsening visual acuity with progressive macular traction.
- Ocriplasmin, a medication that can be injected intravitreally to induce PVD formation and therefore relieve VMT. It is a recombinant protease that targets fibronectin and laminin. Ocriplasmin is successful in releasing VMT in approximately 50 % of cases; however, transient dyschromatopsia and decrease in visual acuity may occur.

82.9 Follow-Up

- Amsler grid for self-monitoring.
- Monitor for progression or development of PVD with resolution.

References and Suggested Reading

1. Bottos JM, Elizalde J, Rodrigues EB, Maia M. Current concepts in vitreomacular traction syndrome. Curr Opin Ophthalmol. 2012;23:195–201.
2. Duker JS, Kaiser PK, Binder S, de Smet MD, Gaudric A, Reichel E, Sadda SR, Sebag J, Spaide RF, Stalmans P. The International Vitreomacular Traction Study Group classification of vitreomacular adhesion, traction and macular hole. Ophthalmology. 2013;120:2611–9.
3. Hikichi T, Yoshida A, Trempe CL. Course of vitreomacular traction syndrome. Am J Ophthalmol. 1995;119(1):55–61.
4. John VJ, Flynn Jr HW, Smiddy WE, Carver A, Leonard R, Tabandeh H, Boyer DS. Clinical course of vitreomacular adhesion managed by initial observation. Retina. 2014;34:442–6. doi:10.1097/IAE.0b013e3182a15f8b.

5. Sharma P, Juhn A, Houston SK, Fineman M, Chiang A, Ho A, Regillo C. Efficacy of intravitreal ocriplasmin on vitreomacular traction and full thickness macular holes. Am J Ophthalmol. 2015;159(5):861–7.e2. doi:10.1016/j.ajo.2015.01.034.
6. Stalmans P, Benz MS, Gandorfer A, Kampik A, Girach A, Pakola S, Haller JA, MIVI-TRUST Study Group. Enzymatic vitreolysis with ocriplasmin for vitreomacular traction and macular holes. N Engl J Med. 2012;367(7):606–15.
7. Steel DHW, Lotery AJ. Idiopathic vitreomacular traction and macular hole: a comprehensive review of pathophysiology, diagnosis and treatment. Eye. 2013;27:S1–21.

Chapter 83
Cystoid Macular Edema

Daniela Santos and Richard Hwang

83.1 Definitions

- *Cystoid macular edema* (CME): macular thickening associated with increased fluid within the sensory retina of the macula, primarily the outer plexiform layer
- *Angiographic cystoid macular edema*: asymptomatic edema and leakage that is apparent only on fluorescein angiography
- *Clinically significant cystoid macular edema*: CME that decreases vision
- *Chronic cystoid macular edema*: clinically significant CME that has persisted for 6 months or more
- *Irvine-Gass syndrome*: CME that develops after cataract surgery
- *Subclinical foveal edema*: edema less than 300 μm, often not seen on clinical exam

83.2 Symptoms

Blurred vision, decreased distance visual acuity, reduced contrast sensitivity, impaired color vision, decreased reading acuity, reduced reading speed, increased metamorphopsia, increased micropsia, ocular irritability, and increased photophobia.

D. Santos, MD • R. Hwang, MD, PhD (✉)
Rocky Mountain Lions Eye Institute, University of Colorado Denver,
Aurora, CO, USA
e-mail: Richard.hwang@ucdenver.edu

C.A. Medina et al. (eds.), *Manual of Retinal Diseases: A Guide to Diagnosis and Management*, DOI 10.1007/978-3-319-20460-4_83

83.3 Signs

- Common: retinal thickening and cystic structures that extend radially from the foveola; blunted foveal reflex
- Additional: inflammatory cells, optic nerve edema, and subretinal fluid in severe cases; lamellar macular hole, epiretinal membrane, and outer retinal atrophy caused by prolonged CME; surgically related CME located around the fovea; diabetic CME seen in patches throughout the macula

83.4 Etiology

Many conditions are associated with CME (Table 83.1).

Table 83.1 Common causes of cystoid macular edema

Postoperative Pseudophakic/Irvine-Gass syndrome	Occurs 6–10 weeks after cataract surgery in 1–6 % of uncomplicated cases
Diabetic retinopathy	
Retinal vein occlusion	
Hypertensive retinopathy	
Retinal telangiectases	Coats's disease, congenital juxtafoveolar capillary telangiectasia
Radiation retinopathy	
Macroaneurysm	
Choroidal neovascularization	Age-related macular degeneration, angioid streaks
Uveitis	Pars planitis, Behcet's disease, vitiliginous chorioretinitis, scleritis, sarcoidosis, collagen vascular disease
Retinal vasculitis	Eales' disease, CMV retinitis, sarcoidosis
Mechanical	Epiretinal membrane, vitreomacular traction
Other associated conditions	Rhegmatogenous retinal detachment, carotid artery occlusion
Central serous chorioretinopathy	
Hereditary retinal dystrophies	retinitis pigmentosa, choroideremia, autosomal dominant cystoid macular edema
Medication	For example, prostaglandin analogues, epinephrine in aphakic patients, niacin
Intraocular tumors	Malignant melanoma, choroidal hemangioma, angiomatosis retinae
Pseudo CME	No leakage on FA: X-linked hereditary retinoschisis, Goldmann-Favre disease, and nicotinic acid maculopathy
Idiopathic	

83.5 Differential Diagnosis

- Macular phototoxicity
- Stage 1 macular hole
- Vitreomacular traction

83.6 Pathophysiology

In macular edema, there is breakdown of the blood-retinal barrier of retinal capillaries resulting in abnormal permeability of the perifoveal retinal capillaries and leakage. Cystoid spaces typically form in Henle's layer that run laterally away from the fovea. Fluid can accumulate in the outer plexiform layer. Cystoid spaces can also form in any inner retinal layer.

The pathogenesis of CME is multifactorial and usually related to the underlying etiology. Inflammatory mediators are felt to play a role in pseudophakic CME. Decreased pericytes, increased basement membrane thickness, and endothelial changes may contribute to increased retinal vascular permeability in diabetic macular edema. Mechanical forces from vitreomacular traction can lead to CME and release of local inflammatory mediators.

83.7 Workup/Testing

Patient history (e.g., diabetes, uveitis, family history, medications, prior surgery, etc.)
Complete ophthalmologic exam
Adjunctive testing

- OCT: sensitive in detecting CME; treatment response usually measured by serial images; evaluation of vitreoretinal interface possible (Fig. 83.1)
- Fluorescein angiography: CME appears as a petaloid pattern (Fig. 83.2).
- Fundus autofluorescence: cystic spaces can appear hyperautofluoresent due to macular pigment thinning

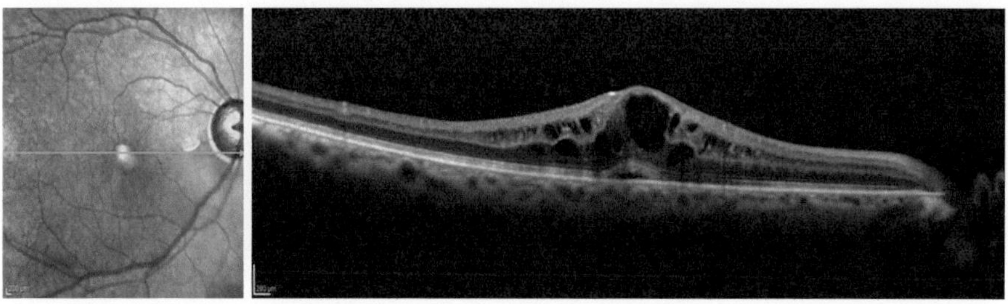

Fig. 83.1 SD-OCT of a right eye demonstrates CME and small amount of subretinal fluid

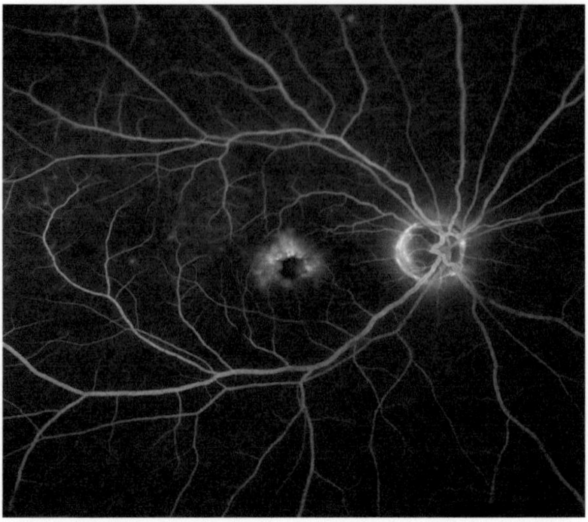

Fig. 83.2 Late-phase fluorescein angiography demonstrates focal flourescein leakage of the perifoveal capillaries and late pooling of the dye in the cystic spaces forming a petaloid pattern

83.8 Prognosis and Management

History and exam are important to identify underlying etiology, which can guide therapy. Depends on the underlying etiology, but most uncomplicated cases of CME resolve spontaneously within a few weeks to months without treatment. Sometimes, resolution of CME may not correlate with improved vision, and prolonged CME can lead to permanent changes in retinal architecture. Treatment options are listed in Table 83.2.

Pseudophakic/Irvine-Gass: occurs 6–10 weeks after cataract surgery in 1–6 % of uncomplicated cataract cases; 95 % resolve spontaneously; risk factors include posterior capsular rupture, vitreous loss, iris prolapse, retained lens fragments, intracapsular extraction, and vitreous strands to wounds; treat if symptomatic; consider YAG vitreolysis for vitreous strands.

83.9 Follow-Up

Most cases resolve spontaneously within a few months. Follow-up in 1–2 months is often recommended to evaluate for efficacy of treatments in uncomplicated cases. When utilizing steroids, IOP checks will be necessary to evaluate for steroid-induced ocular hypertension.

Table 83.2 Treatment options for CME

Topical NSAIDs (dosing often QID for 6–16 weeks) [11, 12]	Ketorolac 0.5 % tid-qid
	Diclofenac 0.1 % tid-qid
	Nepafenac 0.1 % tid
	Flubiprofen 0.03 % qid
	Bromfenac 0.09 % qd-bid
	Fenoprofen 1 % qid
Topical steroids (often used in combination with NSAID) Listed in order of decreasing potency	Difluprednate 0.05 % qid
	Fluorometholone 0.025 %/0.1 % qid (rapid metabolism)[a]
	Dexamethasone 0.1 % qid
	Loteprednol 0.5 % qid[a]
	Rimexolone 1 % qid[a]
	Medrysone 1 % (poor ocular penetration)[a]
	Prednisolone 1 % qid
Sub-tenon steroid (e.g., transeptal, sub-tenon, orbital floor, retrobulbar)	Triamcinolone acetonide 20–40 mg (0.5–1 mL of 40 mg/mL)
Intravitreal steroids	Triamcinolone acetonide (0.05–0.1 mL of 40 mg/mL) 2–4 mg
	Dexamethasone intravitreal implant (Ozurdex) 0.7 mg (32 % eyes with transient >10 mmHg in IOP, peak 60 days after injection; peak effect on retinal thickness and vision at month 3; lasts up to 6 months) [13, 14]
	Fluocinolone acetonide implant (Retisert) 0.59 mg (surgical procedure, lasts 30 months, high rate of cataract progression and elevated IOP)
Systemic steroids	Prednisone 40 mg/day or 1 mg/kg/day with taper
Systemic NSAIDs (e.g., trial for 6 weeks)	Indomethacin 25 mg bid-tid
	Diclofenac 50 mg bid-qid
	Ketorolac 10 mg qid
	Ibuprofen 400–600 mg tid-qid
	Naproxen 250–500 mg bid
	Valdecoxib 10 mg qd
	Celecoxib 100–200 mg bid
	Dosing will need to be adjusted for renal impairment
Carbonic anhydrase inhibitors	Dorzolamide Ophthalmic Solution 2 % tid
	Acetazolamide 250–1000 mg/day
Intravitreal anti-VEGF (e.g., can start with q4 week regimen)	Bevacizumab 1.25 mg
	Ranibizumab 0.5 mg
	Aflibercept 2 mg
Focal laser	For diabetic macula edema, BRVO, macroaneurysm
YAG	Vitreolysis of vitreous strand (with or without wound incarceration)
Vitrectomy +/– membrane peel	For chronic refractory CME or cases associated with vitreoretinal traction or retained lens fragments

[a]Indicates less risk of steroid-induced ocular hypertension

References and Suggested Reading

1. Agarwal A, editor. Gass' atlas of macular diseases. 5th ed. Edinburgh: Elsevier Saunders; 2012.
2. Albert DM, et al. Principles & practice of ophthalmology. 3rd ed. Philadelphia: Saunders; 2008.
3. Guo S, et al. Management of pseudophakic cystoid macular edema. Surv Ophthalmol. 2015;60(2):123–37.
4. Kim SJ, Bressler NM. Optical coherence tomography and cataract surgery. Curr Opin Ophthalmol. 2009;20(1):46–51.
5. Whitmer MT, Kiss S. Cystoid macular edema. In: Yanoff M, Duker JS, editors. Ophthalmology: expert consult. Philadelphia: Elsevier Health Sciences; 2013.
6. Bae JH, Lee CS, Lee SC. Efficacy and safety of intravitreal bevacizumab compared with intravitreal and posterior sub-tenon triamcinolone acetonide for treatment of uveitic cystoid macular edema. Retina. 2011;31(1):111–8.
7. Reis A, et al. Successful treatment of cystoid macular edema with valdecoxib. J Cataract Refract Surg. 2007;33(4):682–5.
8. Hariprasad SM, et al. Treatment of cystoid macular edema with the new-generation NSAID nepafenac 0.1%. Clin Ophthalmol. 2009;3:147–54.
9. Lin JM, et al. Early treatment of severe cystoid macular edema in central retinal vein occlusion with posterior sub-tenon triamcinolone acetonide. Retina. 2007;27(2):180–9.
10. Konstantinidis L, Wolfensberger TJ. Cystoid macular edema. In: Retina. London: Saunders; 2013.
11. Sivaprasad S, Bunce C, Wormald R. Non-steroidal anti-inflammatory agents for cystoid macular oedema following cataract surgery: a systematic review. Br J Ophthalmol. 2005;89(11):1420–2.
12. Warren KA, Bahrani H, Fox JE. NSAIDs in combination therapy for the treatment of chronic pseudophakic cystoid macular edema. Retina. 2010;30(2):260–6.
13. Chan A, Leung LS, Blumenkranz MS. Critical appraisal of the clinical utility of the dexamethasone intravitreal implant (Ozurdex) for the treatment of macular edema related to branch retinal vein occlusion or central retinal vein occlusion. Clin Ophthalmol. 2011;5:1043–9.
14. Haller JA, et al. Dexamethasone intravitreal implant in patients with macular edema related to branch or central retinal vein occlusion twelve-month study results. Ophthalmology. 2011;118(12):2453–60.

Chapter 84
Central Serous Chorioretinopathy

James Lin and Royce W.S. Chen

84.1 Definitions

- Metamorphopsia: the perception of objects as distorted or wavy
- Micropsia: the perception of objects as smaller than their actual size

84.2 Symptoms

- Patients may experience acute onset of blurred or dimmed vision, micropsia, metamorphopsia, paracentral scotoma, and/or decreased color vision.
- Rarely accompanied by migraine-like headache.

84.3 Signs

- Absent foveal reflex
- Serous detachment of the retinal pigment epithelium (RPE).

J. Lin, MD
Department of Ophthalmology, Edward S. Harkness Eye Institute,
Columbia University College of Physicians and Surgeons, New York, NY, USA

R.W.S. Chen, MD (✉)
Department of Ophthalmology, Edward S. Harkness Eye Institute,
Columbia University College of Physicians and Surgeons, New York, NY, USA

Edward S. Harkness Eye Institute, Columbia University Medical Center,
635 W. 165th Street Box 104, New York, NY 10032, USA
e-mail: rc2631@cumc.columbia.edu

C.A. Medina et al. (eds.), *Manual of Retinal Diseases: A Guide to Diagnosis and Management*, DOI 10.1007/978-3-319-20460-4_84

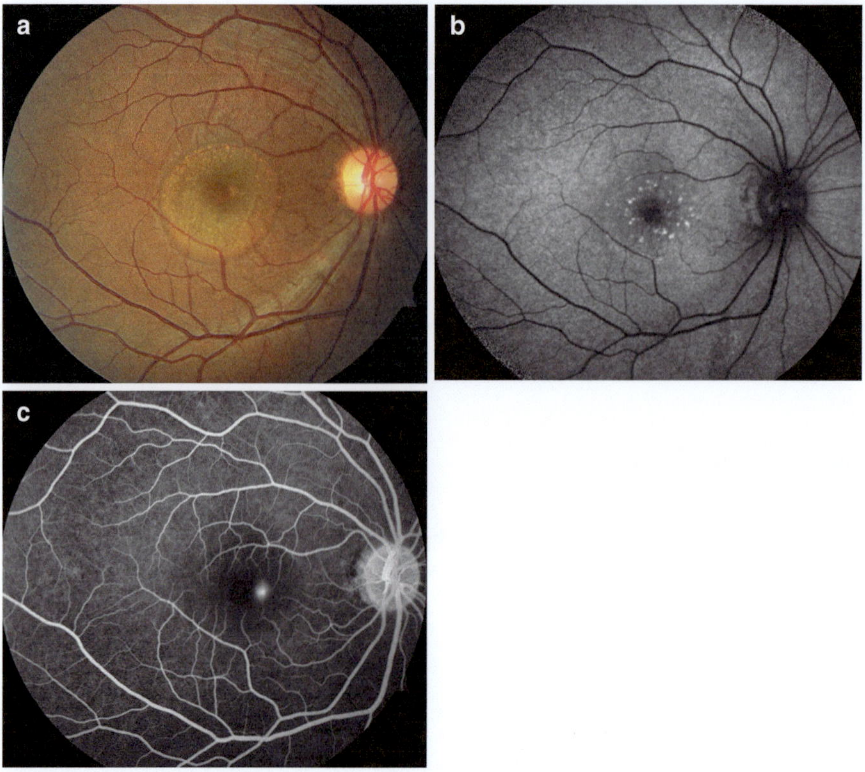

Fig. 84.1 Fundus photograph demonstrating serous detachment of neurosensory retina with yellow subretinal precipitates (**a**). Fundus autofluorescence showing hyperfluorescent dots corresponding to the subretinal precipitates (**b**). Fluorescein angiography of same patient with expansile dot pattern of leakage (**c**)

- Well-circumscribed, serous detachment of the sensory retina (Figs. 84.1 and 84.2).
- Serofibrinous exudate may be present in the area of serous retinal detachment.
- Visual acuity usually ranges from 20/20 to 20/200, but in most patients it is better than 20/30.

84.4 Epidemiology

- Most commonly in healthy men between 25 and 55 years of age
- Male/female ratio of 10:1
- Common in Caucasians, Asians, and Hispanics but rare in African-Americans
- Often bilateral with *asymmetric findings*

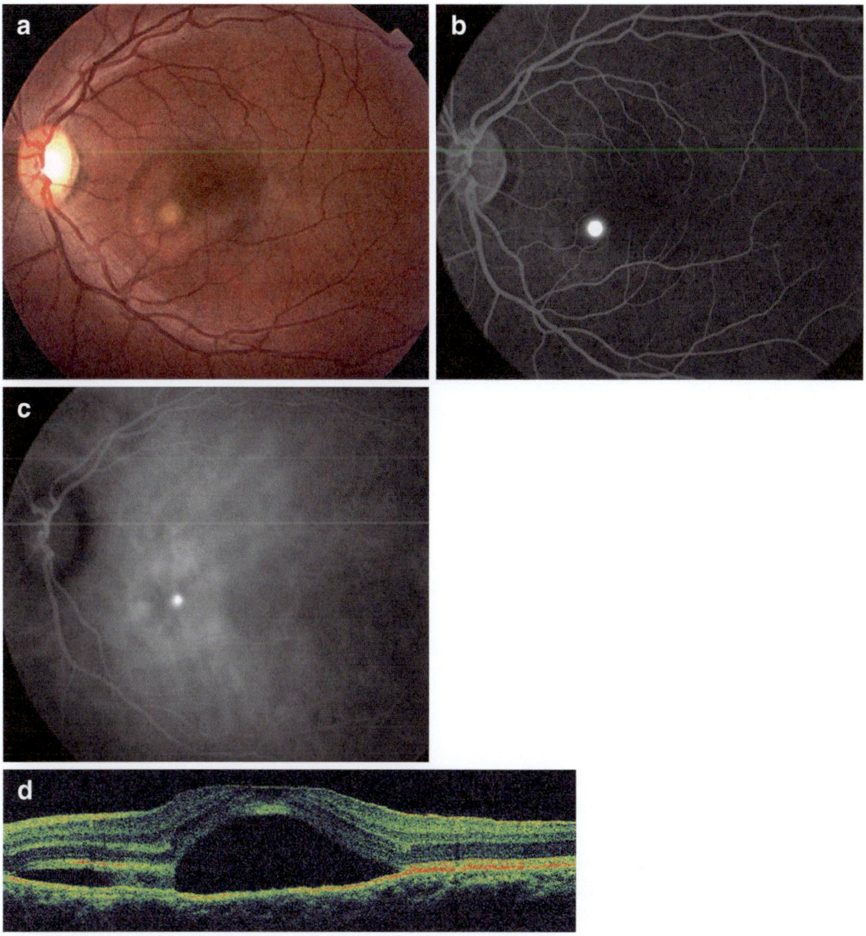

Fig. 84.2 Fundus photograph with area of serous detachment and yellow subretinal fibrinous exudate inferonasal to fovea (**a**). Fluorescein angiogram with expansile dot pattern of hyperfluorescence (**b**). Indocyanine green angiography demonstrating mild inner choroidal staining surrounding a focal hyperfluorescent spot (**c**). Spectral-domain OCT showing serous retinal detachment and subretinal hyperreflectivity nasally, corresponding to the area of subretinal fibrinous exudate (**d**)

84.5 Predisposing Conditions

- Stress
- Anecdotally associated with "type A" personality, hypochondriasis, hysteria, and conversional neurosis
- Exogenous steroid use
- Endogenous hypercortisolism
- Pregnancy

84.6 Differential Diagnosis (Table 84.1)

Table 84.1 Differential diagnosis of central serous chorioretinopathy

Choroidal neovascularization
Macular detachment associated with rhegmatogenous retinal detachment or macular hole
Vogt-Koyanagi-Harada syndrome
Optic nerve pit or coloboma
Choroidal tumors
Intraocular lymphoma
Malignant hypertension
Uveal effusion syndrome
Posterior scleritis

84.7 Etiology

Generally unknown, but associated with endogenously high levels of corticosteroids and treatment of ocular or systemic disease with corticosteroids

84.8 Workup/Testing

- Fluorescein angiography
  - *Expansile dot* pattern is the most common presentation with small, focal, hyperfluorescent leak from choroid through RPE that increases in size and intensity over time (Figs. 84.1 and 84.2).
  - *Smokestack* pattern starts with central spot of hyperfluorescence that spreads vertically and laterally.
  - *Diffuse* pattern occurs when one or more leakage points outside central area develop.
- Optical coherence tomography – increased choroidal thickness accompanied by subretinal fluid and pigment epithelial detachments (Fig. 84.2)
- Fundus autofluorescence (Fig. 84.1)
  - Hypoautofluorescence corresponding to site of RPE leak and pigment mottling in area of RPE disturbance
  - Hyperautofluorescence from "subretinal precipitates" (likely shed photoreceptor outer segments)
- Indocyanine green angiography – choroidal vascular abnormalities including filling delays in choroidal arteries and choriocapillaris, venous dilation, hyperpermeability of choroidal vessels, and multifocal choroidal hyperfluorescent patches (Fig. 84.2)

Table 84.2 Circumstances that may warrant treatment of central serous chorioretinopathy

Serous detachment that persists beyond 3–6 months
Disease recurs in eyes with visual deficits from previous episodes
Permanent visual deficit is present from previous episodes in the fellow eye
Chronic signs such as cystic changes in neurosensory retina or RPE abnormalities
Occupational or other patient needs requiring prompt restoration of vision

84.9 Prognosis and Management

- Visual prognosis is generally good except in chronic recurrent cases and in bullous CSC.
- 80–90 % of eyes with CSC undergo spontaneous resorption of subretinal fluid within 3–4 months.
- Current treatment guidelines recommend observation in most cases, except in the following circumstances (Table 84.2).
- Laser photocoagulation can induce rapid remission but may cause blind spot.
- Verteporfin photodynamic therapy (PDT) – can be used when detachment is too close to center of fovea and may resolve acute leaks of subretinal fluid
- Eplerenone has demonstrated efficacy in some cases of chronic CSC (>4 months).
- CNV may rarely develop in patients with typical CSC.
- Some eyes may have permanently reduced visual acuity, and about 40–50 % of patients experience one or more recurrences.

84.10 Follow-Up

- Examine patient every 6–8 weeks until resolution.
- Follow-up examination within 3–4 weeks if laser photocoagulation is performed to detect post-laser CNV.

References and Suggested Reading

1. Bousquet E, Beydoun T, Zhao M, Hassan L, Offret O, Behar-Cohen F. Mineralocorticoid receptor antagonism in the treatment of chronic central serous chorioretinopathy: a pilot study. Retina. 2013;33:2096–102.
2. Imamura Y, Fujiwara T, Margolis R, Spaide RF. Enhanced depth imaging optical coherence tomography of the choroid in central serous chorioretinopathy. Retina. 2009;29(10):1469–73.
3. Lim JI, Glassman AR, Aiello LP, Chakravarthy U, Flaxel CJ, Spaide RF, Macula Society CSC Collaborative Study Group, Research and Education Committee and Website Committee. Collaborative retrospective macula society study of photodynamic therapy for chronic central

serous chorioretinopathy. Ophthalmology. 2014;121:1073–8. doi:10.1016/j.ophtha.2013.11.040. Epub 2014 Jan 16.
4. Ober MD, Yannuzzi LA, Do DV, Spaide RF, Bressler NM, Jampol LM, Angelilli A, Eandi CM, Lyon AT. Photodynamic therapy for focal retinal pigment epithelial leaks secondary to central serous chorioretinopathy. Ophthalmology. 2005;112(12):2088–94.

Section XII
Toxic Maculopathy

Carlos A. Medina

Chapter 85 Chloroquine/Hydroxychloroquine Toxicity

Carlos A. Medina

85.1 Definitions

- Chloroquine (CQ)
- Hydroxychloroquine (HCQ)

85.2 Symptoms

Decreased vision, abnormal color vision, and nyctalopia

85.3 Signs

- Early: None
- Late: Bull's eye maculopathy, loss of foveal reflex, increased macular pigmentation, arteriolar narrowing, vascular sheathing, peripheral pigmentation, abnormal testing (ERG, EOG), and whorl-like corneal changes

C.A. Medina, MD
Department of Ophthalmology, Bascom Palmer Eye Institute, University of Miami, 900 NW 17th St., Miami, FL 33136, USA
e-mail: camedina2020@gmail.com

C.A. Medina et al. (eds.), *Manual of Retinal Diseases: A Guide to Diagnosis and Management*, DOI 10.1007/978-3-319-20460-4_85

85.4 Dosing

Most patients are routinely given 400 mg of Plaquenil daily. This dose is considered acceptable, except for individuals of short stature (men 5′4″ and shorter and women 5′6″ and shorter) for whom the dose should be determined on the basis of ideal body weight to avoid overdosage:

- Plaquenil 6.5 mg/kg
- Based on lean body weight dosing

85.5 Predisposing Conditions

- Duration of use (>5 years)
- 1000 g cumulative
- Elderly
- Preexisting retinal disease
- Kidney or liver disease

85.6 Differential Diagnosis

Comparison with baseline examination should help rule out any underlying and confounding diagnosis. The differential diagnosis of bull's eye maculopathy should also be included (Table 85.1).

85.7 Etiology

Not well understood but the drugs have acute effects on the metabolism of retinal cells, including the photoreceptors, and bind to melanin in the RPE. This binding may serve to concentrate the agents and contribute to, or prolong, their toxic effects.

Table 85.1 Differential diagnosis of bull's eye maculopathy

Age-related macular degeneration
Benign concentric annular dystrophy
Central areolar choroidal dystrophy
Chloroquine/hydroxychloroquine retinal toxicity
Cone and cone-rod dystrophies
Stargardt disease
Batten disease

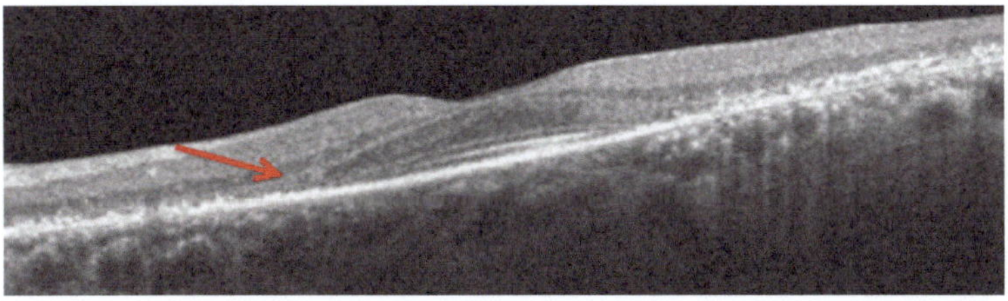

Fig. 85.1 Parafoveal thinning of photoreceptor layers and loss of the inner-outer segment line (*arrow*)

85.8 Workup/Testing

- Baseline testing is recommended within 1 year of start of HCQ and should include white 10–2 automated threshold testing and one of the following:
  - SD-OCT
  - FAF
  - MF-ERG
- Dilated fundus examination should be performed for detection of associated retinal disorders but should not be relied on for screening. Annual screening should begin at 5 years and include:
  - Ocular examination
  - White 10–2 visual field
  - In addition to one or more of the following:
    - Spectral domain OCT (Fig. 85.1)
    - Multifocal ERG
    - Fundus autofluorescence
- Fundus photography is recommended for documentation, especially at baseline, but not sensitive for screening. Time-domain OCT, fluorescein angiography, full-field ERG, Amsler grid, color testing, and EOG are not recommended.

85.9 Prognosis and Management

The goal of screening should be the recognition of toxicity before bull's eye retinopathy is visible on fundus examination, and patients should understand that screening can recognize toxicity early and minimize visual loss, but cannot necessarily prevent all toxicity or guarantee there will be no visual loss. No medical therapy has proven effective in CQ or HCQ toxicity other than cessation of the drug, which is always recommended (if medically acceptable) when toxicity is suspected. Visual prognosis depends on the amount of damage at detection. Progressive damage up to 3 years after discontinuation of treatment has been observed in some patients.

85.10 Follow-Up

Baseline testing should be performed, within one year or starting treatment. Annual screening should start at 5 years with early. Annual screening for patients that have risk factors for developing toxicity such as elderly patiendts and those with pre-existing retinal disease.

References and Suggested Reading

1. Marmor MF. Efficient and effective screening for hydroxychloroquine toxicity. Am J Ophthalmol. 2013;155(3):413–4.
2. Marmor MF, Kellner U, Lai TY, Lyons JS, Mieler WF. Revised recommendations on screening for chloroquine and hydroxychloroquine retinopathy. Ophthalmology. 2011;118(2):415–22.
3. Melles RB, Marmor MF. The risk of toxic retinopathy in patients on long-term hydroxychloroquine therapy. JAMA Ophthalmol. 2014;132(12):1453–60.

Chapter 86
Drug-Induced Toxic Maculopathies

Thalmon R. Campagnoli and William E. Smiddy

86.1 Definitions

Many drugs besides chloroquine and hydroxychloroquine may induce toxic maculopathy. Most toxicity effects are reversible upon discontinuation, resulting in minimal or no visual loss. Understanding the mechanism and pattern of macular toxicity is of great importance to recognize early stages to avoid irreversible vision loss (Table 86.1).

86.2 Symptoms

- Decreased vision
- Central or paracentral visual field changes
- Dyschromatopsia
- Nyctalopia

86.3 Signs

Depends on the drug's toxicity pattern and stage. Usually bilateral

W.E. Smiddy, MD (✉) • T.R. Campagnoli, MD
Department of Ophthalmology, Bascom Palmer Eye Institute, University of Miami,
900 NW 17th St., Miami, FL 33136, USA
e-mail: wsmiddy@med.miami.edu

C.A. Medina et al. (eds.), *Manual of Retinal Diseases: A Guide to Diagnosis and Management*, DOI 10.1007/978-3-319-20460-4_86

Table 86.1 Drugs and patterns of macular toxicity

Pattern	Drugs
RPE disruption	Thioridazine, chlorpromazine, quinine sulfate, clofazimine, deferoxamine, corticosteroid preparations[a], cisplatin and carmustine, denileukin diftitox, ritonavir
Vascular damage	Quinine sulfate, cisplatin and carmustine, talc, oral contraceptives, aminoglycosides, interferon, ergot alkaloids, gemcitabine, denileukin diftitox, imatinib mesylate, cocaine
Cystoid macular edema	Epinephrine, latanoprost, nicotinic acid, paclitaxel/docetaxel, pioglitazone
Retinal folds	Acetazolamide, chlortalidone, ethoxyzolamide, hydrochlorothiazide, metronidazole, sulfa antibiotics, topiramate, triamterene
Crystalline retinopathy	Tamoxifen, canthaxanthin, methoxyflurane, talc, nitrofurantoin, ritonavir
Uveitis	Rifabutin, cidofovir
Miscellaneous	Digoxin, methanol, fludarabine, sildenafil, tadalafil, vardenafil

[a]Toxicity caused by the vehicle in the corticosteroid solution (benzalkonium chloride, myristyl-gamma-picolinium chloride)

Early stage:

- None or minimal fundus changes in the majority of cases.
- Blunted foveal reflex is almost universally observable when fundus changes occur.

Intermediate to late stage:

- Drugs causing disruption of retinal pigment epithelium (RPE) characteristically manifest as RPE atrophy or hyperplasia (intercalated hyperpigmented clumps); these findings may progress and be associated with attenuation of retinal vessels and optic nerve pallor.
- Substances inducing vascular damage (inflammation, constriction) commonly induce microaneurysms, cotton-wool spots, intraretinal hemorrhages, edema, venous beading, capillary nonperfusion, and/or optic disc and retina neovascularization. Retinal whitening, vessels attenuation, and optic disc pallor may ensue if arterial occlusion occurs.
- Cystoid macular edema (CME) classically appears as radially oriented cystoid spaces of clear liquid centered at the macula.
- Macular folds presumably originate from vitreous traction due to anterior shifting of the lens-iris diaphragm caused by certain drugs. Those patients may present with anterior chamber shallowing and symptoms of transient acute myopia.
- Associated signs of uveitis vary widely in degree of vitritis and retinal vasculitis.
- The hallmark of crystalline retinopathy is paramacular crystals typically surrounding the foveal center and may be associated with retinal edema. Those crystals may be deposited in different retinal layers (inner retina, RPE) and may be located along retinal vessels.

Table 86.2 Other toxic ocular effects

Drugs	Ocular effects
Chlorpromazine	Oculogyric crisis, miosis, paralysis of accommodation, crystalline opacities
Deferoxamine	Macular pseudovitelliform detachment, optic neuritis, cataract
Clofazimine	Polychromatic corneal deposits
Cisplatin and carmustine	Ocular pain, chemosis, secondary glaucoma, internal ophthalmoplegia, cavernous sinus syndrome
Imatinib mesylate	Periocular edema
Rifabutin	Anterior uveitis, corneal endothelial deposits
Cidofovir	Anterior uveitis
Drugs causative of retinal folds	Acute myopia, anterior chamber shallowing

Table 86.3 Dosages reported to cause ocular toxicity

Acute toxicity		Chronic toxicity	
Thioridazine	800 mg/day	Quinine sulfate	2 g/day
Quinine sulfate	4 g/day	Clofazimine	200 mg/day; 40 g total
Aminoglycoside[a]	100 μg	Chlorpromazine	2400 mg/day
Rifabutin	300 mg/day	Nicotinic acid	1.5 g/day
Cidofovir[a]	10 μg	Tamoxifen	10 mg/day; 7.7 g total
		Canthaxanthin	19 g total

[a]Intravitreal dose

Other associated ocular changes are sometimes seen in certain drug toxicities (Table 86.2).

86.4 Dosing

Some drugs typically cause toxicity acutely or due to a high total daily dose administered; in theory, those are safer to use for an indeterminate period of time by avoiding overdose. Other drugs induce damage to the macula through cumulative exposure, even if used in recommended doses (Table 86.3).

There is limited knowledge to assume safe dosage limits for some drugs, especially considering the broad range of comorbidities and other factors that may potentially make the retina susceptible to damage even when drugs are used in a recommended dose:

- Oral contraceptives may cause central retinal artery or vein occlusion and should be used cautiously in patients with systemic or retinal vascular disease.
- Heparin overdose may cause scattered retinal hemorrhages completely reversible when dose readjusted.

- Aminoglycosides may obliterate vessels and cause retinal necrosis when injected into the vitreous cavity.
- "Angiographically negative" (nonleaking) CME may occur in nicotinic acid and paclitaxel/docetaxel toxicity.
- Inadvertent benzalkonium chloride or myristyl-gamma-picolinium chloride (contained in some corticosteroid preparations) injection into the eye should prompt immediate surgical removal.
- Methanol can cause optic nerve hyperemia and retina edema within 12–18 h after ingestion. Optic nerve atrophy and irreversible visual loss may ensue if recovery is not evident by 6 days.

86.5 Predisposing Conditions

- Dosing (Table 86.3)
- Duration of use
- Kidney (e.g., methoxyflurane) or liver disease
- Elderly
- Previous retinal pathology
- Use of multiple drugs (drug interaction)

86.6 Differential Diagnosis

Commonly seen retinal pathologies manifesting mainly with RPE and/or vascular changes should be ruled out: age-related macular degeneration, diabetic retinopathy, CME, uveitis, CRVO, BRVO, arterial occlusions, anterior optic neuropathies, macular dystrophies, Stargardt disease, Batten disease, and various others.

86.7 Etiology

Not well understood for a many drugs. Some pathogenic mechanisms include:

- Binding to melanin in the RPE (thioridazine, chlorpromazine)
- Vascular occlusion due to inflammation, thromboembolic event, or mechanical obstruction (talc, interferon, oral contraceptives)
- Direct toxic effect of metabolites to photoreceptors (digoxin), other retinal cells (methanol, fludarabine), or ciliary body (cidofovir)
- Biochemical effects in multiple retinal layers (tamoxifen inhibiting glutamate uptake by RPE cells)
- Interference with phototransduction (sildenafil, tadalafil, vardenafil)

86.8 Workup/Testing

Medical evaluation to assess for systemic disease might be indicated. Retinal vessel attenuation and disc pallor may be early manifestations of quinine toxicity. The most useful tests for diagnosis and/or follow-up are:

- Dilated fundus examination
- Fundus photography; in some instance recommended for documentation, especially at baseline
- Visual field (white 10–2)
- Fluorescein angiography (FA); demonstrate microaneurysms, vascular obstruction or dilation, or areas of capillary nonperfusion or neovascularization
- Spectral-domain OCT (SD-OCT); definitive test for retinal edema and evaluation of RPE and ellipsoid layers abnormalities
- FAF; useful to detect mild RPE toxic signs
- Multifocal electroretinogram (m-ERG)

86.9 Prognosis and Management

- Vision loss is absent or minimal in the majority of cases, at least early on. Substances carrying higher risk for significant, progressive, or irreversible harm include the following: thioridazine, quinine sulfate, clofazimine, corticosteroid preparations, cisplatin and carmustine, talc, oral contraceptives, aminoglycosides, interferon, methanol, fludarabine, sildenafil, and tadalafil.
- Upon discovery of toxicity, the drug should be discontinued if medically acceptable.
- Laser photocoagulation may be indicated if areas of capillary dropout are extensive or if neovascularization occurs.
- CME caused by tamoxifen or paclitaxel/docetaxel seems to respond well to anti-VEGF therapy, allowing continuation of the drug in selected cases. Topical or systemic acetazolamide may be attempted for paclitaxel/docetaxel CME.
- Hemodialysis may be indicated to remove certain drugs from the body (e.g., methanol).
- Prevention of exposure to unintented targets is the key to avoiding toxicity strongly advisable in some instances (e.g., intravitreal aminoglycosides or benzalkonium chloride or myristyl-gamma-picolinium chloride-containing preparations).

86.10 Follow-Up

The follow-up regimen is in accordance with the severity of the toxicity or the therapeutic options available. Once drug use is interrupted and the complications are treated (e.g., CME, neovascularization), a first 6-month interval visit followed by annual ophthalmologic evaluation consisting of dilated fundus examination and ancillary testing is a reasonable approach. It is the authors' recommendation that patients using any of the aforementioned drugs in its normal dosage range should be carefully evaluated and strictly followed in case ocular signs or visual symptoms take place.

References and Suggested Reading

1. Fraunfelder FT, Fraunfelder FW, Chambers WA. Drug-induced ocular side effects. In: Fraunfelder FT, Fraunfelder FW, Chambers WA, editors. Clinical ocular toxicology. 1st ed. Philadelphia: Elsevier Saunders; 2008. p. 45–287.
2. Mittra RA, Mieler WF. Drug toxicity of the posterior segment. In: Ryan SJ, editor. Retina. 5th ed. Philadelphia: Elsevier Saunders; 2013. p. 1532–54.

Section XIII
Uveitis: White Dot Syndromes

Jared E. Knickelbein

Chapter 87
Evaluation of Patients with a White Dot Syndrome

Jared E. Knickelbein, Robert B. Nussenblatt, and H. Nida Sen

87.1 Definitions

The term white dot syndromes (WDS) refers to a group of presumed inflammatory eye diseases that predominantly affect the outer retina, retinal pigment epithelium (RPE), choriocapillaris, choroid, or a combination of these sites. The WDS covered in this section are limited to those that are more commonly seen and include:

- Acute posterior multifocal placoid pigment epitheliopathy (APMPPE)
- Birdshot chorioretinopathy (BCR)
- Multiple evanescent white dot syndrome (MEWDS)
- Multifocal choroiditis and panuveitis (MCP)
- Presumed ocular histoplasmosis syndrome (POHS)
- Punctate inner choroidopathy (PIC)
- Serpiginous choroiditis (SC)

87.2 Symptoms

Symptoms common to most WDS include blurred vision, photopsias, scotomas, and floaters.

J.E. Knickelbein, MD PhD (✉) • R.B. Nussenblatt, MD MPH • H.N. Sen, MD MHS
Laboratory of Immunology, National Eye Institute, National Institutes of Health,
10 Center Dr., Bldg. 10, Room 10D45, Bethesda, MD 20892, USA
e-mail: knickelbeinje@nei.nih.gov

C.A. Medina et al. (eds.), *Manual of Retinal Diseases: A Guide to Diagnosis and Management*, DOI 10.1007/978-3-319-20460-4_87

87.3 Signs

- Variable degrees of anterior chamber and vitreous inflammation.
- Hypopigmented chorioretinal lesions of various size and configuration are seen in most WDS (see table).
- Retinal vasculitis and sequelae of intraocular inflammation, including macular edema (ME), epiretinal membrane (ERM), and choroidal neovascularization (CNV), may be seen.

87.4 Epidemiology

- MCP, MEWDS, PIC, and possibly BCR are more common in women.
- Most WDS is present in people aged 20–60 years.

87.5 Predisposing Conditions

Depends on condition (see Table 87.1):

- APMPPE and MEWDS are associated with viral prodromes.
- MCP, MEWDS, and PIC are associated with myopia.

87.6 Differential Diagnosis

- Syphilis
- Tuberculosis (TB)
- Sarcoidosis
- Lyme
- Bartonella
- Intraocular lymphoma in older individuals

87.7 Etiology

Most WDS is thought to represent autoimmune phenomena possibly with infectious triggers.

Table 87.1 Comparison of white dot syndromes

White dot syndrome	Sex/average age (years)	Laterality	Onset/course	Pertinent associations	Pertinent exam/imaging findings	Treatment
Acute posterior multifocal placoid pigment epitheliopathy (APMPPE)	Female = male 20–30	Bilateral	Acute/self-limited	Viral prodrome; may have cerebral vasculitis	Multiple, cream-colored placoid lesions of variable size; OCT with outer retinal disruption; FA with early hypofluorescence and late hyperfluorescence	Most cases may be observed; systemic corticosteroids for foveal threatening or recurrent disease
Birdshot chorioretinopathy (BCR)	Female > male 40–60	Bilateral	Insidious/chronic	HLA-A29	Deep ovoid cream-colored lesions (up to 1500 μm) radially distributed through posterior pole in "shotgun" pattern; FA may show vascular leakage; ICGA shows hypofluorescent spots more numerous than seen clinically	Immunosuppression or extended-release intravitreal corticosteroid implant
Multifocal choroiditis and panuveitis (MCP)	Female > male 30–40	Bilateral	Insidious/chronic	Myopia; CNV in ~33 %	AC reaction and intense vitritis; multiple to several hundreds discrete lesions of variable size (100–500 μm) at level of RPE or inner choroid scattered through posterior pole and periphery, become "punched-out" with chronicity	Immunosuppression or periocular/intravitreal corticosteroids; anti-VEGF intravitreal injection for CNV

(continued)

Table 87.1 (continued)

White dot syndrome	Sex/average age (years)	Laterality	Onset/course	Pertinent associations	Pertinent exam/imaging findings	Treatment
Multiple evanescent white dot syndrome (MEWDS)	Female > male 20–40	Unilateral	Insidious/ self-limited	Viral prodrome; myopia	Multifocal, small, gray-white perifoveal lesions, "grainy" macula, FA with early hyperfluorescence in "wreath-like" pattern	Most cases may be observed; systemic corticosteroids for aggressive or recurrent disease
Presumed ocular histoplasmosis syndrome (POHS)	Female = male 20–50	Bilateral	Insidious/generally self-limited	Common in Ohio and Mississippi river valleys; CNV in ~5 %	Triad of "punched-out" peripheral choroidal scars, peripapillary atrophy, and absence of anterior or posterior segment inflammation	Most cases may be observed; consider periocular/ intraocular corticosteroids for progressive disease; anti-VEGF intravitreal injection for CNV
Punctate inner choroidopathy (PIC)	Female = male 20–40	Bilateral	Acute/generally self-limited	Caucasian; myopia; CNV common (up to 75 %)	Multiple, small (100–300 μm), well-defined, yellow-white lesions in the outer retina/inner choroid, generally limited to the posterior pole	Most cases may be observed; immunosuppression or periocular/intraocular corticosteroids for foveal threatening or progressive disease; anti-VEGF intravitreal injection for CNV
Serpiginous choroiditis (SC)	Female = male 40–60	Bilateral, asymmetric	Varies/chronic, recurrent	CNV common (up to 25 %)	Helicoid patches of creamy yellow subretinal infiltrates extending from the optic nerve; OCT with outer retinal disruption; FA with early hypofluorescence and late hyperfluorescence	Immunosuppression or periocular/intraocular corticosteroids; anti-VEGF intravitreal injection for CNV

CNV choroidal neovascularization, *OCT* optical coherence tomography, *FA* fluorescein angiography, *ICGA* indocyanine green angiography, *VEGF* vascular endothelial growth factor

87.8 Workup/Testing

Laboratory testing for syphilis, with syphilis IgG and rapid plasma regain (RPR), and TB, with either PPD or TB-specific interferon gamma release assay (e.g., QuantiFERON-TB Gold®) as well as chest X-ray, should be performed to rule out these infectious etiologies. In addition to CXR, serum angiotensin-converting enzyme (ACE; if patient is not on ACE inhibitors) and lysozyme can be obtained to screen for sarcoidosis. Several ophthalmic imaging modalities may be useful in diagnosis and monitoring:

- *Color fundus photography*: Often useful in documenting lesions and in monitoring for progression of disease.
- *Fundus autofluorescence (FAF)*: Especially useful in APMPPE and SC in which active lesions often have a hyperautofluorescent halo and inactive lesions appear hypoautofluorescent.
- *Optical coherence tomography (OCT)*: Useful in determining extent of outer retinal disruption in cases with macular pathology (APMPPE, MEWDS, PIC, SC) and in following reconstitution of outer retinal structures after treatment.
- *Fluorescein angiography (FA)*: Several WDS have distinctive FA patterns (see Table 87.1):
  - APMPPE and SC show early hypofluorescence with late hyperfluorescence.
  - BCR may show retinal vasculitis.
  - MEWDS shows early hyperfluorescence in a "wreath-like" pattern.
  - May be useful in cases of suspected CNV.
- *Indocyanine green angiography* (*ICGA*): May show hypofluorescent spots more numerous than observed clinically in BCR and MEWDS. Late ICG tends to show larger areas of hypofluorescence in most WDS.
- *Visual field testing*: May be useful in documenting scotomas or enlarged blind spot.

87.9 Prognosis and Management

Depends on condition, see Table 87.1 and individual chapters:

- Some WDS, such as APMPPE and MEWDS, are generally self-limited and may not require treatment.
- Others, such as BCR, nearly always require treatment with systemic immunosuppression.

87.10 Follow-Up

Patients should be followed closely (every 2–4 weeks) during acute inflammation, especially if the fovea is threatened. Once quiescence is established, follow-up can be prolonged.

References and Suggested Reading

1. Jampol LM, Becker KG. White spot syndromes of the retina: a hypothesis based on the common genetic hypothesis of autoimmune/inflammatory disease. Am J Ophthalmol. 2003; 135:376–9.
2. Mirza RG, Jampol LM. White spot syndromes and related diseases. In: Schachat AP, Sadda SR, editors. Retina. 5th ed. Amsterdam, The Netherlands: Elsevier; 2013.
3. Nussenblatt RB, Whitecup SM. White-dot syndromes. In: Nussenblatt RB, Whitecup SM, editors. Uveitis: fundamentals and clinical practice. 4th ed. Amsterdam, The Netherlands: Mosby Elsevier; 2010.
4. Quillen DA, Davis JB, Gottlieb JL, et al. The white dot syndromes. Am J Ophthalmol. 2004;137:538–50.

Chapter 88
Multiple Evanescent White Dot Syndrome (MEWDS)

Austin Fox, Jared E. Knickelbein, Robert B. Nussenblatt, and H. Nida Sen

88.1 Definitions

Multiple evanescent white dot syndrome (MEWDS) is an idiopathic inflammatory condition, characterized by multiple white dots in the fundus typically localized to the outer retina, retinal pigment epithelium (RPE), or choroid.

88.2 Symptoms

Acute onset, painless, usually unilateral, blurred vision, scotomas, or photopsias

88.3 Signs

- Visual acuity (VA) may range from 20/20 to 20/200.
- Afferent pupillary defect may be present.
- Anterior chamber is generally quiet.
- Low-grade vitreous cells may be seen.
- Multiple, small, well-defined, gray-white dots (100–200 μm) at the level of the outer retina in the perifoveal area, sparing the fovea.
- Macula with white or orange granularity and abnormal foveal reflex (Fig. 88.1).
- Optic disc edema and hyperemia is common (enlarged blind spot).

A. Fox, BS • J.E. Knickelbein, MD PhD • R.B. Nussenblatt, MD MPH • H.N. Sen, MD MHS (✉)
Laboratory of Immunology, National Eye Institute, National Institutes of Health,
10 Center Dr., Bldg. 10, Room 10N109, Bethesda, MD 20892, USA
e-mail: senh@nei.nih.gov

C.A. Medina et al. (eds.), *Manual of Retinal Diseases: A Guide to Diagnosis and Management*, DOI 10.1007/978-3-319-20460-4_88

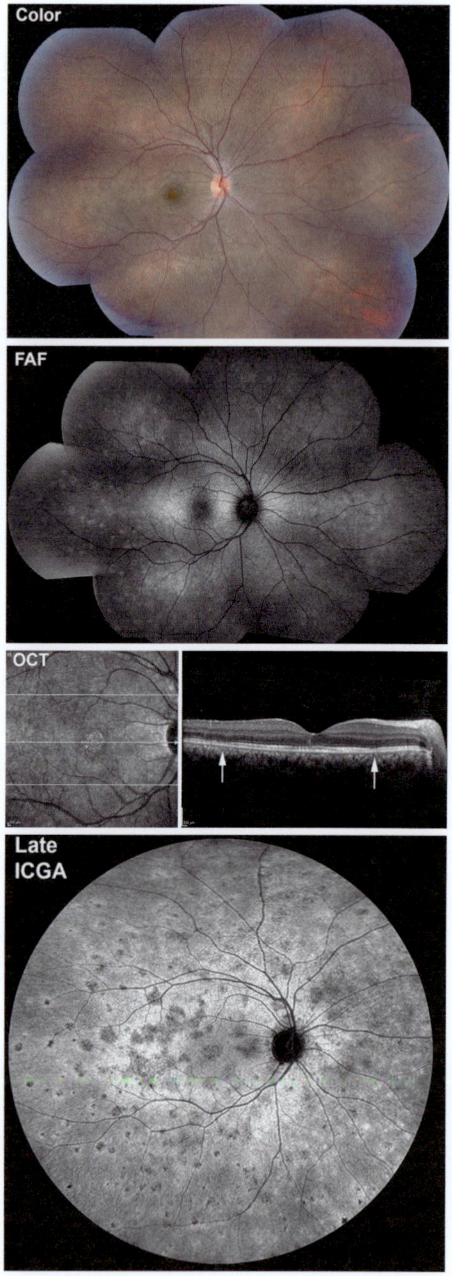

Fig. 88.1 Fundus photograph (*color*), fundus autofluorescence (*FAF*), optical coherence tomography (*OCT*), and late indocyanine green angiography (*ICGA*) image from a 22-year-old moderately myopic male with MEWDS. Note the grainy foveal appearance in the color image; numerous hyperautofluorescent spots in the FAF; disruption of the outer retina, especially the ellipsoid zone (*arrows*), in the OCT; and the numerous hypofluorescent spots in the late ICGA image.

88.4 Epidemiology

MEWDS usually affects individuals in their third to fifth decade (mean age of onset around 28 years) though patients as young as 10 and as old as 67 have been reported. Prevalence is higher in females (3:1). There is no known racial predominance.

88.5 Predisposing Conditions

- Possible association with myopia
- Often preceded by viral or flu-like prodrome

88.6 Differential Diagnosis

- Acute posterior multifocal placoid pigment epitheliopathy (APMPPE)
- Acute macular neuroretinopathy (AMN)
- Acute zonal occult outer retinopathy (AZOOR)
- Acute retinal pigment epitheliitis (Krill's disease)
- Punctate inner choroidopathy (PIC)
- Multifocal choroiditis and panuveitis (MCP)
- Vogt-Koyanagi-Harada (VKH) disease
- Birdshot chorioretinopathy
- Serpiginous choroiditis
- Sarcoidosis
- Syphilis
- Tuberculosis

88.7 Etiology

Not well understood although infectious and autoimmune etiologies have been suggested.

88.8 Workup/Testing

Laboratory testing for syphilis, with syphilis IgG and rapid plasma regain (RPR), and TB, with either PPD or TB-specific interferon gamma release assay (e.g., QuantiFERON-TB Gold®) as well as chest X-ray, should be performed to rule out these infectious etiologies. Several ocular imaging modalities may be useful in diagnosis and monitoring of disease:

- *Fundus autofluorescence (FAF)*: Acute lesions appear hyperfluorescent (Fig. 88.1).
- *Optical coherence tomography (OCT)*: May show disruption of outer retinal structures, especially the ellipsoid zone (Fig. 88.1).
- *Fluorescein angiography (FA)*: Typically shows early hyperfluorescence in "wreath-like" pattern with late staining.
- *Indocyanine green angiography (ICGA)*: Late frames show hypofluorescent lesions generally more numerous than seen clinically or by FA (Fig. 88.1).
- *Electroretinogram (ERG)*: May show reduced a-wave amplitude and reduced early receptor potential amplitudes; ERG returns to baseline with convalescence.
- *Visual field testing*: May show temporal or paracentral scotomas or enlarged blind spot.

88.9 Prognosis and Management

MEWDS is a self-limiting condition, and prognosis is excellent. Episodes last an average of 7 weeks, and most patients return to their baseline visual acuity and experience no further visual symptoms. However, cases of recurrence have been reported. For those with recurrent or persistent disease, systemic treatment (e.g., oral prednisone) should be considered.

88.10 Follow-Up

Patients should be followed closely until symptoms and exam completely resolve.

References and Suggested Reading

1. dell'Omo R, Pavesio CE. Multiple evanescent white dot syndrome (MEWDS). Int Ophthalmol Clin. 2012;52:221–8.
2. Jampol LM, Sieving PA, Pugh D, et al. Multiple evanescent white dot syndrome. I. Clinical findings. Arch Ophthalmol. 1984;102:671–4.
3. Li D, Kishi S. Restored photoreceptor outer segment damage in multiple evanescent white dot syndrome. Ophthalmology. 2009;116:762–70.
4. Nussenblatt RB, Whitecup SM. White-dot syndromes. In: Nussenblatt RB, Whitecup SM, editors. Uveitis: fundamentals and clinical practice. 4th ed. Mosby Elsevier; Amsterdam, the Netherlands 2010.
5. Quillen DA, Davis JB, Gottlieb JL, et al. The white dot syndromes. Am J Ophthalmol. 2004;137:538–50.

Chapter 89
Multifocal Choroiditis and Panuveitis

Jared E. Knickelbein, Robert B. Nussenblatt, and H. Nida Sen

89.1 Definitions

Multifocal choroiditis and panuveitis (MCP) is an idiopathic inflammatory eye disease characterized by discrete variably sized chorioretinal lesions accompanied by an inflammatory reaction in the vitreous and often anterior chamber. Clinically, MCP mimics presumed ocular histoplasmosis syndrome with the exception that MCP is associated with vitreous and often anterior chamber cellular reaction. It is presumed to have an autoimmune etiology. It is more common in young moderately myopic females and is generally bilateral. Secondary complications, such as macular edema, epiretinal membrane (ERM), and choroidal neovascularization (CNV), are important causes of vision loss with MCP.

89.2 Symptoms

Decreased vision, scotomas, and photopsias

J.E. Knickelbein, MD PhD (✉) • R.B. Nussenblatt, MD MPH • H.N. Sen, MD MHS
Laboratory of Immunology, National Eye Institute, National Institutes of Health,
10 Center Dr., Bldg. 10, Room 10D45, Bethesda, MD 20892, USA
e-mail: knickelbeinje@nei.nih.gov

C.A. Medina et al. (eds.), *Manual of Retinal Diseases: A Guide to Diagnosis and Management*, DOI 10.1007/978-3-319-20460-4_89

89.3 Signs

- Anterior chamber reaction and intense vitritis are common.
- Multiple to several hundred discrete lesions of variable size (100–500 um) at the level of the RPE or inner choroid are scattered through the posterior pole and periphery (Fig. 89.1).
- Lesions may be located singly, in clumps, or linearly and become "punched out" in appearance with variable pigment clumping with chronicity.
- Peripapillary atrophy is common and peripapillary CNV may develop.
- Subfoveal CNV occurs in approximately 30 % of eyes.

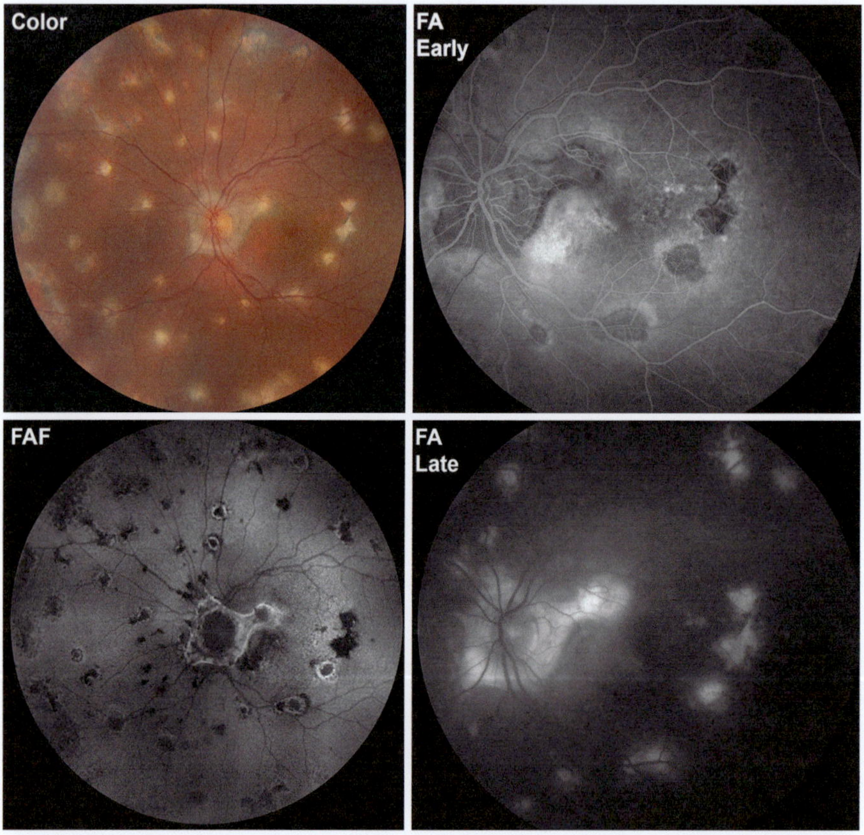

Fig. 89.1 Color fundus photography, fundus autofluorescence (FAF), and fluorescein angiography (FA) images of the left eye of a 29-year-old mildly myopic woman with MCP. Note the scattered lesions of various size (~100–500 μm) and stage with larger and more numerous lesions seen on FAF and FA. FAF also shows hypofluorescent lesions (inactive) as well as lesions with hyperfluorescent ring (mildly active/resolving). FA shows early hypofluorescence with late staining

89.4 Epidemiology

- MCP is approximately three times more common in females.
- The average age of onset is 31–45 years.
- Bilateral in >80 % of cases.

89.5 Predisposing Conditions

- Possible association with moderate myopia
- No systemic manifestations

89.6 Differential Diagnosis

- Presumed ocular histoplasmosis syndrome (POHS)
- Punctate inner choroidopathy (PIC)
- Birdshot chorioretinopathy
- Serpiginous choroiditis
- Ampiginous choroiditis
- Subretinal fibrosis and uveitis syndrome
- Sarcoidosis
- Syphilis
- Tuberculosis (TB)

89.7 Etiology

Unknown, presumed autoimmune etiology

89.8 Workup/Testing

Laboratory testing for syphilis, with syphilis IgG and rapid plasma regain (RPR), and TB, with either PPD or TB-specific interferon gamma release assay (e.g., QuantiFERON-TB Gold®) as well as chest X-ray, should be performed to rule out these infectious etiologies. In addition to CXR, serum angiotensin-converting enzyme (ACE; if patient is not on ACE inhibitors) and lysozyme can be obtained to screen for sarcoidosis. Several ophthalmic imaging modalities may be useful in diagnosis and monitoring:

- *Color fundus photography*: Useful in documenting lesions and in monitoring for progression of disease.
- *Fundus autofluorescence (FAF)*: Active lesions often have a hyperautofluorescent halo, while chronic inactive lesions appear hypoautofluorescent.
- *Fluorescein angiography (FA)*: Acute lesions show early hypofluorescence with late hyperfluorescence, while chronic atrophic lesions demonstrate early hyperfluorescence that fades in the late frames (transmission or "window" defect).
- *Indocyanine green angiography (ICGA)*: Reveals hyperfluorescent lesions that may be more numerous than those seen clinically.
- *Optical coherence tomography (OCT)*: Useful in monitoring for macular edema and ERM.
- *Humphrey visual field (HVF)*: Can show enlargement of the blind spot.

89.9 Prognosis and Management

Visual prognosis is generally good, except in cases when subfoveal CNV develops. Immunosuppression, either systemic or locally, is the mainstay of treatment.

- *Corticosteroids*. Periocular triamcinolone injections may be used, especially in cases of unilateral active disease. Generally, 40 mg of triamcinolone is injected via the sub-Tenon's or orbital floor routes. Alternatively, oral prednisone may be considered. Typical starting doses for active intraocular inflammation are ~1 mg/kg/day. The dose should be tapered by 10 mg every 5–7 days until the range of 20–30 mg/day. Further tapering should be tailored to the clinical response. Calcium and vitamin D supplementation should be prescribed to all patients taking oral corticosteroids.
- *Steroid-sparing agents*: If inadequate response to systemic corticosteroids, additional immunosuppression in the form of antimetabolites (methotrexate, mycophenolate mofetil, or azathioprine), T-cell inhibitors (cyclosporine A or tacrolimus), or anti-TNF biologic agents (infliximab or adalimumab) may be considered. These medications should only be prescribed by clinicians experienced in their use. Routine blood tests are required to monitor for potential toxicity. If needed, a rheumatologist should be consulted to assist in administration of these medications.
- Intravitreal anti-VEGF agents are employed as needed in patients with CNV.

89.10 Follow-Up

Initially, patients should be monitored closely (e.g., every 1–2 weeks) until inflammation is controlled. Follow-up can be prolonged once adequate remission is attained. Patients should be followed routinely long term given the risk of recurrent inflammation and CNV.

References and Suggested Reading

1. Dreyer RF, Gass DJ. Multifocal choroiditis and panuveitis. A syndrome that mimics ocular histoplasmosis. Arch Ophthalmol. 1984;102:1776–84.
2. Jabs DA, Rosenbaum JT, Foster CS, et al. Guidelines for the use of immunosuppressive drugs in patients with ocular inflammatory disorders: recommendations of an expert panel. Am J Ophthalmol. 2000;130:492–513.
3. Kedhar SR, Thorne JE, Wittenberg S, et al. Multifocal Choroiditis with panuveitis and punctate inner choroidopathy: comparison of clinical characteristics at presentation. Retina. 2007;27:1174–9.
4. Michel SS, Ekong A, Baltatzis S, et al. Multifocal choroiditis and panuveitis. Ophthalmology. 2002;109:378–83.
5. Nussenblatt RB, Whitecup SM. White-dot syndromes. In: Nussenblatt RB, Whitecup SM, editors. Uveitis: fundamentals and clinical practice. 4th ed. Amsterdam, The Netherlands: Mosby Elsevier; 2010.
6. Parnell JR, Jampol LM, Yannuzzi LA, et al. Differentiation between presumed ocular histoplasmosis syndrome and multifocal choroiditis with panuveitis based on morphology of photographed fundus lesions and fluorescein angiography. Arch Ophthalmol. 2001;119:208–12.
7. Shakoor A, Vitale AT. Imaging in the diagnosis and management of multifocal choroiditis and punctate inner choroidopathy. Int Ophthalmol Clin. 2012;52:243–56.
8. Spaide RF, Goldberg N, Freund KB. Redefining multifocal choroiditis and panuveitis and punctate inner choroidopathy through multimodal imaging. Retina. 2013;33:1315–24.
9. Thorne JE, Wittenberg S, Jabs DA, et al. Multifocal choroiditis with panuveitis incidence of ocular complications and of loss of visual acuity. Ophthalmology. 2006;113:2310–6.
10. Yeh S, Forooghian F, Wong WT, et al. Fundus autofluorescence imaging of the white dot syndromes. Arch Ophthalmol. 2010;128:46–56.

Chapter 90
Punctate Inner Choroidopathy

Jane S. Kim, Jared E. Knickelbein, Robert B. Nussenblatt, and H. Nida Sen

90.1 Definitions

Punctate inner choroidopathy (PIC) is an uncommon idiopathic inflammatory chorioretinopathy characterized by multiple, small, discrete, yellow-white posterior pole lesions. It is more common in young, moderately myopic females. Choroidal neovascularization (CNV) is a common complication and cause of vision loss.

90.2 Symptoms

- Blurred vision
- Central or paracentral scotomas
- Photopsias
- Floaters
- Photophobia
- Metamorphopsia

J.S. Kim, BS
School of Medicine, University of California, San Diego, La Jolla, CA, USA

Laboratory of Immunology, National Eye Institute, National Institutes of Health,
10 Center Dr., Bldg. 10, Room 10D45, Bethesda, MD 20892, USA

J.E. Knickelbein, MD, PhD • R.B. Nussenblatt, MD, MPH • H.N. Sen, MD, MHS (✉)
Laboratory of Immunology, National Eye Institute, National Institutes of Health,
10 Center Dr., Bldg. 10, Room 10N109, Bethesda, MD 20892, USA
e-mail: senh@nei.nih.gov

C.A. Medina et al. (eds.), *Manual of Retinal Diseases: A Guide to Diagnosis and Management*, DOI 10.1007/978-3-319-20460-4_90

90.3 Signs

- Multiple, small (100–300 μm), well-defined, yellow-white lesions in the outer retina/inner choroid, generally limited to the posterior pole (Fig. 90.1)
- Anterior chamber and vitreous cellular reactions are typically not seen
- CNV is a common complication (up to 75%)
- Other structural complications, such as cataract, epiretinal membrane, and macular edema, are uncommon

90.4 Epidemiology

- More commonly seen among young Caucasian females (20–40 years of age)
- Typically bilateral but may be asymmetric

90.5 Predisposing Conditions

- Moderate myopia

90.6 Differential Diagnosis

- Multifocal choroiditis and panuveitis (MCP)
- Presumed ocular histoplasmosis syndrome (POHS)
- Acute posterior multifocal placoid pigment epitheliopathy (APMPPE)
- Serpiginous choroiditis
- Ampiginous choroiditis
- Birdshot chorioretinopathy
- Subretinal fibrosis and uveitis syndrome
- Acute zonal occult outer retinopathy (AZOOR)
- Sarcoidosis
- Syphilis
- Tuberculosis (TB)

Fig. 90.1 Fundus photograph (color), fluorescein angiogram (*FA*), indocyanine green angiogram (*ICGA*), and optical coherence tomography (*OCT*) of the left eye of a 16-year-old moderately myopic female with PIC. Note the small hypopigmented lesions within and superior to the fovea that are hyperfluorescent early and throughout the FA. On ICGA, lesions are hypofluorescent throughout the angiogram. OCT shows outer retinal hyper-reflectivity and disruption of the normal outer retinal architecture

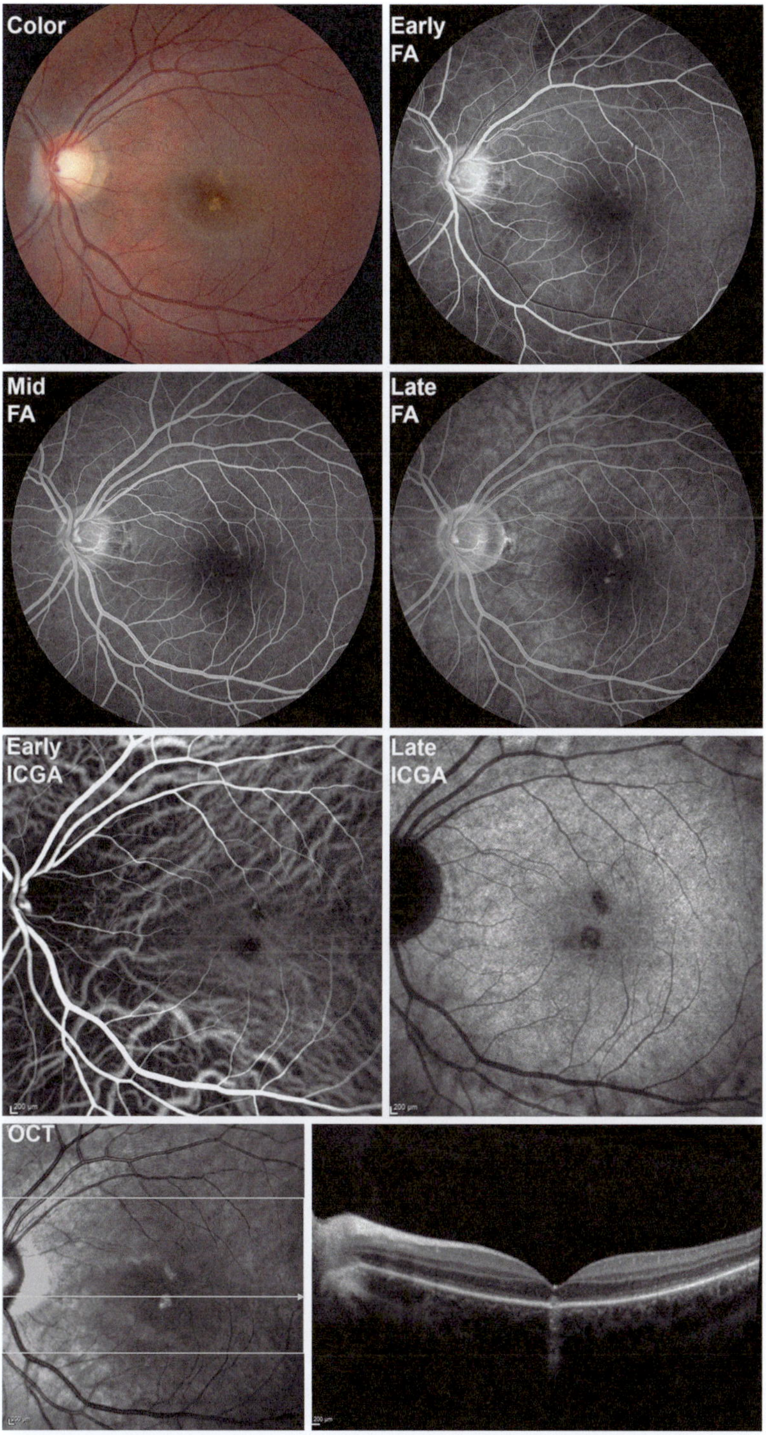
Color
Early FA
Mid FA
Late FA
Early ICGA
Late ICGA
OCT

90.7 Etiology

- Unknown, possible autoimmune etiology

90.8 Workup/Testing

Laboratory testing for syphilis, with syphilis IgG and rapid plasma reagin (RPR), and TB, with either PPD or TB-specific interferon gamma release assay (e.g., QuantiFERON-TB Gold®) as well as chest X-ray (CXR), should be performed to rule out these infectious etiologies. In addition to CXR, serum angiotensin-converting enzyme (ACE; if patient is not on ACE inhibitors) and lysozyme can be obtained to screen for sarcoidosis. Several ophthalmic imaging modalities may be useful in diagnosis and monitoring:

- *Color fundus photography*: Useful in documenting lesions and in monitoring for progression of disease.
- *Fundus autofluorescence (FAF)*: Active lesions often have a hyperautofluorescent halo, while chronic inactive lesions appear hypoautofluorescent.
- *Optical coherence tomography (OCT)*: Acute lesions demonstrate hyper-reflectivity in the outer retina with disruption of the normal outer retinal architecture (Fig. 90.1).
- *Fluorescein angiography (FA)*: Acute lesions may show early hyperfluorescence with late staining or leakage (Fig. 90.1), while chronic atrophic lesions demonstrate early hyperfluorescence that fades in the late frames (transmission or "window" defect).
- *Indocyanine green angiography (ICGA)*: Hypofluorescent spots corresponding to lesions in early, mid, and late phases. Late ICG may demonstrate larger areas of hypofluorescence than seen on fundus exam or FA (Fig. 90.1). CNV shows early hyperfluorescence.
- *Humphrey visual field (HVF)*: Can show central or paracentral scotomas.

90.9 Prognosis and Management

The prognosis for PIC is generally good unless foveal lesions are present or CNV develops. Patients with nonprogressive disease may be observed; however, recent studies have suggested that immunosuppressive therapy (see below) decreases the rate of CNV development. Intravitreal anti-VEGF agents are employed as needed in patients with CNV:

- *Corticosteroids*. Periocular triamcinolone injections may be used, especially in cases of unilateral active disease. Generally, 40 mg of triamcinolone is injected via the sub-Tenon's or orbital floor routes. Alternatively, oral prednisone may be considered. Typical starting dose for active intraocular inflammation is ~1 mg/kg/day.

The dose should be tapered by 10 mg every 5–7 days until the range of 20–30 mg/day is reached. Further tapering should be tailored to clinical response. Calcium and vitamin D supplementation should be prescribed to all patients taking oral corticosteroids.

- *Steroid-sparing agents*: If there is inadequate response to systemic corticosteroids, additional immunosuppression in the form of oral antimetabolites (methotrexate, mycophenolate mofetil, or azathioprine), T-cell inhibitors (cyclosporine A or tacrolimus), or anti-TNF biologic agents (infliximab or adalimumab) may be considered. These medications should only be prescribed by clinicians experienced in their use. Routine blood tests are required to monitor for potential toxicity. If needed, a rheumatologist should be consulted to assist in administration of these medications.

90.10 Follow-Up

Initially, patients should be monitored closely (e.g., every 1–2 weeks) to assure disease is not progressing. Follow-up can be prolonged once adequate remission is attained. Patients should be followed routinely long term given the risk of disease progression and CNV. Self-monitoring with Amsler grid can be helpful in early detection of recurrence.

References and Suggested Reading

1. Amer R, Lois N. Punctate inner choroidopathy. Surv Ophthalmol. 2011;56:36–53.
2. Essex RW, Wong J, Fraser-Bell S, et al. Punctate inner choroidopathy: clinical features and outcomes. Arch Ophthalmol. 2010;128:982–7.
3. Gerstenblith AT, Thorne JE, Sobrin L, et al. Punctate inner choroidopathy: a survey analysis of 77 persons. Ophthalmology. 2007;114:1201–4.
4. Leung TG, Moradi A, Liu D, et al. Clinical features and incidence rate of ocular complications in punctate inner choroidopathy. Retina. 2014;34:1666–74.
5. Nussenblatt RB, Whitecup SM. White-dot syndromes. In: Nussenblatt RB, Whitecup SM, editors. Uveitis: fundamentals and clinical practice. 4th ed. Edinburgh: Mosby Elsevier; 2010.
6. Shakoor A, Vitale AT. Imaging in the diagnosis and management of multifocal choroiditis and punctate inner choroidopathy. Int Ophthalmol Clin. 2012;52:243–56.
7. Watzke RC, Packer AJ, Folk JC, et al. Punctate inner choroidopathy. Am J Ophthalmol. 1984;98:572–84.

Chapter 91
Acute Posterior Multifocal Placoid Pigment Epitheliopathy

David Valent, Jared E. Knickelbein, Robert B. Nussenblatt, and H. Nida Sen

91.1 Definitions

Acute posterior multifocal placoid pigment epitheliopathy (APMPPE) is a condition characterized by multiple large plaque-like posterior pole lesions located at the level of the inner choroid and/or retinal pigment epithelium (RPE). Often, the lesions are transient and follow a viral prodrome suggesting a possible infectious etiology.

91.2 Symptoms

Decreased vision, photopsias, and scotomas; usually bilateral but can present unilaterally with the fellow eye becoming affected days to weeks later

91.3 Signs

- Anterior segment is typically quiet; however, it can present with low-grade non-granulomatous inflammation. The vitreous may have no inflammation or mild to moderate inflammation.

D. Valent, DO (✉)
National Eye Institute, National Institutes of Health,
10 Center Dr., Bldg 10, Rm 10D45, Bethesda, MD, USA
e-mail: drdavevalent@gmail.com

J.E. Knickelbein, MD, PhD • R.B. Nussenblatt, MD, MPH • H.N. Sen, MD, MHS
Laboratory of Immunology, National Eye Institute, National Institutes of Health,
Bethesda, MD, USA

C.A. Medina et al. (eds.), *Manual of Retinal Diseases: A Guide to Diagnosis and Management*, DOI 10.1007/978-3-319-20460-4_91

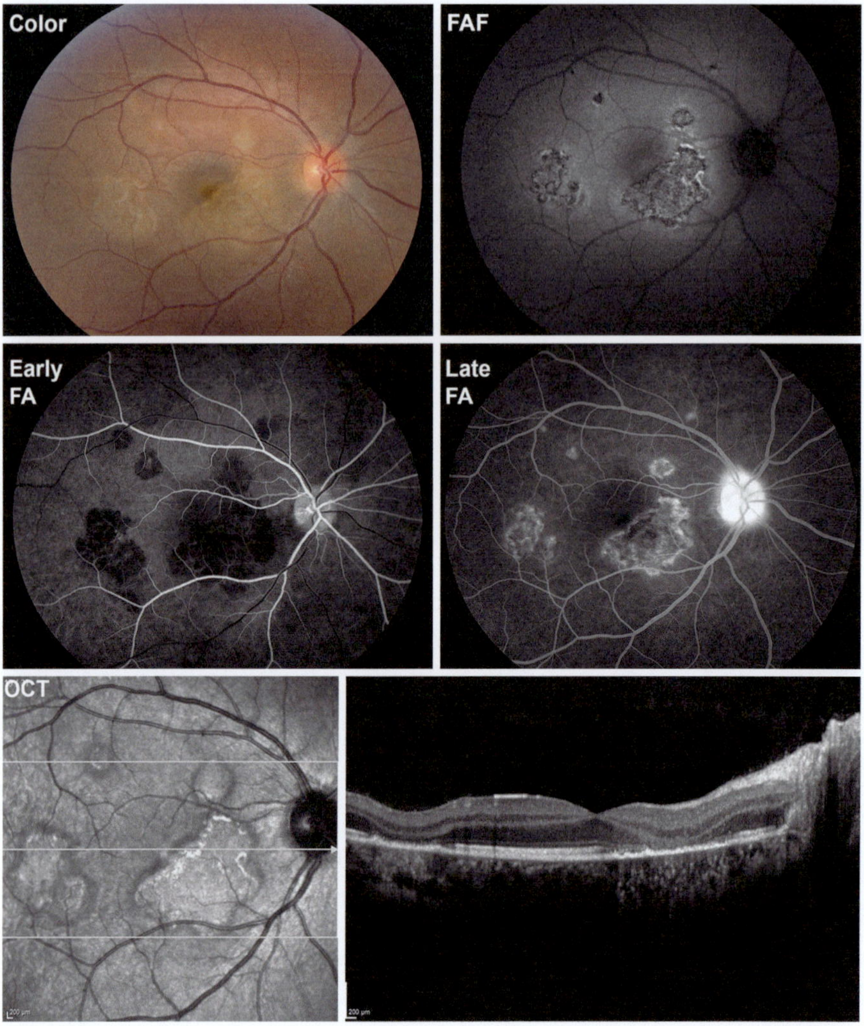

Fig. 91.1 Fundus photograph (color), fundus autofluorescence (*FAF*), fluorescein angiography (*FA*), and optical coherence tomography of the right eye of a 26-year-old woman with APMPEE. Note the creamy placoid lesions affecting the posterior pole. On FAF, the lesions consist of speckled hypo- and hyperautofluorescence. The classic FA pattern shows hypofluorescence of lesions in the early phase with late hyperfluorescence in the late phase. Also note the late disc leakage. OCT shows disruption of the outer retinal architecture

- Funduscopic examination reveals clearly defined multiple yellow-white (cream-colored) placoid lesions in the posterior pole, typically 1–2 disc diameters in size (Fig. 91.1).
- APMPPE can be associated with central nervous system (CNS) vasculitis. Associated symptoms include but are not limited to headache, hearing loss, or meningeal signs.

91.4 Epidemiology

- APMPPE typically affects young patients under the age of 30 but has been reported in older individuals.
- No gender predilection.

91.5 Predisposing Conditions

- Preceding viral or flu-like illness in approximately 1/3 of patients
- Reportedly associated with human leukocyte antigen (HLA)-B2 and (HLA)-DR7

91.6 Differential Diagnosis

- Multiple evanescent white dot syndrome (MEWDS).
- Serpiginous choroiditis.
- Multifocal choroiditis and panuveitis.
- Punctate inner choroidopathy.
- Syphilis.
- Tuberculosis (TB).
- Vogt-Koyanagi-Harada disease.
- Sarcoidosis.
- Behçet's disease.
- In atypical cases (e.g., older age, history of malignancy) with placoid-like lesions, lymphoma must be considered.

91.7 Etiology

Exact etiology is unknown. APMPPE is thought to be secondary to localized areas of choroidal non-perfusion. This ischemia leads to abnormalities in both the retinal pigment epithelium and photoreceptors. The association with a preceding viral or flu-like illness leads some to hypothesize that this could be a focal viral-related infection.

91.8 Workup/Testing

Laboratory testing for syphilis, with syphilis IgG and rapid plasma regain (RPR), and TB, with either PPD or TB-specific interferon gamma release assay (e.g., QuantiFERON-TB Gold®) as well as chest X-ray, should be performed to rule out these infectious etiologies. Several ocular imaging modalities may be useful in diagnosis and monitoring of disease:

- *Color fundus photography*: Useful in documenting lesions and in monitoring for progression of disease.
- *Fundus autofluorescence (FAF)*: Acutely, FAF shows hypoautofluorescence due to blockage or speckled hyper- and hypoautofluorescence corresponding to the staining placoid lesions on late angiography (Fig. 91.1). This may or may not correlate with the lesions visible on fundus examination.
- *Optical coherence tomography (OCT)*: Shows hyper-reflectivity and/or disruption of outer retinal layers, typically with a normal retinal thickness (Fig. 91.1). This hyper-reflectivity is thought to be related to either inflammatory cell infiltration or swelling of the outer retinal cells. The hyper-reflectivity decreases as placoid lesions resolve on fundus examination.
- *Fluorescein angiography (FA)*: FA demonstrates characteristic hypofluorescent lesions in the early phase of the angiogram with late hyperfluorescence of the same areas ("block early, stain late"; Fig. 91.1).
- *Indocyanine green angiography (ICGA)*: Active lesions are hypofluorescent both in the early and late phases of the angiogram. These areas of hypofluorescence may be more numerous than the number of lesions seen on fundoscopy and can resolve with treatment.
- *Humphrey visual field (HVF)*: Can show enlargement of the blind spot.
- *Additional considerations*: With the risk of CNS vasculitis, a thorough review of systems is extremely important. If there is a history of severe headache, hearing loss, or symptoms of meningeal irritation, neuroimaging should be performed.

91.9 Prognosis and Management

Most patients have a good visual prognosis, even without therapy. Some case reports discuss treatment using systemic corticosteroids, but it is difficult to assess the benefit of this treatment. For those with more severe vision loss or fovea-threatening lesions, systemic corticosteroids should be considered. Recurrence of the disease is rare but possible. For those with recurrent APMPPE, ampiginous choroiditis (Fig. 91.2), or persistent placoid choroidopathy, systemic immunosuppression is warranted. If there is evidence of cerebral vasculitis on neuroimaging, intravenous corticosteroid therapy is required with subsequent immunosuppression.

91.10 Follow-Up

These patients should be followed closely for any significant decrease in visual acuity or neurologic symptoms. Visual prognosis is quite good, with most patients returning to baseline visual acuity. However, they can have persistent visual field deficits. The placoid lesions resolve with time, leaving behind a variable degree of pigmentary changes.

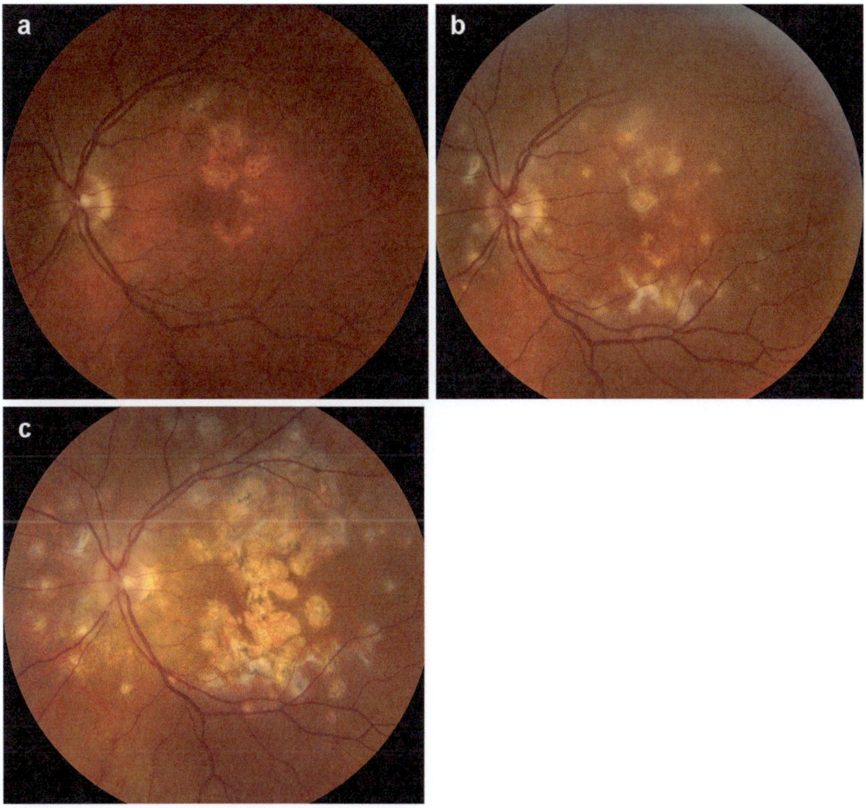

Fig. 91.2 Fundus photographs of a patient with ampiginous choroidopathy. The initial presentation (**a**) with 3-year (**b**) and 7-year (**c**) follow-up. Note the multiple lesions that expand in size and number over time

References and Suggested Reading

1. Abu-Yaghi NE, Hartono SP, Hodge DO, Pulido JS, Bakri SJ. White dot syndromes: a 20-year study of incidence, clinical features, and outcomes. Ocul Immunol Inflamm. 2011;19: 426–30.
2. Comu S, Verstraeten T, Rinkoff JS, Busis NA. Neurological manifestations of acute posterior multifocal placoid pigment epitheliopathy. Stroke. 1996;27:996–1001.
3. Gass JD. Acute posterior multifocal placoid pigment epitheliopathy. Arch Ophthalmol. 1968;80:177–85.
4. Jones NP. Acute posterior multifocal placoid pigment epitheliopathy. Br J Ophthalmol. 1995;79:384–9.
5. Nussenblatt RB, Whitecup SM. White-dot syndromes. In: Nussenblatt RB, Whitecup SM, editors. Uveitis: fundamentals and clinical practice. 4th ed. Amsterdam, the Netherlands: Mosby Elsevier; 2010.

6. Spaide RF. Autofluorescence imaging of acute posterior multifocal placoid pigment epitheliopathy. Retina. 2006;26:479–82.
7. Steiner S, Goldstein DA. Imaging in the diagnosis and management of APMPPE. Int Ophthalmol Clin. 2012;52:211–9.
8. Williams DF, Mieler WF. Long-term follow-up of acute multifocal posterior placoid pigment epitheliopathy. Br J Ophthalmol. 1989;73:985–90.
9. Wolf MD, Folk JC, Panknen CA, Goeken NE. HLA-B7 and HLA-DR2 antigens and acute posterior multifocal placoid pigment epitheliopathy. Arch Ophthalmol. 1990;108:698–700.

Chapter 92
Serpiginous Choroidopathy

David Valent, Jared E. Knickelbein, Robert B. Nussenblatt, and H. Nida Sen

92.1 Definitions

Serpiginous choroidopathy, also known as serpiginous choroiditis, geographic choroiditis, geographic choroidopathy, or macular geographic helicoid choroidopathy, classically presents with a helicoid peripapillary lesion that spreads outward from the disc in a "serpentine" fashion. Multifocal lesions are not typical but have been reported. Active lesions present as patches of creamy yellow subretinal infiltrates. The overlying retina is typically edematous. The periphery tends to be spared from these lesions. The inflammatory lesion tends to resolve over 6–8 weeks, leaving an area of atrophy, involving both the retinal pigment epithelium (RPE) and choriocapillaris. Patients can present with lesions in different stages of resolution. There are variants including macular serpiginous choroiditis, relentless placoid chorioretinitis, and ampiginous choroiditis, with FA and ICG findings similar to classic serpiginous choroidopathy but present and behave in different manners as follows:

- *Macular serpiginous choroiditis*: Serpiginous lesion sparing in the peripapillary area
- *Ampiginous choroidopathy or relentless placoid chorioretinitis*: Aggressive variant with recurrent activity including new lesions extending into the periphery and with characteristics initially resembling APMPPE

D. Valent, DO (✉)
National Eye Institute, National Institutes of Health,
10 Center Dr, Bldg 10, Rm 10D45, Bethesda, MD, USA
e-mail: drdavevalent@gmail.com

J.E. Knickelbein, MD, PhD • R.B. Nussenblatt, MD, MPH • H.N. Sen, MD, MHS
Laboratory of Immunology, National Eye Institute, National Institutes of Health,
Bethesda, MD, USA

C.A. Medina et al. (eds.), *Manual of Retinal Diseases: A Guide to Diagnosis and Management*, DOI 10.1007/978-3-319-20460-4_92

92.2 Symptoms

- Blurred vision
- Metamorphopsia
- Central or pericentral scotomas

92.3 Signs

- Typically, no inflammation seen in the anterior segment. If present, mild non-granulomatous anterior chamber inflammation can be seen during disease activity.
- Minimal vitreous inflammation may be present.
- Helicoid peripapillary lesion that spreads outward from the disc in a "serpentine" fashion (Fig. 92.1).
- Active lesions present as patches of creamy yellow subretinal infiltrates typically at the border of a preexisting area of atrophy (Fig. 92.2).

92.4 Epidemiology

- Serpiginous is a rare cause of uveitis, representing less than 5 % of posterior uveitis cases in the United States.
- There does not appear to be any racial predilection.
- Average age of onset is 43–59 years (range from late teens to 60s).
- Some reports indicate a slightly higher incidence in men.

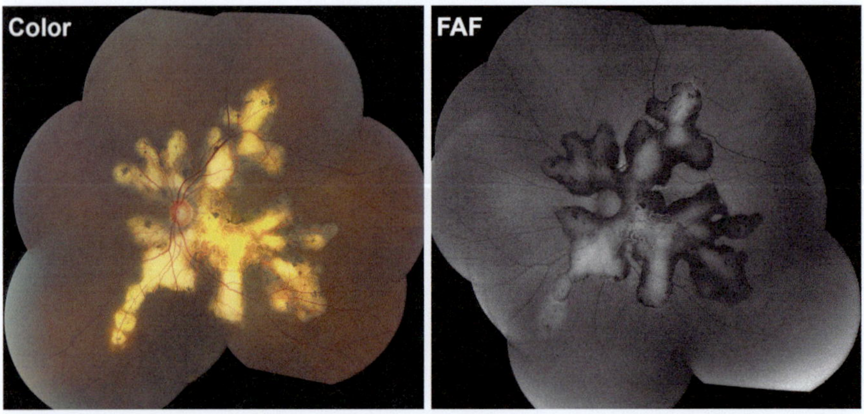

Fig. 92.1 Color fundus photograph (color) and fundus autofluorescence (*FAF*) of the left eye of a 49-year-old Hispanic man with quiescent serpiginous choroidopathy. Note the helicoid pattern of chorioretinal scarring extending from the optic nerve. FAF shows hypoautofluorescence of the lesion borders

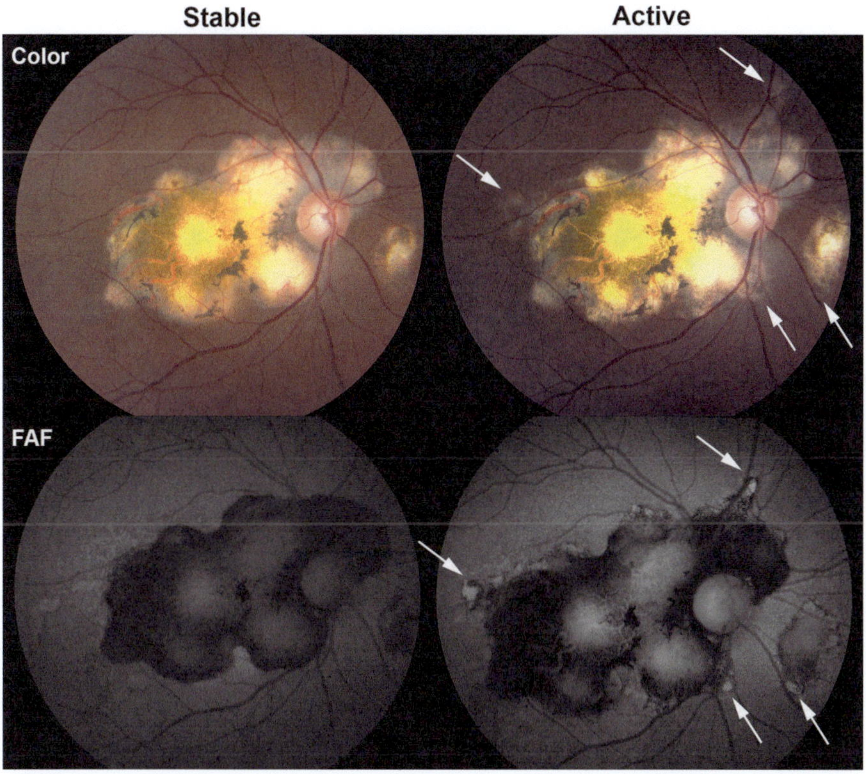

Fig. 92.2 Color fundus photographs (color) and fundus autofluorescence (*FAF*) of the right eye of the same patient from Fig. 92.1. The *left column* shows images from a visit when the serpiginous lesions were stable. The *right column* shows images from a follow-up visit when the disease was active. Note the multiple areas of new activity at the border of the preexisting lesion that appear white-yellow on the color photos and hyperautofluorescent on FAF (*arrows*)

92.5 Predisposing Conditions

- Reports of infectious associations, including *Mycobacterium tuberculosis* and *Herpes simplex virus*, although these are not proven
- There is a possible association with human leukocyte antigen (HLA)-B7

92.6 Differential Diagnosis

- Acute posterior multifocal placoid pigment epitheliopathy (APMPPE)
- Multifocal choroiditis and panuveitis (MCP)
- Presumed ocular histoplasmosis syndrome (POHS)
- Tuberculosis (TB)

- Syphilis
- Sarcoidosis
- Choroidal ischemia

92.7 Etiology

- Unknown
- Hypotheses include autoimmune, infectious, or vascular etiologies.

92.8 Workup/Testing

Laboratory testing for syphilis, with syphilis IgG and rapid plasma regain (RPR), and TB, with either PPD or TB-specific interferon gamma release assay (e.g., QuantiFERON-TB Gold®) as well as chest X-ray, should be performed to rule out these infectious etiologies. In addition to CXR, serum angiotensin-converting enzyme (ACE; if patient is not on ACE inhibitors) and lysozyme can be obtained to screen for sarcoidosis. Several ophthalmic imaging modalities may be useful in diagnosis and monitoring:

- *Color fundus photography*: Useful in documenting lesions and in monitoring for progression of disease.
- *Fundus autofluorescence (FAF)*: In the acute phase, lesions will be diffusely hyperautofluorescent. Atrophic lesions will appear hypoautofluorescent with distinct margins. The presence of hyperautofluorescence at the edge of an atrophic lesion often indicates new activity (Fig. 92.1).
- *Optical coherence tomography (OCT)*: Acute lesions show hyper-reflectivity involving the outer retina with disruption of the normal outer retinal architecture. With time, outer retinal hyper-reflectivity dissipates with development of outer retina and RPE atrophy.
- *Fluorescein angiography (FA)*: Active lesions show early blockage with late hyperfluorescence, while chronic atrophic lesions demonstrate early hyperfluorescence that fades in the late frames (transmission or "window" defect).
- *Indocyanine green angiography (ICGA)*: Hypofluorescent areas corresponding to the lesions are present throughout the angiogram. Typically, ICGA shows many more lesions than seen clinically.

92.9 Prognosis and Management

Recurrences are common and typically occur at the border of preexisting chorioretinal scars. With each recurrence, there is further extension of the area of atrophy and corresponding scotoma. Visual acuity is directly correlated to involvement of the fovea. Systemic immunosuppression is the mainstay of treatment. Local treatment can be considered in some patients (see below). Intravitreal anti-VEGF agents are employed as needed in patients with CNV:

- *Corticosteroids*. Periocular triamcinolone injections may be used, especially in cases of unilateral active disease. Generally, 40 mg of triamcinolone is injected via the sub-Tenon's or orbital floor routes. Intravitreal triamcinolone and the fluocinolone acetonide implant have also been reported to be effective in unilateral active disease. Alternatively, oral prednisone may be considered. Typical starting dose for active intraocular inflammation is ~1 mg/kg/day. The dose should be tapered by 10 mg every 5–7 days until the range of 20–30 mg/day. Further tapering should be tailored to the clinical response. Calcium and vitamin D supplementation should be prescribed to all patients taking oral corticosteroids.
- *Steroid-sparing agents*: If there is inadequate response to systemic corticosteroids, additional immunosuppression in the form of oral antimetabolites (methotrexate, mycophenolate mofetil, or azathioprine), T-cell inhibitors (cyclosporine A or tacrolimus), or anti-TNF biologic agents (infliximab or adalimumab) may be considered. These medications should only be prescribed by clinicians experienced in their use. Routine blood tests are required to monitor for potential toxicity. If needed, a rheumatologist should be consulted to assist in administration of these medications.

92.10 Follow-Up

Acutely, these patients should be monitored closely for resolution of the active lesion. More stable lesions should still be followed due to the high incidence of recurrence. Some patients may be asymptomatic despite recurrent disease activity. Monitoring these patients with imaging, including color photographs and FAF, at regular intervals can help diagnose early reactivation. Self-monitoring between visits with Amsler grid may be helpful.

References and Suggested Reading

1. Bansal R, Gupta A, Gupta V. Imaging in the diagnosis and management of serpiginous choroiditis. Int Ophthalmol Clin. 2012;52:229–36.
2. Gallagher MJ, Yilmaz T, Cervantes-Castaneda RA, et al. The characteristic features of optical coherence tomography in posterior uveitis. Br J Ophthalmol. 2007;91:1680–5.
3. Golchet PR, Jampol LM, Wilson D, et al. Persistent placoid maculopathy: a new clinical entity. Ophthalmology. 2007;114:1530–40.
4. Jyotirmay B, Jafferji SS, Sudharshan S, Kalpana B. Clinical profile, treatment, and visual outcome of ampiginous choroiditis. Ocul Immunol Inflamm. 2010;18:46–51.
5. Khanamiri HN, Rao NA. Serpiginous choroiditis and infectious multifocal serpiginoid choroiditis. Surv Ophthalmol. 2013;58:203–32.
6. Lim WK, Buggage RR, Nussenblatt RB. Serpiginous choroiditis. Surv Ophthalmol. 2005;50: 231–44.

7. Nussenblatt RB, Whitecup SM. Serpiginous choroidopathy. In: Nussenblatt RB, Whitecup SM, editors. Uveitis: fundamentals and clinical practice. 4th ed. Amsterdam, the Netherlands: Mosby Elsevier; 2010.
8. Seth RK, Gaudio PA. Treatment of serpiginous choroiditis with intravitreous fluocinolone acetonide implant. Ocul Immunol Inflamm. 2008;16:103–5.
9. Vasconcelos-Santos DV, Rao PK, Davies JB, Sohn EH, Rao NA. Clinical features of tuberculous serpiginouslike choroiditis in contrast to classic serpiginous choroiditis. Arch Ophthalmol. 2010;128:853–8.
10. Yeh S, Forooghian F, Wong WT, et al. Fundus autofluorescence imaging of the white dot syndromes. Arch Ophthalmol. 2010;128:46–56.

Chapter 93
Birdshot Chorioretinopathy

Jesia Hasan, Jared E. Knickelbein, Robert B. Nussenblatt, and H. Nida Sen

93.1 Definition

Birdshot chorioretinopathy, also known as vitiliginous chorioretinitis, is a nongranulomatous idiopathic posterior uveitic entity.

93.2 Symptoms

Decreased vision, floaters, photopsias, and nyctalopia

93.3 Signs

- Quiet to low-grade inflammation in the anterior chamber.
- Mild to moderate vitritis.
- Bilateral deep ovoid cream-colored lesions (up to 1500 μm) radially distributed in the posterior pole and mid-periphery, often best observed with the indirect ophthalmoscope (Fig. 93.1).
- Retinal vascular leakage.
- Macular edema.
- Optic nerve head inflammation may be seen.

J. Hasan, MD (✉) • J.E. Knickelbein, MD, PhD • R.B. Nussenblatt, MD, MPH
H.N. Sen, MD, MHS
Laboratory of Immunology, National Eye Institute, National Institutes of Health,
10 Center Dr., Bldg. 10, Room 10D45, Bethesda, MD 20892, USA
e-mail: knickelbeinje@nei.nih.gov

C.A. Medina et al. (eds.), *Manual of Retinal Diseases: A Guide to Diagnosis and Management*, DOI 10.1007/978-3-319-20460-4_93

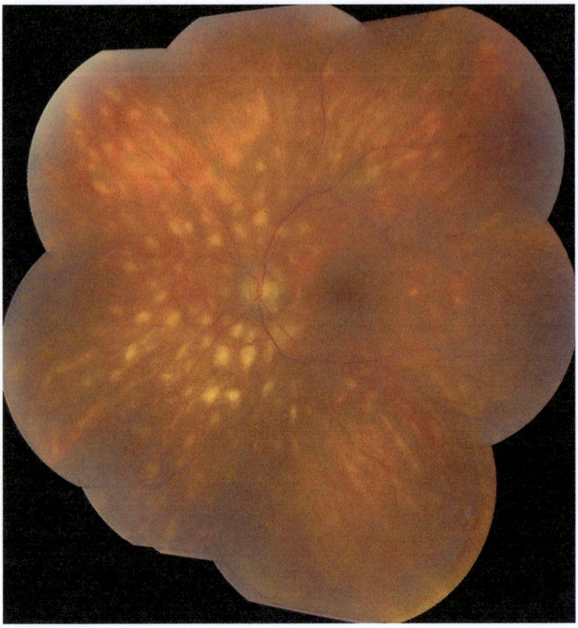

Fig. 93.1 Color fundus photograph of the left eye of a 54-year-old Caucasian woman with birdshot chorioretinopathy. Note the deep ovoid cream-colored lesions radially distributed through the posterior pole

93.4 Epidemiology

- Accounts for approximately 1–8 % of posterior uveitis cases.
- Average age of presentation is approximately 50 years.
- More common in patients with Northern European ancestry.
- Possible slight female preponderance.

93.5 Predisposing Conditions

- Strong association with human leukocyte antigen (HLA)-A29
- Generally considered to be an isolated ocular disease

93.6 Differential Diagnosis

- Multifocal choroiditis and panuveitis (MCP)
- Presumed ocular histoplasmosis syndrome (POHS)
- Posterior scleritis
- Pars planitis
- Sarcoidosis
- Syphilis

- Tuberculosis (TB)
- Vogt-Koyanagi-Harada (VKH) disease (chronic stage)
- Sympathetic ophthalmia
- Intraocular lymphoma

93.7 Etiology

Idiopathic, presumed T-cell-mediated autoimmune disease

93.8 Workup/Testing

Laboratory testing for syphilis, with syphilis IgG and rapid plasma regain (RPR), and TB, with either PPD or TB-specific interferon gamma release assay (e.g., QuantiFERON-TB Gold®) as well as chest X-ray, should be performed to rule out these infectious etiologies. In addition to CXR, serum angiotensin-converting enzyme (ACE; if patient is not on ACE inhibitors) and lysozyme can be obtained to screen for sarcoidosis. HLA testing for the A29 haplotype can aid in the diagnosis, although ~6 % of the Caucasian population is HLA-A29 positive. Several ophthalmic imaging modalities may be useful in diagnosis and monitoring:

- *Color fundus photography*: Useful in documenting lesions and in monitoring for progression of disease.
- *Fundus autofluorescence (FAF)*: Hypoautofluorescence representing areas of retinal pigment epithelium (RPE) atrophy may not correspond to the location of clinically observed lesions. Hypofluorescent lesions on FAF may be more numerous than seen on exam. Macular hypoautofluorescence has been associated with poorer visual acuity.
- *Fluorescein angiography (FA)*: Birdshot lesions may show early hypofluorescence and mild hyperfluorescence in the late phase. FA is more useful in assessing the degree of retinal vasculitis and optic nerve head leakage.
- *Optical coherence tomography (OCT)*: Useful in assessing for macular edema and visualizing outer retinal changes in areas of lesions.
- *Indocyanine green angiography (ICGA)*: Often shows hypofluorescent spots more numerous than clinically apparent lesions.
- *Full-field electroretinogram (ERG)*: Can detect altered retinal function (prolonged 30-Hz flicker implicit time and reduced scotopic B-wave amplitude) despite good visual acuity. Useful in following disease evolution and response to treatment.
- *Goldmann visual field (GVF)*: Can identify scotomata, particularly noted in the I-4 isopter, which may be reversible with therapy. Useful in following disease evolution and response to treatment.

93.9 Prognosis and Management

The disease course is characterized by a chronic and progressive nature, while it may be self-limited in a small proportion of patients. Central retinal function and visual acuity may be maintained until late in the disease and thus can be misleading in terms of severity of the disease. Therefore, it is necessary to screen patients for disease progression with FA, ERG, and GVF even if central visual acuity remains good and inflammation appears quiet clinically. Systemic immunosuppression is the mainstay of treatment:

- *Corticosteroids*: Treatment with systemic corticosteroids (1 mg/kg/day oral prednisone with a slow taper) is recommended. Adjunctive periocular corticosteroids (e.g., 20–40 mg triamcinolone) can be used to manage flares. The intravitreal fluocinolone acetonide implant should be considered in cases where systemic therapy is either contraindicated, not tolerated, or insufficient.
- *Steroid-sparing agents*: Early introduction of corticosteroid-sparing immunomodulatory therapy is recommended. Antimetabolites (methotrexate, mycophenolate mofetil, or azathioprine), T-cell inhibitors (cyclosporine A or tacrolimus), or anti-TNF biologic agents (infliximab or adalimumab) may be considered. These medications should only be prescribed by clinicians experienced in their use. Routine blood tests are required to monitor for potential toxicity. If needed, a rheumatologist should be consulted to assist in administration of these medications.

93.10 Follow-Up

During active disease, patients should be followed closely (e.g., every 2–4 weeks) until inflammation is controlled. During periods of quiescence, follow-up can be prolonged. Patients should be followed routinely long term given the risk of recurrent or progressive inflammation.

References and Suggested Reading

1. Agarwal A. Inflammatory diseases of the retina. In: Agarwal A, editor. Gass' atlas of macular diseases. 5th ed. Amsterdam, The Netherlands: Saunders Elsevier; 2012.
2. Faia LJ. Gender differences in birdshot chorioretinopathy and the white dot syndromes: do they exist? J Ophthalmol. 2014;2014:146768.
3. Jabs DA, Rosenbaum JT, Foster CS, et al. Guidelines for the use of immunosuppressive drugs in patients with ocular inflammatory disorders: recommendations of an expert panel. Am J Ophthalmol. 2000;130:492–513.

4. Levinson RD, Brezin A, Rothova A, et al. Research criteria for the diagnosis of birdshot chorioretinopathy: results of an international consensus conference. Am J Ophthalmol. 2006;141: 185–7.
5. Nussenblatt RB, Whitecup SM. Birdshot retinochoroidopathy. In: Nussenblatt RB, Whitecup SM, editors. Uveitis: fundamentals and clinical practice. 4th ed. Amsterdam, The Netherlands: Mosby Elsevier; 2010.
6. Shao EH, Menezo V, Taylor SR. Birdshot chorioretinopathy. Curr Opin Ophthalmol. 2014;25:488–94.
7. Thorne JE, Jabs DA, Peters GB, et al. Birdshot retinochoroidopathy: ocular complications and visual impairment. Am J Ophthalmol. 2005;140:45–51.
8. Tomkins-Netzer O, Taylor SR, Lightman S. Long-term clinical and anatomic outcome of birdshot chorioretinopathy. JAMA Ophthalmol. 2014;132:57–62.
9. Yeh S, Forooghian F, Wong WT, et al. Fundus autofluorescence imaging of the white dot syndromes. Arch Ophthalmol. 2010;128:46–56.

Chapter 94
Ocular Histoplasmosis

Padmini Kaushal, Jared E. Knickelbein, Robert B. Nussenblatt, and H. Nida Sen

94.1 Definitions

Ocular histoplasmosis, also referred to as presumed ocular histoplasmosis syndrome (POHS), is an inflammatory eye disease associated with systemic infection with the fungus *Histoplasma capsulatum.*

94.2 Symptoms

Painless vision loss, metamorphopsia, and central scotomas

94.3 Signs

- Classic triad (Fig. 94.1):
  - Round or oval-shaped "punched-out" peripheral choroidal scars referred to as "histo spots"
  - Peripapillary pigment atrophy
  - Absence of anterior chamber or vitreous inflammation

P. Kaushal, MD (✉)
National Eye Institute, National Institutes of Health,
10 Center Dr., Bldg. 10, Room 10D45, Bethesda, MD 20892, USA
e-mail: knickelbeinje@nei.nih.gov

J.E. Knickelbein, MD, PhD • R.B. Nussenblatt, MD, MPH • H.N. Sen, MD, MHS
Laboratory of Immunology, National Eye Institute, National Institutes of Health,
Bethesda, MD, USA

C.A. Medina et al. (eds.), *Manual of Retinal Diseases: A Guide to Diagnosis and Management*, DOI 10.1007/978-3-319-20460-4_94

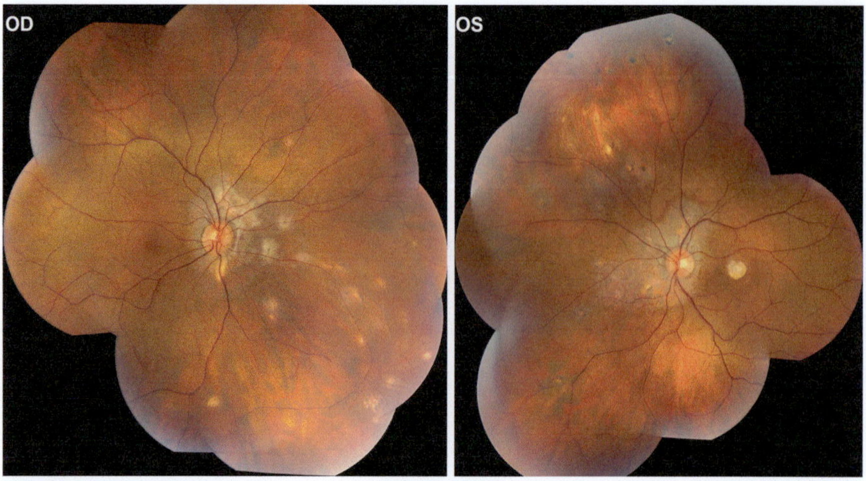

Fig. 94.1 *Right* (OD) and *left* (OS) eyes of a 42-year-old man with POHS. Note the peripheral "punched-out" lesions and peripapillary atrophy in both eyes. Also note the foveal disciform scar from CNV in the left eye

- Occasionally, a linear streak of pigmented lesions also is seen near the equator.
- Choroidal neovascularization (CNV) can occur in approximately 5 % and is the leading cause of vision loss.

94.4 Epidemiology

- There is no gender predilection.
- Generally seen in patients between 20 and 50 years of age.
- Typically bilateral but may be asymmetric.

94.5 Predisposing Conditions

- More common in regions endemic for *H. capsulatum*, such as the Ohio and Mississippi river valleys in the United States (4.4 % of individuals).
- Associated with human leukocyte antigen (HLA)-B7 and HLA-DRw2.
- In patients with POHS, smoking is a strong risk factor for development of CNV.

94.6 Differential Diagnosis

- Multifocal choroiditis and panuveitis (MCP)
- Punctate inner choroidopathy (PIC)
- Acute posterior multifocal placoid pigment epitheliopathy (APMPPE)

- Serpiginous choroiditis
- Ampiginous choroiditis
- Birdshot chorioretinopathy
- Subretinal fibrosis and uveitis syndrome
- Acute zonal occult outer retinopathy (AZOOR)
- Sarcoidosis
- Syphilis
- *Mycobacterium tuberculosis* (TB)

94.7 Etiology

POHS is considered "presumed" ocular histoplasmosis because a causal relationship with the fungus *Histoplasma capsulatum* has not been definitively proven. Skin testing for delayed-type hypersensitivity reactions against *H. capsulatum* antigen is positive in most patients diagnosed with POHS. POHS may represent an autoimmune response triggered by fungal infection.

94.8 Workup/Testing

POHS is a clinical diagnosis with the diagnosis made based upon the identification of classic fundus findings. Often, patients have a positive reaction to *H. capsulatum* antigen skin testing. However, this is not required to make the diagnosis and is rarely done. Serologic testing for *Histoplasma* antibody is not very helpful. Laboratory testing for syphilis, with syphilis IgG and rapid plasma regain (RPR), and TB, with either PPD or TB-specific interferon gamma release assay (e.g., QuantiFERON-TB Gold®) as well as chest X-ray, should be performed to rule out these infectious etiologies. It should be noted that prior histoplasmosis infection can cause calcified hilar lymphadenopathy. In addition to CXR, serum angiotensin-converting enzyme (ACE; if patient is not on ACE inhibitors) and lysozyme can be obtained to screen for sarcoidosis. Several ophthalmic imaging modalities may be useful in diagnosis and monitoring:

- *Color fundus photography*: Useful in documenting lesions and in monitoring for progression of disease.
- *Fundus autofluorescence* (*FAF*): Active lesions often have a hyperautofluorescent halo, while chronic inactive lesions appear hypoautofluorescent.
- *Fluorescein angiography* (*FA*): Acute lesions show early hypofluorescence with late hyperfluorescence, while chronic atrophic lesions demonstrate early hyperfluorescence that fades in the late frames (transmission or "window" defect). FA is also useful in identifying CNV.
- *Indocyanine green angiography* (*ICGA*): Reveals hypofluorescent spots that may be more numerous than those seen clinically.
- *Optical coherence tomography* (*OCT*): Useful in monitoring CNV.

94.9 Prognosis and Management

In the absence of CNV, most patients are asymptomatic and do not require treatment. Intravitreal anti-VEGF agents are employed as needed in patients with CNV. Photodynamic therapy with verteporfin may also be considered. Patients who smoke should be counseled on cessation. In some patients, lesions may enlarge or new lesions may occur. Periocular or intravitreal corticosteroids should be considered if lesions threaten the fovea or cause symptoms.

94.10 Follow-Up

Patients with POHS should be followed routinely with dilated fundus exams to monitor disease. Use of an Amsler grid should be encouraged. Patients with CNV require closer follow-up depending on their response to treatment.

References and Suggested Reading

1. Ehlers JP, Hawkins BS, Schachat AP. Ocular histoplasmosis. In: Schachat AP, Sadda SR, editors. Retina. 5th ed. Amsterdam, the Netherlands: Elsevier; 2013.
2. Nussenblatt RB, Whitecup SM. Ocular histoplasmosis. In: Nussenblatt RB, Whitecup SM, editors. Uveitis: fundamentals and clinical practice. 4th ed. Amsterdam, the Netherlands: Mosby Elsevier; 2010.
3. Parnell JR, Jampol LM, Yannuzzi LA, et al. Differentiation between presumed ocular histoplasmosis syndrome and multifocal choroiditis with panuveitis based on morphology of photographed fundus lesions and fluorescein angiography. Arch Ophthalmol. 2001;119:208–12.
4. Ramaiya K, Blinder K, Ciulla T, et al. Ranibizumab versus photodynamic therapy for presumed ocular histoplasmosis syndrome. Ophthalmic Surg Lasers Imaging Retina. 2013;44:17–21.
5. Thuruthumaly C, Yee DC, Rao PK. Presumed ocular histoplasmosis. Curr Opin Ophthalmol. 2014;25:508–12.

Section XIV
Uveitis: Non White Dot Syndromes

Jared E. Knickelbein

Chapter 95
Behçet's Disease

Austin Fox, Jared E. Knickelbein, Robert B. Nussenblatt, and H. Nida Sen

95.1 Definitions

Behçet's disease (BD) is a systemic vasculitis characterized by recurrent uveitis, oral aphthous ulcers, and genital ulcers.

95.2 Symptoms

- *Ocular*: Acute-onset, recurrent, reduced vision, redness, associated ocular pain, floaters, and photophobia
- *Extraocular*: Painful oral and genital ulcers, arthralgia, abdominal pain, chest pain, hemoptysis, nausea, bloating, and diarrhea

95.3 Signs

Ocular Behçet's disease typically presents with nongranulomatous ocular inflammation.

- *Anterior segment*: Scleritis, episcleritis, conjunctivitis with conjunctival ulcers, subconjunctival hemorrhage, keratitis, iridocyclitis with hypopyon (migratory and "cold"), and fine keratic precipitates.

A. Fox, BS • J.E. Knickelbein, MD, PhD
R.B. Nussenblatt, MD, MPH • H.N. Sen, MD, MHS (✉)
Laboratory of Immunology, National Eye Institute, National Institutes of Health, 10 Center Dr., Bldg. 10, Room 10 N109, Bethesda, MD 20892, USA
e-mail: senh@nei.nih.gov

C.A. Medina et al. (eds.), *Manual of Retinal Diseases: A Guide to Diagnosis and Management*, DOI 10.1007/978-3-319-20460-4_95

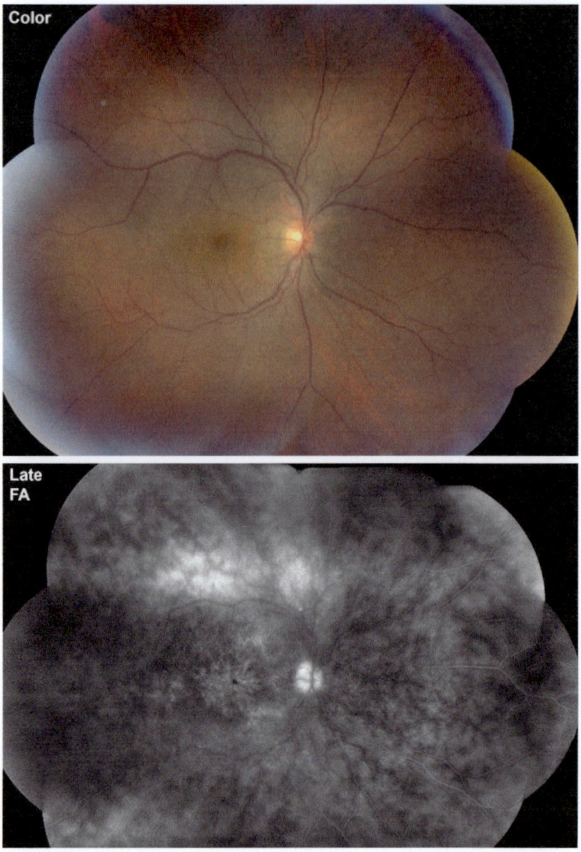

Fig. 95.1 Fundus photograph (color) and late fluorescein angiogram (FA) of a 28-year-old man with ocular Behçet's disease. Note the diffuse retinal vascular leakage

- *Posterior uveitis:* Retinal vasculitis (Fig. 95.1), vitritis, focal necrotizing retinitis, retinal hemorrhage and edema, branch or central retinal vein occlusion, and optic neuritis.
- *Extraocular*: Oral aphthous ulcers (most common, 98 %), genital ulcers (75–85 %), skin lesions (90 %), positive pathergy test, erythema nodosum, folliculitis, arthritis, pericarditis, vascular disease, and central nervous system vasculitis.
- Complications may include cataract, peripheral anterior synechiae, posterior synechiae, iris atrophy, neovascularization, and secondary glaucoma.

95.4 Epidemiology

BD usually presents in the second–fourth decade of life but can manifest at any age. There is a higher prevalence in Middle Eastern, Mediterranean, and Eastern Asian countries. In countries along the ancient Silk Road, there is higher prevalence of BD in males. Contrarily, BD is more common in females in Western Europe and the United

States. In addition, male sex has been associated with poorer visual outcome and higher mortality. Panuveitis and neurologic involvement are more common in males, while anterior uveitis and mucocutaneous manifestations are more common in females.

95.5 Predisposing Conditions

- Lineage of Middle Eastern, Mediterranean, Eastern Asian, Japanese descent
- Human leukocyte antigen (HLA)-B51
- First-degree relative with BD

95.6 Differential Diagnosis

- Viral retinitis (CMV, VZV, HSV)
- Systemic lupus erythematosus (SLE)-associated retinal vasculitis
- Granulomatosis with polyangiitis (GPA) (formerly known as Wegener's granulomatosis)
- Polyarteritis nodosa (PAN)
- Sarcoidosis
- Syphilis
- Tuberculosis (TB)
- HLA-B27-associated anterior uveitis with hypopyon

95.7 Etiology

Not fully understood, though autoimmune, infectious, and environmental etiologies have been suggested. BD is characterized by leukocytoclastic vasculitis and perivascular inflammation with recurrent retinal vaso-occlusive episodes, which may lead to retinal ischemia and irreversible blindness. BD can affect all vessels (arterial and venous) of all sizes.

95.8 Workup/Testing

BD is a clinical diagnosis as there are no specific imaging, laboratory, or histologic findings. Definitive diagnosis may be difficult given the systemic nature of the disease and the possibility of manifestations at different times during the clinical course. See Table 95.1 for proposed diagnostic criteria from the International Study Group for Behçet's Disease.

Table 95.1 Diagnostic criteria for Behçet's disease: International Study Group for Behçet's Disease

Recurrent oral ulceration	
Minor or major aphthous lesions or herpetiform-like lesions at least three times within a 12-month period. Noted by the physician or patient	
Plus 2 other criteria	
Recurrent genital ulceration	Aphthous ulceration or scar noted by the physician or patient
Eye lesions	Anterior and/or posterior uveitis, cells in the vitreous, or retinal vasculitis noted by an ophthalmologist
Skin lesions	Erythema nodosum, pseudofolliculitis, or papulopustular lesions
	OR
	Acneiform nodules in postadolescent patient not receiving corticosteroid therapy
	Noted by the physician or patient
Positive pathergy test	Read by a physician at 24–48 h

Adapted from *Lancet* [2]

Laboratory testing for syphilis with syphilis IgG and rapid plasma reagin (RPR) and TB, with either PPD or TB-specific interferon gamma release assay (e.g., QuantiFERON-TB Gold®) as well as chest X-ray, should be performed to rule out these infectious etiologies. In addition to CXR, serum angiotensin-converting enzyme (ACE; if patient is not on ACE inhibitors) and lysozyme can be obtained to screen for sarcoidosis. HLA testing for the B51 haplotype can aid in the diagnosis. Pathergy test (pinprick test; positive if papule >2 mm diameter at 24–48 h) can also be useful. Neurologic symptoms should prompt neuroimaging (to assess for CNS vasculitis) and lumbar puncture, which may show cerebrospinal fluid (CSF) pleocytosis.

Several ophthalmic imaging modalities may be useful in diagnosis and monitoring:

- *Color fundus photography*: Useful in documenting areas of retinitis and in monitoring for progression of disease.
- *Fluorescein angiography (FA)*: With posterior segment involvement, it can show diffuse retinal vascular leakage, leakage from the optic disc, late staining of the vasculature, possible neovascularization, and areas of non-perfusion. Areas of necrotizing retinitis may show late staining.
- *Optical coherence tomography (OCT)*: Useful in assessing for macular edema.

95.9 Prognosis and Management

BD is typically episodic characterized by acute exacerbations followed by remission. BD with posterior segment and neurologic involvement is often difficult to treat and carries the greatest morbidity and mortality. Irreversible blindness or death may result if left untreated. Systemic immunosuppression is the mainstay of treatment:

- *Corticosteroids*: Treatment with systemic corticosteroids (1 mg/kg/day oral prednisone with a slow taper or 1,000 mg/day intravenously for 3 days followed by oral taper) is recommended to gain initial control of inflammation. Adjunctive periocular (e.g., 20–40 mg triamcinolone) or intravitreal (2–4 mg preservative-free triamcinolone) can be used to manage uveitis flares, but systemic treatment is essential given the systemic nature of the disease.
- *Steroid-sparing agents*: Early introduction of corticosteroid-sparing immunomodulatory therapy is recommended. Antimetabolites (methotrexate, mycophenolate mofetil, or azathioprine), T-cell inhibitors (cyclosporine A or tacrolimus), or anti-TNF biologic agents (infliximab or adalimumab) can be used. Anti-TNF agents have been successfully used in BD. Type I interferons are also used. These medications should only be prescribed by clinicians experienced in their use. Routine blood tests are required to monitor for potential toxicity. Patients with BD should be comanaged with rheumatologists or other specialists depending on organ system involvement.

95.10 Follow-Up

Patients should be followed up on a patient-specific basis depending on disease manifestations and the treatment regimens.

References and Suggested Reading

1. Behçet's Disease Research Committee of Japan, Behçet's disease: guide to diagnosis of Behçet's disease. Jpn J Ophthalmol. 1974;18:291–4.
2. Criteria for diagnosis of Behçet's disease. International Study Group for Behçet's Disease. Lancet. 1990;335:1078–80.
3. Evereklioglu C. Current concepts in the etiology and treatment of Behçet disease. Surv Ophthalmol. 2005;50:297–350.
4. Nussenblatt RB, Whitcup SM. Uveitis: fundamentals and clinical practice. 4th ed. Amsterdam, the Netherlands: Mosby; 2010. p. 332–54.
5. Tugal-Tutkun I, Onal S, Altan-Yaycioglu R, et al. Uveitis in Behçet disease: an analysis of 880 patients. Am J Ophthalmol. 2004;138:373–80.

Chapter 96
Posterior Scleritis

Jane S. Kim, Jared E. Knickelbein, Robert B. Nussenblatt, and H. Nida Sen

96.1 Definitions

Posterior scleritis is inflammation of the sclera posterior to the ora serrata or extra-ocular muscle insertions. Posterior scleritis may be present in patients with associated anterior scleritis or it may present in the absence of anterior scleral inflammation.

96.2 Symptoms

- Periocular pain, often described as deep and boring and exacerbated with eye movements
- Binocular diplopia
- Eye redness if anterior sclera involved
- Decreased vision

96.3 Signs

Possible findings include:

- Proptosis
- Ocular motility defect

J.S. Kim, BS
University of California, San Diego, School of Medicine, La Jolla, CA, USA

Laboratory of Immunology, National Eye Institute, National Institutes of Health, Bethesda, MD, USA

J.E. Knickelbein, MD, PhD • R.B. Nussenblatt, MD, MPH • H.N. Sen, MD, MHS (✉)
Laboratory of Immunology, National Eye Institute, National Institutes of Health, 10 Center Dr., Bldg. 10, Bethesda, MD 20892, USA
e-mail: senh@nei.nih.gov

C.A. Medina et al. (eds.), *Manual of Retinal Diseases: A Guide to Diagnosis and Management*, DOI 10.1007/978-3-319-20460-4_96

- Elevated intraocular pressure due to anterior rotation of the ciliary body causing angle closure
- Keratitis in cases of associated anterior scleritis
- Scleral hyperemia, thickening, and/or nodules
- Vitritis
- Retinal vasculitis
- Macular edema
- Exudative retinal detachment
- Choroidal effusion
- Choroidal and/or retinal folds
- Optic disk edema

96.4 Epidemiology and Predisposing Conditions

- Accounts for up to 13 % of scleritis cases (anterior scleritis is much more common)
- More commonly seen among middle-aged females
- Associated with rheumatoid arthritis, granulomatosis with polyangiitis, and other systemic vasculitides

96.5 Differential Diagnosis

- Rheumatoid arthritis (RA)
- Systemic lupus erythematosis (SLE)
- Granulomatosis with polyangiitis (GPA)
- Polyarteritis nodosa (PAN)
- Orbital pseudotumor
- Uveal effusion syndrome
- Vogt-Koyanagi-Harada (VKH) syndrome
- Sarcoidosis
- Tuberculosis (TB)
- Carotid-cavernous fistula
- Choroidal hemangioma
- Choroidal melanoma
- Choroidal lymphoma
- Metastasis

96.6 Etiology

Posterior scleritis may be idiopathic or occur secondary to systemic conditions, e.g., rheumatoid arthritis, granulomatosis with polyangiitis, and systemic lupus erythematosus. Exact etiology remains unknown.

96.7 Workup/Testing

Thorough history and exam should be conducted to assess for possible systemic inflammatory disease. Laboratory testing should be performed to assess for systemic inflammatory disease:

- Complete blood count (CBC)
- Basic metabolic panel (BMP)
- Erythrocyte sedimentation rate (ESR)
- C-reactive protein (CRP)
- Rheumatoid factor (RF)
- Anti-cyclic citrullinated peptide (anti-CCP) antibodies
- Anti-neutrophil cytoplasmic antibodies (c- and p-ANCA)
- Anti-nuclear antibodies (ANA)
- Urine analysis

Testing for TB with either PPD or TB-specific interferon gamma release assay (e.g., QuantiFERON-TB Gold®) as well as chest X-ray (CXR) may be considered. In addition to CXR, serum angiotensin-converting enzyme (ACE; if patient is not on ACE inhibitors) and lysozyme can be obtained to screen for sarcoidosis. Computed tomography (CT) of the orbits may be obtained to assess for orbital inflammation. Several ophthalmic imaging modalities may be useful in diagnosis and monitoring:

- *Optical coherence tomography (OCT)*: Can show macular edema and subretinal fluid
- *Enhanced depth imaging (EDI) OCT*: Can show choroidal thickening
- *B-scan ultrasonography:* Can show scleral thickening, scleral nodules, retrobulbar edema, and T-sign (retrobulbar edema surrounding the optic nerve; Fig. 96.1)

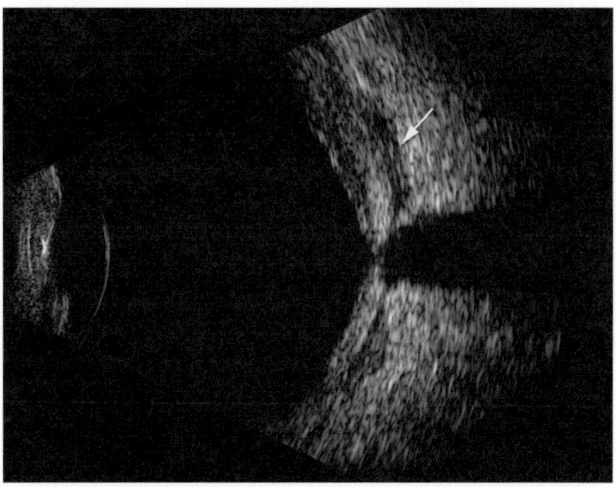

Fig. 96.1 B-scan ultrasound image demonstrating retrobulbar hypoechogenicity in sub-Tenon's space surrounding the optic nerve (T-sign, *arrow*) (Image courtesy of the Bascom Palmer Eye Institute Ultrasonography Department, Eddy Mesa, MD)

96.8 Prognosis and Management

Severity of visual impairment is variable, but it can be severe, depending on the extent of complications. Treatment of any underlying systemic inflammatory disease should be undertaken by the appropriate medical specialist. While mild cases of anterior scleritis may be treated with systemic nonsteroidal anti-inflammatory drugs, posterior scleritis generally requires systemic immunosuppression. Typically oral prednisone is started at a dose of ~1 mg/kg/day with subsequent taper. If inadequate response to systemic corticosteroids, additional immunosuppression in the form of antimetabolites (methotrexate, mycophenolate mofetil, or azathioprine), T-cell inhibitors (cyclosporine A or tacrolimus), or anti-TNF biologic agents (infliximab or adalimumab) should be considered. These medications should only be prescribed by clinicians experienced in their use. Routine blood tests are required to monitor for potential toxicity. If needed, a rheumatologist should be consulted to assist in administration of these medications.

References

1. Benson WE, Shields JA, Tasman W, et al. Posterior scleritis. A cause of diagnostic confusion. Arch Ophthalmol. 1979;97:1482–6.
2. Calthorpe CM, Watson PG, McCartney AC. Posterior scleritis: a clinical and histological survey. Eye. 1988;2:267–77.
3. Benson WE. Posterior scleritis. Surv Ophthalmol. 1988;32:297–316.
4. McCluskey PJ, Watson PG, Lightman S, et al. Posterior scleritis: clinical features, systemic associations, and outcome in a large series of patients. Ophthalmology. 1999;106:2380–6.
5. Wakefield D, Di Girolamo N, Thurau S, et al. Scleritis: immunopathogenesis and molecular basis for therapy. Prog Retin Eye Res. 2013;35:44–62.

Chapter 97
Vogt-Koyanagi-Harada Syndrome

Laurence Jaworski, Jared E. Knickelbein, Robert B. Nussenblatt, and H. Nida Sen

97.1 Definitions

Vogt-Koyanagi-Harada (VKH) syndrome is a rare multisystem autoimmune disease affecting the eyes, brain, inner ear, and skin.

97.2 Symptoms

Ocular symptoms can include photophobia, pain, redness, and blurry vision. Prodromal systemic symptoms often mimic a viral illness with headaches, tinnitus, difficulty in hearing, neck stiffness, weakness, and nausea.

L. Jaworski, MD, FRCSC (✉)
Laboratory of Immunology, National Eye Institute, National Institutes of Health, 10 Center Dr., Bethesda, MD 20892, USA

Centre Hospitalier de l'Université de Montréal (CHUM), Université de Montréal, 1560, rue Sherbrooke Est, Montréal, Québec H2L 4 M1, Canada
e-mail: laurence.jaworski@umontreal.ca

J.E. Knickelbein, MD, PhD • R.B. Nussenblatt, MD, MPH • H.N. Sen, MD, MHS
Laboratory of Immunology, National Eye Institute, National Institutes of Health, Bethesda, MD, USA

C.A. Medina et al. (eds.), *Manual of Retinal Diseases: A Guide to Diagnosis and Management*, DOI 10.1007/978-3-319-20460-4_97

97.3 Signs

The disease can be divided into four phases:

1. Prodromal phase: Usually without ocular finding, but optic neuritis and cranial nerve palsies have been reported. CSF analysis can show pleocytosis.
2. Uveitic phase: Bilateral granulomatous panuveitis (primarily a choroiditis) with exudative retinal detachments with or without optic disc swelling (Fig. 97.1). Occasionally, ciliary body swelling can cause a shallow anterior chamber with an elevated IOP.
3. Convalescent phase: Signs of depigmentation including vitiligo, poliosis, and sunset glow fundus as well as Dalen-Fuchs-like lesions can occur 2–6 months after the onset of disease (Fig. 97.2). Pigmentary changes in the posterior pole are also common.
4. Chronic recurrent phase: Recurrences usually manifest as anterior uveitis. Glaucoma, cataract, subretinal neovascular membrane, and subretinal fibrosis can occur.

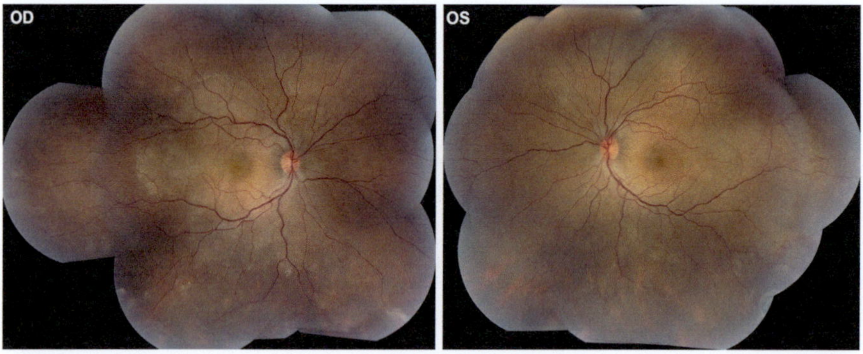

Fig. 97.1 Color fundus photographs of the right (**a**) and left (**b**) eyes demonstrating choroiditis with exudative retinal detachments in an 18-year-old African American woman with VKH

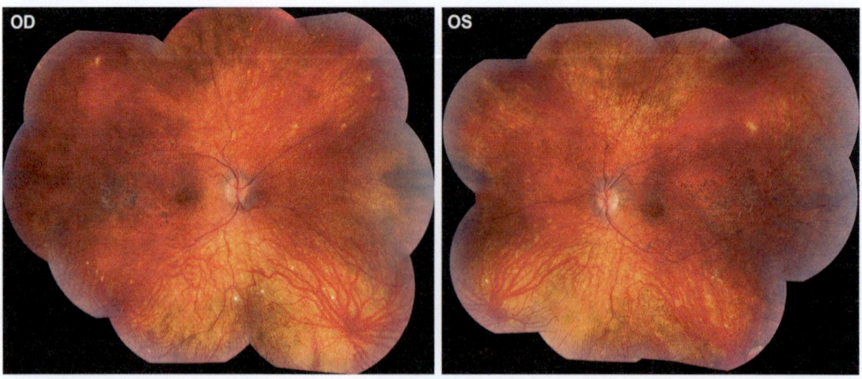

Fig. 97.2 Color fundus photographs of the right (**a**) and left (**b**) eyes demonstrating sunset glow fundus with pigment migration and Dalen-Fuchs-like lesions in the same patient eight months later

97.4 Epidemiology

It is estimated that 1–4 % of all uveitis cases in the United States are caused by VKH. The incidence is higher in South America, Asia, and the Middle East. VKH affects mostly individuals from 20 to 50 years old and is more common in women (79 %), except in Japan where it is more common in men.

97.5 Predisposing Conditions

- Dark skin pigmentation
- Native American ancestry
- HLA-DRB1*0405 and some other less common haplotypes

97.6 Differential Diagnosis

- Sympathetic ophthalmia
- Sarcoidosis
- Syphilis
- Tuberculosis (TB)
- Posterior scleritis
- Acute posterior multifocal placoid pigment epitheliopathy (APMPPE)
- Idiopathic uveal effusion syndrome
- Central serous chorioretinopathy

97.7 Etiology

The exact cause of VKH remains unknown. It is thought to be a T-cell-mediated process directed against melanocytes. The targeted antigen may be tyrosinase or a tyrosinase-related protein.

97.8 Workup/Testing

VKH is a clinical diagnosis (Table 97.1). Systemic manifestations must be present in order to diagnose a "definite VKH" case. Thus, an isolated ocular disease can only be diagnosed as "probable VKH." Definite diagnoses are subdivided into incomplete (in which eye findings plus either neurologic or skin findings are present) and complete (when all criteria are met). Laboratory testing for syphilis, with syphilis IgG and rapid plasma reagin (RPR) and TB, with either PPD or TB-specific

Table 97.1 Revised diagnostic criteria for VKH

1. No history of penetrating ocular trauma or surgery preceding the initial onset uveitis
2. No clinical or laboratory evidence suggestive of other ocular disease entities
3. Bilateral ocular involvement (a or b must be met, depending on the stage of disease when the patient is examined)
(A) *Early manifestations*
(1) Evidence of diffuse choroiditis (+/– anterior uveitis, vitreous cells, or optic disc hyperemia), which may manifest as one of the following:
(a) Focal areas or subretinal fluid
(b) Bullous serous retinal detachments
(2) With equivocal fundus findings, both of the flowing must be present as well:
(a) Focal areas of delay in choroidal perfusion, multifocal areas of pinpoint leakage, large placoid areas of hyperfluorescence, pooling within subretinal fluid, and optic nerve staining by FA
(b) Diffuse choroidal thickening without evidence of posterior scleritis by ultrasonography
(B) *Late manifestations*
(1) History suggestive of prior presence of findings from 3a, and either both 2 and 3 below, or multiple signs from 3
(2) Ocular depigmentation: Sunset glow fundus and/or Sugiura's sign (perilimbal vitiligo)
(3) Other ocular signs:
(a) Nummular chorioretinal depigmented scars
(b) RPE clumping and/or migration
(c) Recurrent or chronic anterior uveitis.
4. Neurologic/auditory findings (may have resolved by time of examination)
(A) Meningismus (malaise, fever, headache, nausea, abdominal pain, stiffness of the neck and back, or a combination of these factors; headache alone is not sufficient to meet definition of meningismus, however)
(B) Tinnitus
(C) CSF pleocytosis
5. Integumentary finding (not preceding onset of CNS or ocular disease)
(A) Alopecia
(B) Poliosis
(C) Vitiligo
Complete VKH: criteria 1–5 must be present
Incomplete VKH: criteria 1–3 and either 4 or 5 must be present
Probable VKH/isolated eye disease: criteria 1–3 must be present

Adapted from *Am J Ophthalmol* 2001;131:647–52

interferon gamma release assay (e.g., QuantiFERON-TB Gold®) as well as chest X-ray, should be performed to rule out these infectious etiologies. In addition to CXR, serum angiotensin-converting enzyme (ACE; if patient is not on ACE inhibitors) and lysozyme can be obtained to screen for sarcoidosis. Several ophthalmic imaging modalities may be useful in diagnosis and monitoring:

- *Optical coherence tomography (OCT)*: Can show elevation of the neural retina with subretinal fluid and "fibrin-like" material.

- *Enhanced depth imaging (EDI) OCT* and *B-scan ultrasonography*: Can show choroidal thickening.
- *Fluorescein angiography (FA)*: During acute disease, typically shows disc leakage as well as early pinpoint areas of hyperfluorescence with subsequent accumulation of dye in areas of exudative retinal detachment.
- *Indocyanine green angiography (ICGA)*: During acute disease, shows hypofluorescent spots indicative of choroidal granulomas.
- If neurologic symptoms are present, consider neuroimaging and lumbar puncture with cerebrospinal fluid (CSF) analysis, especially in atypical cases.
- Audiology testing may reveal subclinical neurosensory hearing loss.

97.9 Prognosis and Management

With the use of high-dose systemic corticosteroids and sometimes immunomodulatory agents, the prognosis of VKH has improved over the past decades. Early and aggressive systemic corticosteroid treatment is very important, and prolonged systemic corticosteroid treatment has been associated with fewer recurrences and better prognosis. Neurology and/or ear, nose, and throat (ENT) consultations should be obtained when neurologic and/or auditory symptoms are present. The following treatment regimens can be used:

- High-dose oral corticosteroids (~1 mg/kg/day) with gradual taper over 6 months or more or pulse IV methylprednisolone (up to 1 g daily × 3 days) followed by oral steroids (~1 mg/kg/day) with gradual taper over the course of 6 months or more.
- Topical steroids and cycloplegics should be used as needed for anterior chamber inflammation.
- Periocular (sub-Tenon's or orbital floor) triamcinolone injections (20–40 mg) can be useful adjuncts.
- In patients unresponsive or intolerant to systemic steroids, immunomodulatory agents should be considered. Cyclosporine, azathioprine, methotrexate, and mycophenolate mofetil have all been reported for treatment of VKH. In case of failure with these drugs, biologic (anti-TNF) or cytotoxic agents could also be considered.

97.10 Follow-Up

Initial investigation and treatment may require hospitalization. Patients should be followed closely initially (e.g., daily to every week) to monitor treatment response and side effects. As the inflammation subsides, the follow-up can be prolonged to monthly. Oral prednisone taper should be adjusted according to the clinical findings and extended over a minimum of 6 months. Patients should also be monitored regularly after discontinuation of prednisone to ensure a timely diagnosis and management of recurrent inflammation or other complications (e.g., glaucoma, cataract, neovascular membrane) if they occur.

References and Suggested Reading

1. Al Dhahri H, Al Rubaie K, Hemachandran S, et al. Patterns of uveitis in a University-based Tertiary Referral Center in Riyadh, Saudi Arabia. Ocul Immunol Inflamm. 2014;24:1–9.
2. Bykhovskaya Thorne JE, Kempen JH, et al. Vogt-Koyanagi-Harada disease: clinical outcomes. Am J Ophthalmol. 2005;140:674–8.
3. Goto H, Rao PK, Rao NA. Vogt-Koyanagi-Harada disease. In: Schachat AP, Sadda SR, editors. Retina. 5th ed. Amsterdam, the Netherlands: Elsevier; 2013.
4. Liberman P, Gauro F, Berger O, et al. Causes of uveitis in a Tertiary Center in Chile: a cross-sectional retrospective review. Ocul Immunol Inflamm. 2014;1:1–7.
5. Nakayama M, Keino H, Okada AA, et al. Enhanced depth imaging optical coherence tomography of the Choroid in Vogt-Koyanagi-Harada disease. Retina. 2012;32:2061–9.
6. Nussenblatt RB, Whitecup SM. Vogt-Koyanagi-Harada syndrome. In: Nussenblatt RB, Whitecup SM, editors. Uveitis: fundamentals and clinical practice. 4th ed. Amsterdam, the Netherlands: Mosby Elsevier; 2010.
7. Pan D, Hirose T. Vogt-Koyanagi-Harada syndrome: review of clinical features. Semin Ophthalmol. 2011;26:312–5.
8. Read RW, Holland GN, Rao NA, et al. Perspective – revised diagnostic criteria for Vogt-Koyanagi-Harada disease: report of an International Committee on Nomenclature. Am J Ophthalmol. 2001;131:647–52.
9. Read RW, Yu F, Accorinti M, et al. Evaluation of the effect on outcomes of the route of administration of corticosteroids in acute Vogt-Koyanagi-Harada disease. Am J Ophthalmol. 2006;142:119–24.
10. Sakata VM, da Silva FT, Hirate CE, et al. Diagnosis and classification of Vogt-Koyanagi-Harada disease. Autoimmun Rev. 2014;13:550–5.

Chapter 98
Ocular Sarcoidosis

Laurence Jaworski, Jared E. Knickelbein, Robert B. Nussenblatt, and H. Nida Sen

98.1 Definitions

Sarcoidosis is a multisystemic granulomatous inflammatory disease with possible pulmonary (most common), cardiac, digestive, renal, rheumatologic, neurologic, dermatologic, and ocular involvement. The eyes, one of the most common extrapulmonary sites, ocular adnexa, and orbit can all be affected. Ocular findings occur in 15–50 % of patients with sarcoidosis. The following syndromes are associated with sarcoidosis:

- *Löfgren's syndrome* presents with fever, erythema nodosum, arthritis, and bilateral hilar adenopathy with or without anterior uveitis.
- *Heerfordt's syndrome* (uveoparotid fever) presents with fever, parotid swelling, uveitis, and facial nerve palsy.

L. Jaworski, MD, FRCSC (✉)
Laboratory of Immunology, National Eye Institute, National Institutes of Health,
10 Center Dr., Bethesda, MD 20892, USA

Centre Hospitalier de l'Université de Montréal (CHUM), Université de Montréal,
1560, rue Sherbrooke Est, Montréal, QC H2L 4 M1, Canada
e-mail: laurence.jaworski@umontreal.ca

J.E. Knickelbein, MD, PhD • R.B. Nussenblatt, MD, MPH • H.N. Sen, MD, MHS
Laboratory of Immunology, National Eye Institute, National Institutes of Health,
10 Center Dr., Bethesda, MD 20892, USA

C.A. Medina et al. (eds.), *Manual of Retinal Diseases: A Guide to Diagnosis and Management*, DOI 10.1007/978-3-319-20460-4_98

98.2 Symptoms

Common ocular symptoms are photophobia, pain, redness, and blurred vision. Foreign body sensation, ocular discomfort, eyelid edema, proptosis, and diplopia can also occur. Systemic symptoms include fever, malaise, fatigue, weight loss, difficulty breathing, skin nodules (erythema nodosum), arthritis, and facial palsy, although many patients can be entirely asymptomatic.

98.3 Signs

Uveitis is the most common ocular manifestation (30–70 %). Typically, sarcoid uveitis is bilateral and granulomatous, but it may also be non-granulomatous in a large proportion of patients. The anterior chamber (AC) is the most common anatomic location of inflammation in sarcoidosis, but it can also present as intermediate, posterior, or panuveitis. Specific signs depending on anatomic location are:

- *Orbital disease*: Exophthalmia, vision loss, and limitation of eye movement.
- *Lacrimal gland involvement*: Enlargement of the gland and keratoconjunctivitis sicca.
- *Anterior segment disease*: Eyelid and conjunctival granulomas, scleral nodules, scleritis, interstitial keratitis, band keratopathy, AC cells and flare, keratic precipitates that are often granulomatous or "mutton fat" (Fig. 98.1), iris nodules (Koeppe, pupillary margin; Busacca, iris surface; Berlin, angle), anterior and posterior synechiae, increased IOP, and cataract.

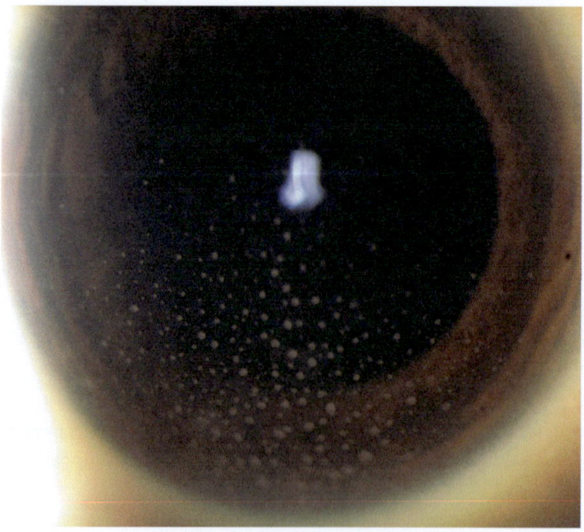

Fig. 98.1 Granulomatous "mutton-fat" keratic precipitates

- *Posterior segment disease*: Vitritis with or without snowballs sometimes linearly distributed and described as a "string of pearls," chorioretinitis (Fig. 98.2), retinal phlebitis that can appear as "candle-wax drippings" (Fig. 98.3), vascular occlusions, retinal neovascularization, and granulomas of optic nerve head (Fig. 98.4) or choroid.

Large choroidal granulomas can rarely be associated with exudative retinal detachment. Macular edema is common, and epiretinal membrane (ERM) can develop.

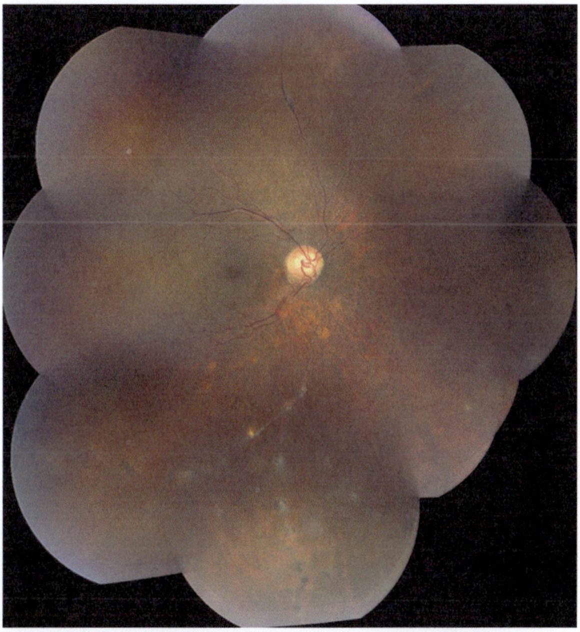

Fig. 98.2 Multifocal chorioretinal scars with vascular and glaucomatous optic nerve head changes in chronic ocular sarcoidosis

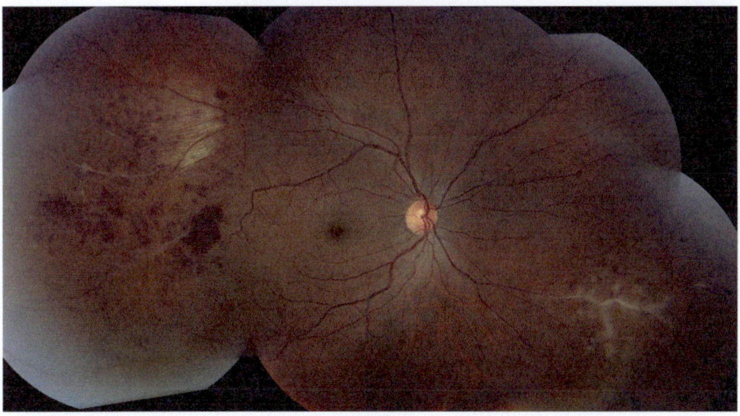

Fig. 98.3 Active vasculitis and retinal hemorrhage in ocular sarcoidosis

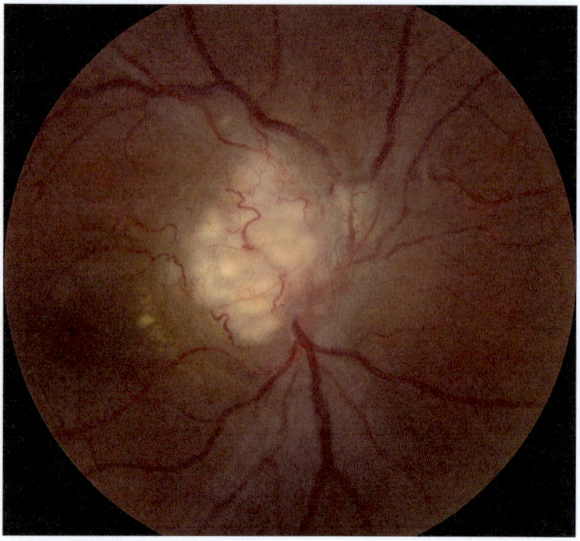

Fig. 98.4 Optic nerve head granuloma in a patient with sarcoidosis

98.4 Epidemiology

It is estimated that biopsy-proven sarcoidosis is the underlying diagnosis in about 5 % of all uveitis cases. Sarcoidosis can affect people of all ages and all races, but the disease is more prevalent in blacks compared to whites. Females represent approximately 60 % of cases. The peak incidence is between the ages of 20–40 years old. African Americans with ocular sarcoidosis tend to present at a younger age than Caucasian patients, in whom the onset of uveitis can commonly be observed after the age of 50 years old.

98.5 Predisposing Conditions

- African American heritage or Scandinavian origin
- Family history of sarcoidosis (5x elevated risk if first- or second-degree relative with sarcoidosis)

98.6 Differential Diagnosis

The differential diagnosis for sarcoidosis is broad and includes:

- Infectious etiologies including tuberculosis (TB), syphilis, *Bartonella*, Lyme, and herpesviruses (e.g., HSV, VZV, CMV)
- Behçet's disease

- Birdshot chorioretinopathy
- Acute posterior multifocal placoid pigment epitheliopathy (AMPPE)
- Serpiginous choroidopathy
- Multifocal choroiditis and panuveitis (MCP)
- Vogt-Koyanagi-Harada (VKH) syndrome
- Sympathetic ophthalmia (SO)
- Pars planitis
- Juvenile idiopathic arthritis (JIA)-associated uveitis or Blau syndrome in children
- Masquerade syndromes (e.g., intraocular lymphoma or metastasis) especially in patients over the age of 50 years

98.7 Etiology

The exact cause of sarcoidosis remains unknown. It is thought to be a T cell-mediated process and involves the formation of noncaseating granulomas. Genetic inheritance, including HLA-DRB1 and some other haplotypes, infectious organisms, and exposure to environmental agents have all been suggested as etiologies or triggers.

98.8 Workup/Testing

There is no single diagnostic test specific for sarcoidosis. Recently, uveitis specialists participating in the first International Workshop on Ocular Sarcoidosis (IWOS) proposed diagnostic criteria that allow for diagnosis of presumed ocular sarcoidosis in the absence of biopsy (see reference 7 for full criteria). The following should be considered for a patient suspected of having sarcoidosis:

- *A complete history and ocular examination*, including a gonioscopy and dilated retinal exam, should be performed.
- *Laboratory testing* for syphilis, with syphilis IgG and rapid plasma reagin (RPR), and TB, with either PPD or TB-specific interferon gamma release assay (e.g., QuantiFERON-TB Gold®) as well as chest X-ray, should be performed to rule out these infectious etiologies. Serum angiotensin-converting enzyme (ACE; if patient is not on ACE inhibitors) and lysozyme level can be elevated, although normal levels do not exclude the diagnosis (ACE elevated in 60 % and lysozyme elevated in 76 % of sarcoidosis patients).
- *Chest X-ray* usually shows hilar adenopathy, and sometimes interstitial lung anomalies, but will be normal for approximately 10 % of patients with sarcoidosis.
- *Thoracic computed tomography (CT)* should be considered when there is a strong clinical suspicion of sarcoidosis in cases with negative chest X-ray.

- *Gallium scan* can also be helpful in the diagnosis (positive in ~50 %).
- *Tissue biopsy* documenting classic noncaseating granuloma remains the gold standard for diagnosis. It can be done on conjunctival nodules, but is more frequently performed on skin, lungs, or lymph node specimens. Random conjunctival biopsy has very low yield and is not recommended.
- *Ocular imaging*, including fundus photography, optical coherence tomography (OCT), fluorescein angiography (FA), and indocyanine green angiography (ICGA), may be useful in diagnosis and monitoring of the abovementioned signs.

98.9 Prognosis and Management

Visual prognosis is worse in eyes developing chronic intraocular inflammation and in eyes with posterior segment involvement. The development of secondary glaucoma also confers poor prognosis. Oral corticosteroids are the mainstay of sarcoidosis treatment, but patients who are systemically asymptomatic or have a mild disease can be treated locally as needed. The following steps should be considered:

- Request a pulmonology or internal medicine consultation to ensure that a proper systemic investigation is performed. Pulmonary function testing and/or bronchoscopy with bronchoalveolar lavage can help in establishing the diagnosis. Neurology, cardiology, and dermatology consults should be requested based on review of systems if needed.
- Anterior segment inflammation can be managed with topical steroids (e.g., prednisolone acetate 4–8 times per day adjusted for amount of inflammation) and cycloplegics alone. When the posterior segment is involved, systemic corticosteroids (up to 1 mg/kg/day) are generally required. One should keep in mind that this treatment might mask systemic findings so, whenever possible, it should be postponed until a biopsy is obtained.
- Periocular (sub-Tenon's or orbital floor) triamcinolone injections (20–40 mg) can be useful adjuncts in patients intolerant to systemic therapy.
- In patients unresponsive or intolerant to systemic steroids, or when steroids cannot be successfully tapered to low doses (e.g., <7.5 mg/day), immunomodulatory agents should be considered. Methotrexate, azathioprine, mycophenolate mofetil, cyclosporine, and anti-TNF-α agents, such as infliximab and adalimumab, have all been reported to be beneficial in the treatment of sarcoidosis.
- Macular edema should be treated aggressively with topical, local, and/or systemic treatments. If a concomitant epiretinal membrane affecting vision is present, pars plana vitrectomy with epiretinal membrane peeling can be considered once inflammation has been quiescent for a prolonged period.

98.10 Follow-Up

Patients should be followed closely initially (e.g., daily to q 1 week depending on the amount of inflammation) until the inflammation subsides. Once quiescence is established, follow-up can be prolonged. Patients should also be monitored regularly after discontinuation of treatment to ensure a timely diagnosis and management of recurrent inflammation or other complications (e.g., glaucoma, cataract) if they occur.

References and Suggested Reading

1. Birnbaum AD, Oh FS, Chakrabarti A, et al. Clinical features and diagnostic evaluation of biopsy-proven ocular sarcoidosis. Arch Ophthalmol. 2011;129:409–13.
2. Bonfioli AA, Orefice F. Sarcoidosis. Semin Ophthalmol. 2005;20:177–82.
3. Bui KM, Garcia-Gonzalez JM, Patel SS, et al. Directed conjunctival biopsy and impact of histologic sectioning methodology on the diagnosis of ocular sarcoidosis. J Ophthalmic Inflamm Infect. 2014;4:8.
4. Herbort CP, Rao NA, Mochizuki M, et al. International criteria for the diagnosis of ocular sarcoidosis: results of the first international workshop on ocular sarcoidosis (IWOS). Ocul Immunol Inflamm. 2009;17:160–9.
5. Jamilloux Y, Kodjikian L, Broussolle C, et al. Sarcoidosis and uveitis. Autoimmun Rev. 2014;13:840–9.
6. Kawagoe T, Mizuki N. Sarcoidosis. Curr Opin Ophthalmol. 2011;22:502–7.
7. Sarcoidosis. In: Nussenblatt RB, Whitecup SM, editors. Uveitis: fundamentals and clinical practice, 4th ed. Edinburgh: Mosby: Elsevier; 2010.
8. Sepah YJ, Jabs DA, Nguyen QD. Sarcoidosis. In: Schachat AP, Sadda SR, editors. Retina, 5th ed. Amsterdam, The Netherlands: Elsevier; 2013.
9. Thomas KW, Hunninghake GW. Sarcoidosis. JAMA. 2003;289:3300–3.

Chapter 99
Sympathetic Ophthalmia

Padmini Kaushal, Jared E. Knickelbein, Robert B. Nussenblatt, and H. Nida Sen

99.1 Definitions

Sympathetic ophthalmia (SO) is a rare bilateral but asymmetric granulomatous panuveitis occurring classically after penetrating ocular trauma, but it can also occur after ocular surgery, including vitrectomy, cryotherapy, and cyclophotocoagulation. A prospective study from England and Ireland reported a minimum estimated incidence of 0.03 cases per 100,000 people per year. The injured eye is referred to as the exciting eye; the fellow eye is the sympathizing eye. Typically, the exciting eye has more severe inflammation. The time to development of SO varies, but approximately 90 % of patients develop the disease within 1 year of injury.

99.2 Symptoms

Decreased vision, photophobia, floaters.

P. Kaushal, MD (✉) • J.E. Knickelbein, MD, PhD • R.B. Nussenblatt, MD, MPH
H.N. Sen, MD, MHS
National Eye Institute, National Institutes of Health,
10 Center Dr., Bldg. 10, Room 10D45, Bethesda, MD 20892, USA
e-mail: knickelbeinje@nei.nih.gov

C.A. Medina et al. (eds.), *Manual of Retinal Diseases: A Guide to Diagnosis and Management*, DOI 10.1007/978-3-319-20460-4_99

99.3 Signs

- Varying degrees of anterior chamber inflammation ranging from mild non-granulomatous reaction to severe granulomatous anterior uveitis with mutton-fat keratic precipitates.
- Moderate to severe vitritis.
- Papillitis may be seen.
- Multiple serous retinal detachments.
- White-yellowish lesions (Dalen-Fuchs nodules) at the level of the choroid in the mid-peripheral fundus (Fig. 99.1).
- Rarely, extraocular findings similar to Vogt-Koyanagi-Harada disease, such as alopecia, poliosis, vitiligo, and sensorineural hearing loss can be present.

99.4 Predisposing Conditions

- Ocular trauma – either accidental or iatrogenic (e.g. intraocular surgery)
- Possible association with human leukocyte antigens HLA-DR4, HLA-DRw53, and HLA-DQw3

99.5 Differential Diagnosis

- Vogt-Koyanagi-Harada (VKH) disease
- Behçet's disease

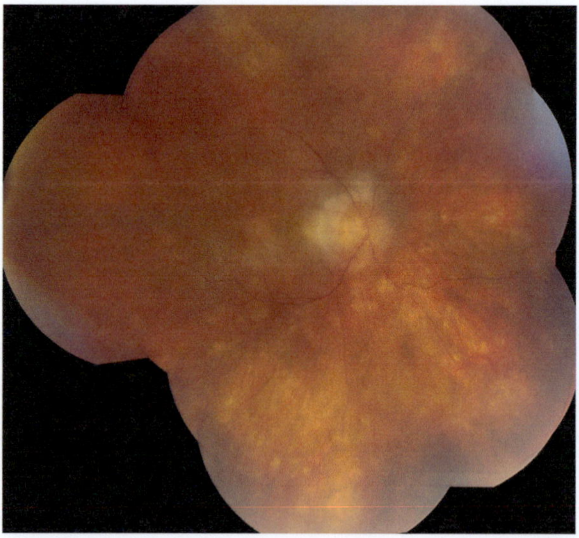

Fig. 99.1 Fundus photo of the right eye of a 54-year-old man approximately 1 year after pars plana vitrectomy for post-cataract surgery endophthalmitis. Note the scattered deep white-yellowish lesions (Dalen-Fuchs nodules)

- Sarcoidosis
- Syphilis
- Tuberculosis (TB)
- Post-operative endophthalmitis
- Phacoanaphylactic uveitis

99.6 Etiology

Thought to involve autosensitization with release of intraocular antigens at the time of injury that leads to an adaptive immune response against the released antigens.

99.7 Workup/Testing

The diagnosis is based on history and clinical examination. A history of ocular trauma, either accidental or surgical, is necessary for the diagnosis. Laboratory testing for syphilis, with syphilis IgG and rapid plasma reagin (RPR), and TB, with either PPD or TB-specific interferon gamma release assay (e.g. QuantiFERON-TB Gold®) as well as chest X-ray, should be performed to rule out these infectious etiologies. In addition to CXR, serum angiotensin converting enzyme (ACE; if patient is not on ACE inhibitors) and lysozyme can be obtained to screen for sarcoidosis. Several ophthalmic imaging modalities may be useful in diagnosis and monitoring:

- *Optical coherence tomography (OCT)*: Can show elevation of the neural retina with subretinal fluid in cases with serous retinal detachment. Areas corresponding to choroidal granulomas or Dalen-Fuchs nodules can show hyper-reflectivity and disruption of the outer retina.
- *Fluorescein angiography (FA)*: During acute disease, may show disc leakage as well as early pinpoint areas of hyperfluorescence with subsequent accumulation of dye in areas of exudative retinal detachment. Dalen-Fuchs nodules are typically hypofluorescent early and stain late during acute disease. Chronically, they appear as transmission defects with early and persistent hyperfluorescence.
- *Indocyanine green angiography (ICGA)*: During acute disease, shows hypofluorescent spots indicative of choroidal granulomas.
- *B-scan ultrasonography*: May show choroidal thickening most commonly around the optic nerve as well as exudative retinal detachment.

99.8 Prognosis and Management

Overall, SO has a poor prognosis with approximately half of patients experiencing 20/40 visual acuity or worse vision. Classically, enucleation within 14 days of injury had been thought of as the only way to prevent SO from developing. However, since ocular surgical techniques have improved, primary enucleation is done less often. Once SO develops, secondary enucleation of the injured eye does not seem lead to an improvement in visual acuity or overall prognosis. Systemic immunosuppression is the mainstay of treatment:

- *Corticosteroids*: Systemic corticosteroids are the mainstay of treatment. Oral prednisone is typically started at a dose of ~1 mg/kg/day. For severe inflammation, intravenous methylprednisolone at a dose of 1000 mg/day for 3 days may be administered followed by oral prednisone taper. The dose of oral prednisone should be tapered by 10 mg every 5–7 days until the range of 20–30 mg/day. Further tapering should be tailored to the clinical response. Calcium and vitamin D supplementation should be prescribed to all patients taking oral corticosteroids. Alternatively, in some cases, local corticosteroid therapies in the form periocular (e.g. 20–40 mg of triamcinolone via the sub-Tenon's or orbital floor routes) or intravitreal (e.g. 2–4 mg of preservative-free triamcinolone) injections can be used.
- *Steroid-sparing agents*: If inadequate response to systemic corticosteroids or if corticosteroids cannot be tapered without a flare-up, additional immunosuppression in the form of antimetabolites (methotrexate, mycophenolate mofetil, or azathioprine), T-cell inhibitors (cyclosporine A or tacrolimus), or anti-TNF biologic agents (infliximab or adalimumab) is needed. These medications should only be prescribed by clinicians experienced in their use. Routine blood tests are required to monitor for potential toxicity. If needed, a rheumatologist should be consulted to assist in the administration of these medications.

References and Suggested Reading

1. Arevalo JF, Garcia RA, Al-Dhibi HA, et al. Update on sympathetic ophthalmia. Middle East Afr J Ophthalmol. 2012;19:13–21.
2. Chu XK, Chan CC. Sympathetic ophthalmia: to the twenty-first century and beyond. J Ophthalmic Inflamma Infect. 2013;3:49.
3. Kilmartin D, Dick A, Forrester J. Prospective surveillance of sympathetic ophthalmia in the UK and Republic of Ireland. Br J Ophthalmol. 2000;84:259–63.
4. Power WJ, Foster CS. Update on sympathetic ophthalmia. Int Ophthalmol Clin. 1995;35:127–37.
5. Sympathetic ophthalmia. In: Nussenblatt RB, Whitecup SM, editors. Uveitis: fundamentals and clinical practice, 4th ed. Mosby: Elsevier; 2010.
6. Vasconcelos-Santos, DV, Narsing AR. Sympthetic ophthalmia. In: Schachat AP, Sadda SR, editors. Retina. 5th ed. Amsterdam, The Netherlands: Elsevier; 2013.

Chapter 100
Pars Planitis

Jesia Hasan, Jared E. Knickelbein, Robert B. Nussenblatt, and H. Nida Sen

100.1 Definition

Intermediate uveitis is defined as an intraocular inflammation primarily involving the vitreous cavity. It is often accompanied by peripheral retinal vascular leakage. Pars planitis defined as intermediate uveitis with snowbank or snowball formation in the absence of infectious or systemic disease.

100.2 Epidemiology

Pars planitis typically presents in individuals aged 15–40 years, without a race or gender predilection. It is often bilateral but asymmetric.

100.3 Symptoms

- Floaters.
- Blurred vision.
- Redness, pain, and photophobia are common in children but rare in adults.

J. Hasan, MD (✉) • J.E. Knickelbein, MD, PhD • R.B. Nussenblatt, MD, MPH
H.N. Sen, MD, MHS
Laboratory of Immunology, National Eye Institute, National Institutes of Health,
10 Center Dr., Bethesda, MD, 20892, USA
e-mail: jesia.hasan@gmail.com

C.A. Medina et al. (eds.), *Manual of Retinal Diseases: A Guide to Diagnosis and Management*, DOI 10.1007/978-3-319-20460-4_100

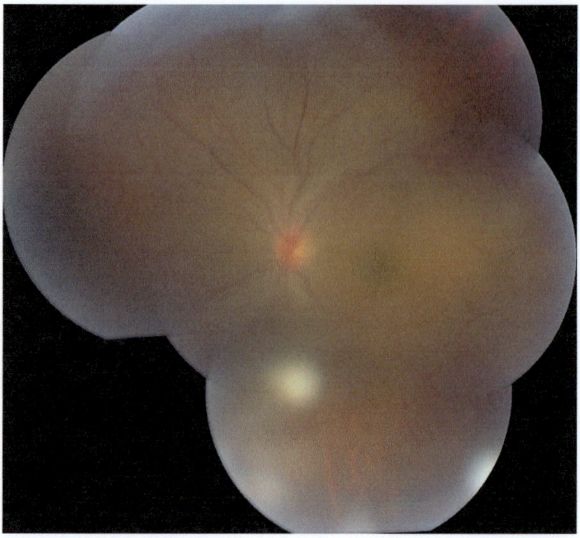

Fig. 100.1 The left eye of a patient with vitreous haze and snowballs

100.4 Signs

- Quiet to low-grade inflammation in the anterior chamber
- Predominant cellular reaction in the vitreous cavity
- Snowballs – yellow-white aggregates of inflammatory cells in the inferior vitreous (Fig. 100.1)
- Snowbanks – yellow-gray exudates along the ora serrata that usually require scleral depression to be seen
- Cystoid macular edema (CME)
- Sheathing and/or occlusion of small retinal venules
- Peripheral retinal neovascularization
- Vitreous hemorrhage
- Rhegmatogenous retinal detachment from vitreous traction
- Cyclitic membranes
- Epiretinal membrane

100.5 Etiology

By definition, pars planitis is idiopathic.

100.6 Differential Diagnosis

Intermediate uveitis has been linked to a number of infectious and inflammatory disorders:

- Sarcoidosis
- Multiple sclerosis
- Inflammatory bowel disease
- Tubulointerstitial nephritis and uveitis syndrome (TINU)
- Intraocular lymphoma
- Retinoblastoma
- Lyme disease
- Syphilis
- Toxocariasis
- Cat scratch disease
- Epstein-Barr virus infection
- HTLV-1 Infection
- Hepatitis C infection
- Tuberculosis (TB)

100.7 Workup/Testing

Laboratory testing for syphilis, with syphilis IgG and rapid plasma reagin (RPR), and TB, with either PPD or TB-specific interferon gamma release assay (e.g., QuantiFERON-TB Gold®) as well as chest X-ray, should be performed to rule out these infectious etiologies. In addition to CXR, serum angiotensin converting enzyme (ACE; if patient is not on ACE inhibitors) and lysozyme can be obtained to screen for sarcoidosis. Serologic testing for Lyme disease in those exposed to an endemic area or reporting a history of a tick bite should be ordered with confirmatory western blot if initial enzyme-linked immunosorbent assay (ELISA) is positive. Unilateral inflammation in younger patients should prompt testing for *Toxocara* serology. Neurologic history and evaluation, including an MRI scan, are recommended if there is any suspicion for multiple sclerosis. In older patients, evaluation for intraocular lymphoma should be considered (diagnostic vitrectomy for cytology and IL-10/IL-6 cytokine analysis, neuroimaging, and lumbar puncture). Several ophthalmic imaging modalities may be useful in diagnosis and monitoring:

- *Fluorescein angiography (FA)*: Identifies areas of retinal vasculitis such as vascular leakage and staining of vessel walls. Wide-angle FA is especially helpful in these cases.

- *Optical coherence tomography (OCT)*: Useful in assessing the presence and extent of macular edema.
- *B-scan ultrasonography*: Can demonstrate extent of vitreous debris and reveal cyclitic membranes obscured by media opacities. Anterior segment ultrasound [ultrasound biomicroscopy (UBM)] can be useful in identifying cyclitic membranes.

100.8 Prognosis and Management

A small fraction of cases are benign and self-limited. Most patients experience a chronically active course or periods of exacerbations and remissions. Seventy-five percent of patients maintain visual acuity of 20/40 or better. Secondary complications include cataract, glaucoma, CME, retinal neovascularization, vitreous hemorrhage, and tractional or rhegmatogenous retinal detachment.

In pars planitis, where no underlying condition is identified, a stepwise approach is employed to control inflammation. Mild cases in the absence of CME and with only minimal peripheral small vessel leakage may be observed. Decline in visual acuity, presence of CME, or retinal vasculitis should prompt immunosuppressive treatment:

- *Corticosteroids*: Periocular or intraocular triamcinolone injections may be used, especially in cases of asymmetric or unilateral disease. Generally, 40 mg of triamcinolone is injected via the sub-Tenon's or orbital floor routes, or 4 mg of preservative-free triamcinolone is injected intravitreally. Alternatively, oral prednisone may be considered. Typical starting dose for active intraocular inflammation is ~1 mg/kg/day. The dose should be tapered by 10 mg every 5–7 days until the range of 20–30 mg/day. Further tapering should be tailored to the clinical response. Calcium and vitamin D supplementation should be prescribed to all patients taking oral corticosteroids.
- *Steroid-sparing agents*: If inadequate response to systemic corticosteroids, additional immunosuppression in the form of antimetabolites (methotrexate, mycophenolate mofetil, or azathioprine), T-cell inhibitors (cyclosporine A or tacrolimus), or anti-TNF biologic agents (infliximab or adalimumab) may be considered. These medications should only be prescribed by clinicians experienced in their use. Routine blood tests are required to monitor for potential toxicity. If needed, a rheumatologist should be consulted to assist in the administration of these medications.
- *Peripheral retinal photocoagulation/cryotherapy*: Have been reported to be effective; treatment should avoid snowbanks, which may contract and give rise to retinal tears.
- *Pars plana vitrectomy*: May be considered in refractory cases and for secondary complications. In such cases, perioperative immunosuppression is important.

100.9 Follow-Up

During active disease, patients should be followed closely (e.g., every 1–4 weeks). During periods of quiescence, follow-up can be prolonged to every 3–6 months.

References and Suggested Reading

1. Donaldson MJ, Pulido JS, Herman DC, et al. Pars planitis: a 20-year study of incidence, clinical features, and outcomes. Am J Ophthalmol. 2007;144:812–7.
2. Intermediate uveitis. In: Nussenblatt RB, Whitecup SM, editors. Uveitis: fundamentals and clinical practice, 4th ed. Mosby: Elsevier; 2010.
3. Stavrou P, Baltatzis S, Letko E, et al. Pars plana vitrectomy in patients with intermediate uveitis. Ocul Immunol Inflamm. 2001;9:141–51.

Section XV
Infectious Diseases

Ella H. Leung

Chapter 101
Posterior Manifestations of HIV/AIDS

Ella H. Leung

101.1 Definitions

- Human immunodeficiency virus (HIV)
- Acquired immune deficiency syndrome (AIDS): CD4 < 200 cells/μL, CD4 percentage <14 %, or AIDS-defining illness

101.2 Symptoms

Decreased vision, floaters, decreased contrast sensitivity, loss of visual field, photopsias, and scotomas

101.3 Signs

101.3.1 Noninfectious

HIV retinopathy (CD4 < 50): Cotton wool spots, intraretinal hemorrhages, and microvascular changes (microaneurysms, telangiectasias, non-perfusion, vascular occlusion, the Roth spots)

E.H. Leung, MD
Department of Ophthalmology, Bascom Palmer Eye Institute, University of Miami, 900 NW 17th Street, Miami, FL 33136, USA
e-mail: ehleung@med.miami.edu

C.A. Medina et al. (eds.), *Manual of Retinal Diseases: A Guide to Diagnosis and Management*, DOI 10.1007/978-3-319-20460-4_101

Immune recovery uveitis (IRU, CD4>100 or CD4 increases by >50): Uveitis (iritis, vitritis), cystoid macular edema (CME), optic disc edema, and epiretinal membrane
Intraocular lymphoma (CD4<500): Yellow-white subretinal infiltrates

101.3.2 Infectious Retinitis

Viral

- *Cytomegalovirus retinitis* (CD4<50): Hemorrhagic, perivascular, or granular retinal necrosis and retinitis, minimal vitritis
- *Acute retinal necrosis* (CD4 usually >50): Panuveitis, well-demarcated areas of retinitis, vitritis, occlusive vasculitis, and papillitis. VZV>HSV. May have viral keratitis
- *Progressive outer retinal necrosis* (CD4<50): Rapidly progressive necrotizing retinitis, retinal whitening, minimal vasculitis, and minimal vitritis. HSV>VZV. May have viral keratitis

Parasitic

- *Toxoplasmosis gondii* (CD4<200): Focal or multifocal necrotizing retinitis with vitritis, no retinal hemorrhages
- *Syphilis* (CD4<200): Uveitis, optic neuritis, retinitis, and chorioretinitis. *See* Chap. 114*: Syphilitic chorioretinitis*

Bacterial

Mycobacterium tuberculosis (CD4<200): Uveitis (posterior, anterior, panuveitis), retinitis, optic neuritis, focal or diffuse choroiditis, choroidal tubercules, retinal periphlebitis, and endophthalmitis

Fungal

- *Candida albicans:* Fluffy white lesions with satellites in the retina and/or choroid, sometimes associated with endogenous infection
- *Cryptococcus neoformans* (CD4<50): Chorioretinitis, endophthalmitis, papilledema, and retrobulbar neuritis, usually associated with CNS infection
- *Pneumocystis carinii/Pneumocystis jirovecii* (*PCP*, CD4<200): Bilateral yellow lesions in the choroid, minimal vitritis, usually associated with disseminated systemic disease

101.4 Epidemiology

Up to 70–90 % of patients with HIV/AIDS will develop ocular manifestations.

101.5 Predisposing/Associated Conditions

- Not on highly active antiretroviral therapy (HAART)/combination antiretroviral therapy (CART)/antiretroviral therapy (ART)
- Immunosuppression/low CD4 count
- Systemic infection

101.6 Differential Diagnosis

Sarcoidosis, Vogt-Koyanagi-Harada syndrome, lymphoma, HLA-B27, juvenile idiopathic arthritis, and systemic lupus erythematosus

101.7 Etiology

- Noninfectious: unclear etiology of IRU, possible from an improved ability to mount an immune response to antigens from CMV, VZV, mycobacteria, HSV, etc. (Fig. 101.1).
- Infectious: microorganism invasion, resulting in inflammation and necrosis

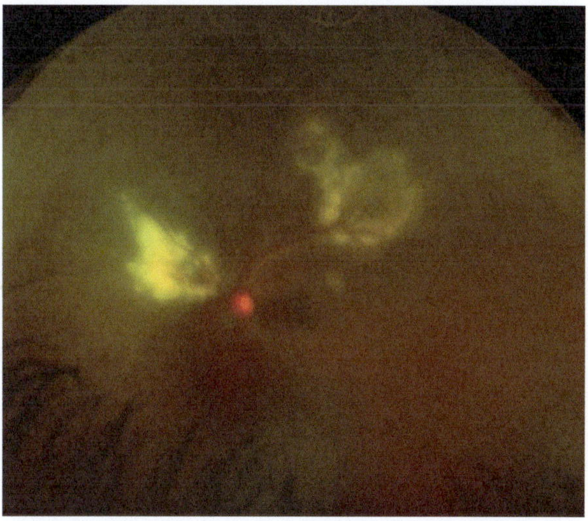

Fig. 101.1 Optos fundus photo of a patient with CMV retinitis and a CD4 count of 8 cells/µl. Note the retinal perivascular retinal whitening and necrosis

101.8 Workup/Testing

- Dilated fundus exam if any visual symptoms
- Imaging:
  - Fundus photographs
  - Optical coherence tomography (OCT)
  - Fluorescein angiography
- Labs: CD4 count
  - If unclear diagnosis: biopsy with cytology or polymerase chain reaction (e.g., CMV, VZV, HSV, toxoplasmosis, etc.)
  - If suspect TB: PPD, CXR, and quantiFERON Gold
  - If suspect syphilis: enzyme immunoassay (EIA)/chemiluminescence immunoassay (CIA)
  - If suspect lymphoma or syphilis: consider lumbar puncture or vitreous biopsy

101.9 Prognosis and Management

Depends on etiology

101.9.1 For All HIV/AIDS Patients

Consult infectious disease specialist to start *HAART*: 2 nucleoside reverse transcriptase inhibitors and 1 non-nucleoside reverse-transcriptase inhibitors (e.g., tenofovir + emtricitabine + efavirnez)

101.9.2 Noninfectious Etiologies

- HIV Retinopathy: HAART
- IRU: Periocular, topical, and intraocular steroids
- Lymphoma: Refer to oncologist for radiation/chemotherapy

101.9.3 Infectious Etiologies

- CMV: *Please see* Chap. 111: *CMV retinitis*
- ARN: *Please see* Chap. 110: *ARN*
- PORN: *Please see* Chap. 109*: PORN*

- Toxoplasmosis: *Please see* Chap. 108: *Toxoplasmosis*
- Syphilis: *Please see* Chap. 114: *Syphilitic chorioretinitis*
- Tuberculosis: rifampin 500–600 mg per day + isoniazid (INH) 5 mg/kg/day + pyrimethamine 25–30 mg/kg/d + ethambutol 15 mg/kg/day × 2 months → then rifampin and INH × 4–7 more months
- Candida: fluconazole 6–12 mg/kg/day PO or IV or amphotericin B 0.7–1 mg/kg/day IV × 6–12 weeks, possible intravitreal amphotericin B 5–10 mg
- Cryptococcus (choroiditis without meningitis): fluconazole 400 mg/day + flucytosine 100–150 mg/day × 10 weeks then maintenance therapy
- PCP: Bactrim DS or pentamidine 4 mg/kg/d IV × 3 weeks, then PO q12 h prophylaxis until CD4 > 200

101.10 Follow-Up

Depends on the etiology, but frequent follow-up may be necessary initially until the patient is stabilized and the diagnosis is certain.

- HIV retinopathy: baseline eye exam and follow-up every 3 months while CD4 < 50; lesions may spontaneously resolve over weeks to months.
- IRU: weekly follow-up until resolution
- Lymphoma: monthly follow-up
- CMV/ARN/PORN: *please* see Chaps. 109, 110, and 111.
- Toxoplasmosis: every 3–5 days, then as indicated by clinical exam
- Syphilis: *please* see Chap. 114
- TB: monthly until significant clinical improvement; monitor for medication toxicity
- *Candida*: weekly until resolution
- *Cryptococcus*: weekly until resolution
- PCP: monthly until resolution (usually 1–3 months)

References and Suggested Reading

1. Becker KN, Becker NM. Ocular manifestations seen in HIV. Dis Mon. 2014;60(6):268–75.
2. Cunningham Jr ET, Margolis TP. Ocular manifestations of HIV infection. N Engl J Med. 1998;339(4):236–44.
3. International Council of Ophthalmology. ICO International Clinical Guideline, ocular HIV/AIDS related diseases. 2011. Available at http://www.icoph.org/resources/88/ICO-International-Clinical-Guideline-Ocular-HIVAIDS-Related-Diseases-.html.
4. Jabs DA, Van Natta ML, Holbrook JT, Kempen JH, Meinert CL, Davis MD. Studies of the Ocular Complications of AIDS Research Group. Longitudinal study of the ocular complications of AIDS: 1. Ocular diagnoses at enrollment. Ophthalmology. 2007;114(4):780–6.
5. Panel on Antiretroviral Guidelines for Adults and Adolescents. Guidelines for the use of antiretroviral agents in HIV-1-infected adults and adolescents. Department of Health and Human Services. Available at http://aidsinfo.nih.gov/ContentFiles/AdultandAdolescentGL.pdf.

Chapter 102
Toxoplasmosis

Tahira Mathen and Yuguang He

102.1 Definitions

Infection caused by the intracellular protozoan parasite *Toxoplasmosis gondii*. It is the most common cause of posterior uveitis.

102.2 Systemic Signs and Symptoms

- Immunocompetent hosts: 80–90 % are asymptomatic

  May have fevers, chills, headaches, pharyngitis, myalgias, cervical or generalized lymphadenopathy (20–30 % of immuncompetent patients), or hepatosplenomegaly

- HIV+ (CD4 usually <100):

  CNS disease most common: encephalitis: headaches, confusion, focal neurologic deficits, and seizures
  Other: pneumonitis and chorioretinitis most common

- Congenital toxoplasmosis:

  Classic triad of chorioretinitis, hydrocephalus, and intracranial calcifications is found in <10 % of infants with toxoplasmosis.

T. Mathen, MD (✉) • Y. He, MD
Department of Ophthalmology, University of Texas Southwestern Medical Center, 5323 Harry Hines Boulevard, Dallas, TX 75390, USA
e-mail: tahiramathen@gmail.com

C.A. Medina et al. (eds.), *Manual of Retinal Diseases: A Guide to Diagnosis and Management*, DOI 10.1007/978-3-319-20460-4_102

Others: jaundice, hepatomegaly, splenomegaly, thrombocytopenia, anemia, seizures, abnormal CSF, microcephaly, sensorineural hearing loss, and mental retardation.

102.3 Ocular Symptoms and Signs

- Congenital:

  Unilateral or bilateral scar ± active retinochoroiditis, frequently in the macula.
  May have microphthalmia, retinal detachment, or optic atrophy.
  Cataract and glaucoma are less common than in congenital rubella.

- Adults and older children:

  Blurred vision and floaters are most common symptoms
  Focal, white chorioretinitis with overlying vitritis adjacent to a chorioretinal scar is classic for reactivation of toxoplasmosis (cannot distinguish between reactivation of congenital or acquired disease). ± anterior uveitis, optic disc edema, vasculitis, and arteriolar occlusion

102.4 Epidemiology

- Congenital toxoplasmosis occurs in 1 in 10,000 live births in the USA.
- Nine percent of people in the USA and 78 % in Brazil are seropositive for toxoplasma. Cats are the only animals in which *T. gondii* can complete its life cycle.
- Four modes of transmission to humans:

  1. Ingestion of oocytes from soil contaminated by cat feces.
  2. Ingestion of tissue cysts in undercooked meat from an infected animal.
  3. Vertical transmission from mother to fetus: increased risk with increased gestational age at time of maternal infection; however likelihood of serious sequelae such as stillbirth or neurologic injury is higher at lower gestational age.
  4. Blood transfusion or organ transplantation from an infected donor.

102.5 Predisposing Conditions

HIV+, usually when CD4 < 100

102.6 **Differential Diagnosis** (Tables 102.1 and 102.2)

Table 102.1 Differential diagnosis of congenital toxoplasmosis

Herpes
CMV
Rubella
Congenital lymphocytic choriomeningitis
Chorioretinal coloboma

Table 102.2 Differential diagnosis of toxoplasmosis in adults

Syphilis
Tuberculosis
Endogenous endophthalmitis (bacterial or fungal)
Necrotizing herpetic retinitis
Sarcoidosis
Toxocariasis
Neuroretinitis
DUSN
Behcet's disease
Multifocal choroiditis and panuveitis

102.7 Workup/Testing

- Immunocompetent patients and pregnant women: check IgM/IgG.

  IgM: positive within 1 week after infection.

    Perform first in babies (IgG crosses placenta and may represent maternal infection).
    IgM does not exclude congenital infection: if negative or equivocal, check IgA and IgE (more sensitive) and repeat during first year of life.

  IgG positive 2–4 weeks after initial infection, positive for life, may help rule out disease if negative.
  Commercially available serologic tests for toxoplasmosis vary in sensitivity and specificity. If the diagnosis is in doubt, consider checking a confirmatory test through the Palo Alto Medical Foundation (PAMF) Toxoplasma Serology Laboratory, which is the reference lab for the CDC.

- HIV: Check IgM/IgG (but less likely to be positive). Check MRI brain for multiple ring-enhancing lesions
- Fetus: infection may be diagnosed with ultrasound (nonspecific abnormalities) and PCR of amniotic fluid
- Atypical cases: check PCR of aqueous or check Goldmann-Witmer coefficient (>3 suggests infection)

102.8 Prognosis and Management (Table 102.3)

Table 102.3 Treatment of ocular toxoplasmosis

Standard adult therapy	
Pyrimethamine	100 mg daily for 2 days then 25–50 mg daily Significant adverse effect: leukopenia Check WBC and platelets q1–2 weeks while on treatment
Folinic acid	5 mg daily (increase up to 25 mg PO daily if pyrimethamine-induced leukopenia occurs)
Sulfadiazine	4 mg daily for 2 days, then 1 g QID
± Prednisone	1 mg/kg daily; start after the third day of antibiotic therapy Taper based on clinical response Avoid without concurrent antibiotic therapy and in immunocompromised patients
Alternative therapy	
Systemic	*Intravitreal*
Trimethoprim-sulfamethoxazole (160 mg/800 mg BID)[a] or Pyrimethamine + folinic acid + clindamycin (300 mg QID) or Pyrimethamine + folinic acid + azithromycin (500 mg daily)	Clindamycin 1 mg/0.1 ml and dexamethasone 400 μg/ 0.1 mL
[a]Combination oral trimethoprim-sulfamethoxazole with intravitreal clindamycin is frequently used	
Maintenance therapy in HIV+ patients	
Trimethoprim-sulfamethoxazole	160 mg/800 mg every other day
or	
Pyrimethamine and	12.5–25 mg PO daily and
Sulfadiazine and	500 mg daily and
Folinic acid	5 mg daily
Consider discontinuing therapy in asymptomatic patients who maintain CD4 > 200 for 6 months	
Treatment for pregnant women	
Spiramycin (preferred)	1 g TID without food until delivery Available in the USA to pregnant women through compassionate use pathway if an Investigational New Drug number is obtained from the FDA
or	
Pyrimethamine and	25 mg PO daily *and*
Sulfadiazine and	1 g PO 4 times a day *and*
Folinic acid	5–25 mg PO daily
Treatment for congenital toxoplasmosis	
Pyrimethamine	2 mg/kg (maximum 50 mg/dose) once daily for 2 days Then 1 mg/kg (maximum 25 mg/dose) once daily for 6 months Then 1 mg/kg (maximum 25 mg/dose) every other day to complete 1 year of therapy and
Sulfadiazine	100 mg/kg per day divided in two doses every day for 1 year and
Folinic acid	10 mg three times per week during and for 1 week after pyrimethamine therapy

Immunocompetent:
May observe small, extramacular lesions (many self-limited and heal after 1–2 months; scars become hyperpigmented or atrophic with white center from underlying sclera). Antibiotic therapy is usually given for 4–6 weeks based on clinical response (Fig. 102.1).

Immunosuppressed patients, pregnant women, and congenital infection: Treatment is mandatory (Fig. 102.2)

102.9 Follow-Up

- Congenital toxoplasmosis: any infant with toxoplasmosis should be screened for ocular manifestations every 3 months until 18 months of life and then every 6–12 months.
- All patients: follow-up for late complications such as retinal holes, retinal detachments, and subretinal neovascularization.

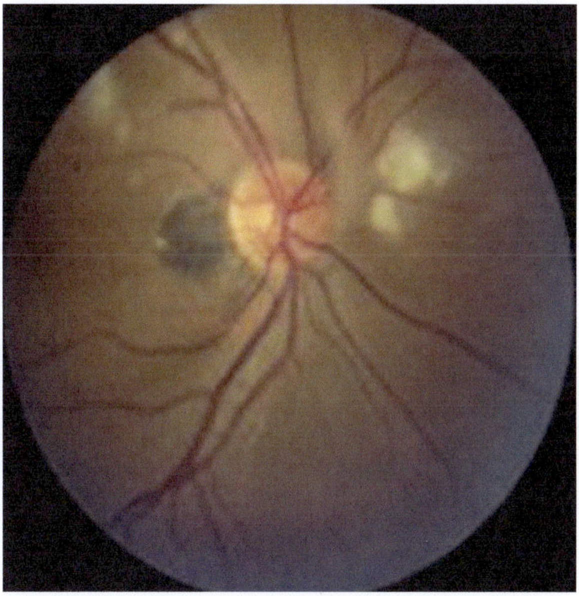

Fig. 102.1 Focal retinitis and vitritis adjacent to an old scar

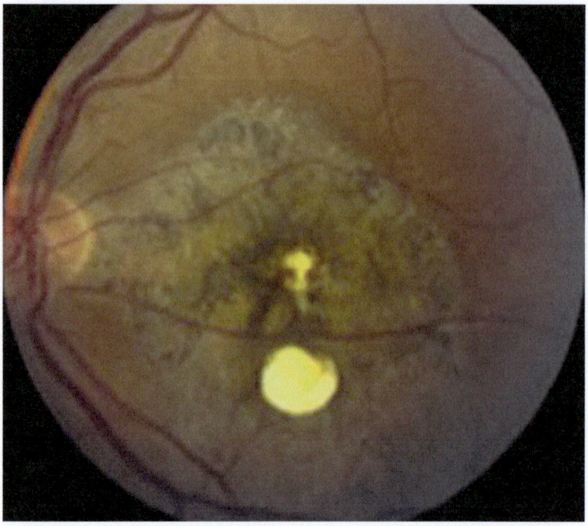

Fig. 102.2 Large atrophic macular scar

References and Suggested Reading

1. Gilbert R, Petersen E. Toxoplasmosis and pregnancy. In: Post TW, editor, UpToDate. Waltham: UpToDate. Accessed Mar 2015.
2. Guerina N, Lee J, Lynfield R. Congenital toxoplasmosis: treatment, outcome, and prevention. In: Post TW editor. UpToDate. Waltham: UpToDate. Accessed Mar 2015.
3. Harrell M, Carvounis P. Current treatment of toxoplasma retinochoroiditis: an evidence-based review. J Ophthalmol. 2014;2014:273506.
4. Heller H. Toxoplasmosis in immuncompetent hosts. In: Post TW editor. UpToDate. Waltham: UpToDate. Accessed Mar 2015.
5. Kim S, Scott IU, Brown GC, Brown MM, Ho AC, Ip MS, Recchia FM. Interventions for toxoplasma retinochoroiditis. Ophthalmology. 2013;120(2):371–8.
6. Palo Alto Medical Foundation Toxoplasma Serology Laboratory. http://www.pamf.org/serology.
7. Remington JS. Toxoplasmosis in the adult. Bull N Y Acad Med. 1974;50(2):211.
8. Tenter AM, Heckeroth AR, Weiss LM. Toxoplasma gondii: from animals to humans. Int J Parasitol. 2000;30(12–13):1217.
9. Vasconcelos-Santos DV. Ocular manifestations of a systemic disease: toxoplasmosis. Curr Opin Ophthalmol. 2012;23:543–50.
10. Vasconcelos-Santos DV, Dodds EM, Orefice F. Review for disease of the year: differential diagnosis of ocular toxoplasmosis. Ocular Immunol Inflamm. 2011;19(3):171–9.

Chapter 103
Progressive Outer Retinal Necrosis

Meenakashi Gupta

103.1 Definitions

- Progressive outer retinal necrosis (PORN)
- Acute retinal necrosis (ARN)

103.2 Symptoms

- Decreased or blurred vision, constriction of visual field, and ocular pain
- Rarely may have floaters

103.3 Signs

- Rapidly progressive necrotizing retinitis characterized by early patchy multifocal retinal lesions that appear deep on fundoscopy (Fig. 103.1). Posterior pole may be involved early in disease (Fig. 103.2). Multifocal lesions quickly progress to confluence and to full-thickness retinal involvement.
- Perivascular "clearing" in which perivascular edema and necrosis are cleared first.
- Tissue may appear unaffected but is not spared.
- Absence of vascular inflammation.

M. Gupta, MD
Retina Service, New York Eye and Ear Infirmary of Mount Sinai,
310 E 14th Street, New York, NY 10003, USA
e-mail: meenakashi.gupta@gmail.com

C.A. Medina et al. (eds.), *Manual of Retinal Diseases: A Guide to Diagnosis and Management*, DOI 10.1007/978-3-319-20460-4_103

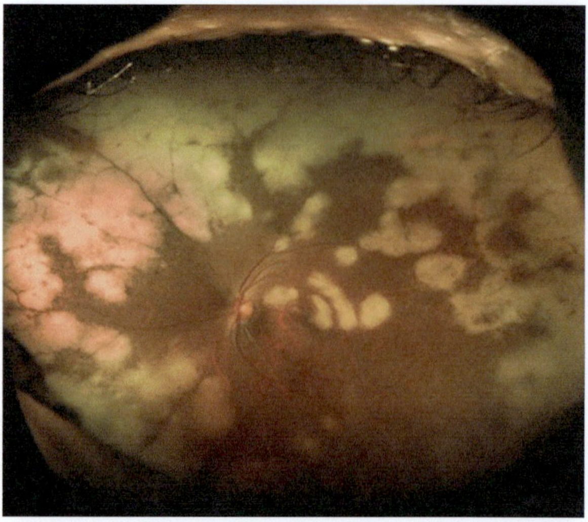

Fig. 103.1 Affected eye in patient with HIV highlighting clear media and coalescing multifocal retinal lesions with deep appearance typical of PORN

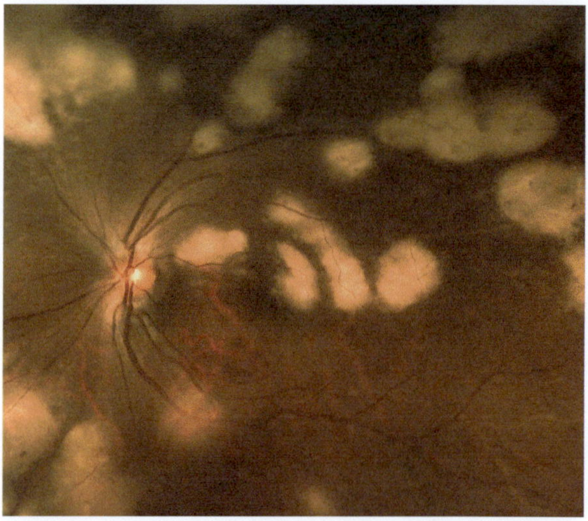

Fig. 103.2 Magnified view of posterior pole with macular lesions that are often seen early in disease course

- Minimal to no vitreous inflammation.
- Disease may be bilateral.
- May have previous or concurrent history of cutaneous zoster.

103.4 Epidemiology

- First described in 1990 in 2 patients with HIV. The majority of cases have been described in patients with advanced stages of HIV/AIDs (CD4+ T lymphocytes ≤50 cells/mm^3).

- With introduction of HAART therapy, HIV-related cases have declined. More recently, cases have been described in patients on immunosuppressive therapy.

103.5 Predisposing Conditions

- Severely immunocompromised status
- Cases have been described due to:

  Infection (HIV/AIDs)
  Immunosuppressive therapy following stem cell transplantation, for autoimmune disorders, malignancy, and other conditions (including corticosteroids, cyclosporine, mycophenolate mofetil, azathioprine, alkylating agents, cytotoxic agents, DNA synthesis inhibitors)
  Immune defects (CD4 lymphocytopenia)

103.6 Inheritance

None

103.7 Differential Diagnosis

- Acute retinal necrosis (ARN tends to have more vasculitis, more vitritis, often has later involvement of the macula, and is more likely to affect immunocompetent individuals than PORN.)
- Cytomegalovirus retinitis (CMV retinitis has more hemorrhages and does not respond to acyclovir.)
- Syphilis chorioretinitis

103.8 Etiology

- Most commonly due to VZV infection.
- Early disease appears to involve the outer retina on clinical exam.
- Histopathology and recent OCT evaluations suggest that primary site of necrosis may actually be the inner retina with destruction of the outer retinal layers occurring subsequently.

103.9 Workup/Testing

- PCR of aqueous and/or vitreous for VZV, HSV1, HSV2, and CMV
- Serology for syphilis: RPR, VDRL, and FT-ABS
- WBC and CD4 count
- HIV test

103.10 Prognosis and Management

- Patients require immediate antiviral therapy.
- Systemic treatment is needed to protect the other eye and prevent central nervous system involvement.
- Optimal treatment has been difficult to define.
  Several different regimens for systemic treatment and/or intravitreal therapy have been described (Table 103.1).
- Recent studies have shown improved visual outcomes with combination systemic and intravitreal antiviral therapy.
  Utility of laser demarcation to decrease rate of retinal detachment remains controversial.
- Treatment of underlying systemic condition is essential.
- Long-term suppressive antiviral therapy is necessary in patients who are unable to achieve immune reconstitution.
- Poor prognosis with severe vision loss developing from widespread retinal necrosis, ischemic optic neuropathy, and high rate of retinal detachment.
- Bilateral involvement may develop in first few weeks after initial diagnosis.

103.11 Follow-Up

- Patients should be followed closely, initially every few days until the condition improves or stabilizes.
- Both eyes need to be examined as bilateral disease is common.

Table 103.1 Antiviral therapy of progressive outer retinal necrosis

	Systemic			Intravitreal	
	Acyclovir	Foscarnet	Ganciclovir	Foscarnet	Ganciclovir
Dose	*Induction* 10–20 mg/kg every 8 h *Maintenance* 800 mg po 5 times daily (Oral valacyclovir has also been used for maintenance)	*Induction* 60–90 mg/kg IV every 8 h *Maintenance* 90–130 mg/kg once daily	*Induction* 5 mg/kg IV every 12 h *Maintenance* 5 mg/kg daily (Oral valganciclovir has also been used for induction and/or maintenance)	2.4 mg/0.1 mL (1.2 mg/0.05 mL dosing has also been used)	2 mg/0.05 mL (Implants have also been used)
Duration	Induction dosing at least 2–3 weeks followed by maintenance dosing until completely healed			Injection 2–3 times per week for 2–3 weeks followed by maintenance therapy 1–2 times per week as indicated until retinitis is stabilized	
Notes	One or more systemic agents used in combination with intravitreal therapy			One or more intravitreal agents used in combination with systemic therapy	

References and Suggested Reading

1. Benz MS, Glaser JS, Davis JL. Progressive outer retinal necrosis in immunocompetent patients treated initially for optic neuropathy with systemic corticosteroids. Am J Ophthalmol. 2003;135(4):551–3.
2. Bryan RG, Myers FL. Progressive outer retinal necrosis in a patient with rheumatoid arthritis. Arch Ophthalmol. 1998;116(9):1249.
3. Coisy S, Ebran JM, Milea D. Progressive outer retinal necrosis and immunosuppressive therapy in myasthenia gravis. Case Rep Ophthalmol. 2014;5(1):132–7.
4. Engstrom Jr RE, Holland GN, Margolis TP, Muccioli C, Lindley JI, Belfort Jr R, Holland SP, Johnston WH, Wolitz RA, Kreiger AE. The progressive outer retinal necrosis syndrome: a variant of necrotizing herpetic retinopathy in patients with AIDS. Ophthalmology. 1994;101: 1488–502.
5. Forster DJ, Dugel PU, Frangieh GT, et al. Rapidly progressive outer retinal necrosis in the acquired immunodeficiency syndrome. Am J Ophthalmol. 1990;110(4):341–8.
6. Gupta M, Jardeleza MS, Kim I, Durand ML, Kim L, Lobo AM. Varicella zoster virus necrotizing retinitis in two patients with idiopathic CD4 lymphocytopenia. Ocul Immunol Inflamm. 2015;15:1–5.
7. Margo CE, Friedman SM. Progressive outer retinal necrosis (PORN): a catchy acronym but is the anatomy correct? The salient observation of Lorenz E. Zimmerman, MD. JAMA Ophthalmol. 2014;132(5):651–2.
8. Njoo FL, Rothova A, Van Der Lelij A. Progressive outer retinal necrosis in a patient with cutaneous non-Hodgkin's T cell lymphoma (Sezary syndrome). Br J Ophthalmol. 1998;82(10): 1218–9.
9. Scott IU, Luu KM, Davis JL. Intravitreal antivirals in the management of patients with acquired immunodeficiency syndrome with progressive outer retinal necrosis. Arch Ophthalmol. 2002;120(9):1219–22.
10. Shinoda K, Inoue M, Ishida S, et al. Progressive outer retinal necrosis in a patient with nephrotic syndrome. Ophthalmic Surg Lasers. 2001;32(1):67–72.

Chapter 104
Acute Retinal Necrosis

Mitul C. Mehta and Baruch D. Kuppermann

104.1 Definitions

1994 Executive Committee of the American Uveitis Society:

1. One or more foci of retinal necrosis with discrete borders located in the peripheral retina
2. Rapid progression in the absence of antiviral therapy
3. Circumferential spread
4. Evidence of occlusive vasculopathy with arterial involvement
5. A prominent inflammatory reaction in the vitreous and anterior chambers (Fig. 104.1)

104.2 Symptoms

Rapid decline in vision, floaters, pain, red eye, and neurologic symptoms

M.C. Mehta, MD, MS (✉) • B.D. Kuppermann, MD, PhD
Gavin Herbert Eye Institute, University of California, Irvine,
850 Health Sciences Rd, Irvine, CA 92697-4375, USA
e-mail: mcmehta@uci.edu

C.A. Medina et al. (eds.), *Manual of Retinal Diseases: A Guide to Diagnosis and Management*, DOI 10.1007/978-3-319-20460-4_104

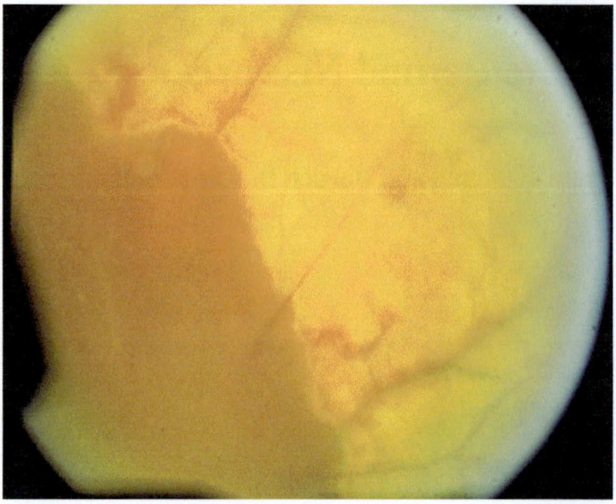

Fig. 104.1 Retinal necrosis, showing retinal whitening and attenuation of blood vessels. Notice the sclerotic blood vessel in the non-necrotic retina (Courtesy of Dr. Baruch D. Kuppermann)

104.3 Signs

- Iritis (either granulomatous or not)
- Scleritis/episcleritis
- Vitritis
- Retinal whitening and necrosis
- Vascular occlusions
- Retinal breaks and detachments
- Papillitis
- Bilateral in 20–33 % (second eye usually within 6 weeks)

104.4 Etiology

Viral retinitis: VZV > HSV > CMV

104.5 Demographics

- Often immunocompetent people but can be induced by immunosuppression
- No race or sex predilection
- Average age at presentation VZV, 52.4 years; HSV-1, 44.3 years; and HSV-2, 24.3 years

104.6 Differential Diagnosis (Table 104.1)

Table 104.1 Differential diagnosis of acute retinal necrosis

Infectious	Autoimmune	Neoplastic
Syphilis	Sarcoidosis	Intraocular lymphoma
Toxoplasmosis	Behçet's disease	
Tuberculosis		
Endophthalmitis (fungal/bacterial)		

104.7 Workup/Testing

- PCR of intraocular fluid (AC or vitreous for definitive diagnosis): check VZV, HSV 1 and 2, CMV, and toxoplasma (Fig. 104.2).
- CBC w/ differential.
- Rule out other infections: toxoplasma IgG/IgM, RPR/VDRL, FTA-ABS or TPPA, PPD/QuantiFERON Gold, and ACE/lysozyme.
- Check pupils for a relative afferent pupillary defect (RAPD).
- Consider neuroimaging (associated with encephalitis).
- Consider fluorescein angiography to identify vascular occlusive disease.
- Consider HIV testing.
- Fundus photography (especially wide angle) can help to follow progression.

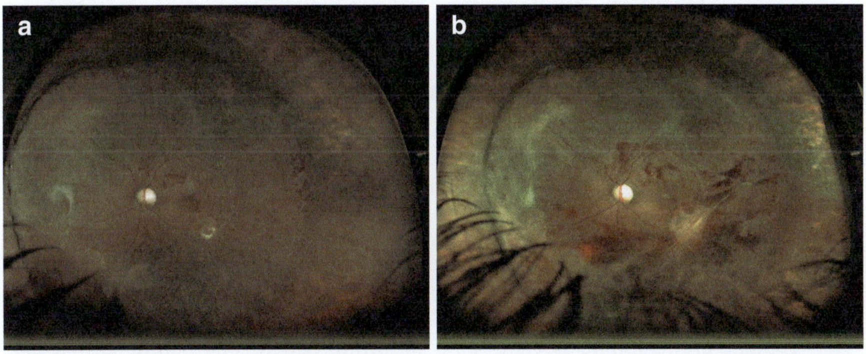

Fig. 104.2 This is a patient's postoperative days 1 (**b**) and 21 (**a**), respectively, with a VZV-ARN-related retinal detachment after pars plana vitrectomy, scleral buckle, endolaser, silicone oil tamponade, and intravitreal foscarnet injection. Notice the progressive preretinal fibrosis and retinal hemorrhages despite aggressive treatment. After multiple surgeries the patient ultimately was left with a blind, hypotonous eye; however due to early systemic treatment, she never developed viral disease in the other eye (Courtesy of Dr. Mitul C. Mehta)

104.8 Prognosis and Management

Prognosis is poor due to the risk of retinal detachment, macular, and optic nerve involvement. There is significant risk for bilateral involvement if systemic antiviral treatment is not started early.

- Treat immunocompetent patients for at least 3–4 months.
- Treat immunocompromised patients for longer.
- Systemic antiviral treatment.
  - IV acyclovir (10–15 mg/mk/day divided in 3 doses) × 7 days followed by oral acyclovir 800 mg 5× per day is the traditional treatment.
  - Oral valacyclovir (2g TID), valganciclovir (900 mg BID), and famciclovir (500 mg TID) to obtain high serum concentrations without hospital admission.
- Intravitreal treatment (if sight threatening or not responding to systemic treatment).
  - Foscarnet 2.4 mg/0.1 mL (undiluted from IV solution) can be used in acyclovir resistant VZV or HSV.
  - Ganciclovir 2 mg/0.1 mL given 2–3× per week.
  - Ganciclovir implant gives sustained concentration of 1 mcg/hour for 8 months (typically used for CMV in immunocompromised patients).
- Laser photocoagulation.
  - Controversial, confluent treatment posterior to necrosis to prevent spread
- Retinal surgery.
  - Rhegmatogenous retinal detachment in up to 75 % of patients can have tractional component.
  - Pars plana vitrectomy, lensectomy, endolaser, fluid-air exchange, and long-acting gas or silicone oil tamponade have shown success in retinal reattachment.
- Ancillary treatment.
  - Oral prednisone (after starting systemic antiviral treatment) 0.5 mg/kg/day
  - Topical prednisolone acetate 1 % or difluprednate ophthalmic drops and cycloplegic drops to treat anterior chamber inflammation

104.9 Follow-Up

Monitor daily in the acute period with scleral depressed examination as small peripheral retinal holes can lead to retinal detachment.

References

1. Flaxel CJ, Yeh S, Lauer AK. Combination systemic and intravitreal antiviral therapy in the management of acute retinal necrosis syndrome (an American Ophthalmological Society thesis). Trans Am Ophthalmol Soc. 2013;111:133–44.
2. Holland GN. Standard diagnostic criteria for the acute retinal necrosis syndrome. Executive Committee of the American Uveitis Society. Am J Ophthalmol. 1994;117:663–7.
3. Lau CH, Missotten T, Salzmann J, Lightman SL. Acute retinal necrosis features, management and outcomes. Ophthalmology. 2007;114:756–62.
4. Luu KK, Scott IU, Chaudhry NA, Verm A, Davis JL. Intravitreal antiviral injections as adjunctive therapy in the management of immunocompetent patients with necrotizing herpetic retinopathy. Am J Ophthalmol. 2000;129:811–3.
5. Van Gelder RN, Willig JL, Holland GN, et al. Herpes Simplex virus type 2 as a cause of acute retinal necrosis syndrome in young patients. Ophthalmology. 2001;108:869–76.
6. Wong RW, Jumper JM, McDonald HR, Johnson RN, Fu A, Lujan BJ, Cunningham ET. Emerging concepts in the management of acute retinal necrosis. Br J Ophthalmol. 2013;97:545–52.

Chapter 105
Cytomegalovirus Retinitis

Tahira Mathen

105.1 Definitions

CMV retinitis is the most common ocular opportunistic infection in patients with AIDS.

105.2 Symptoms

- Blurred vision, floaters, photopsias, and scotomata
- May also have symptoms of systemic CMV including fever, arthralgia, pneumonitis, colitis, esophagitis, encephalitis, and hepatitis

105.3 Signs

Adults

- White, intraretinal infiltration or necrosis and retinal hemorrhages along the vascular arcades in the posterior pole (Fig. 105.1).
- Perivascular sheathing.
- Level of vitritis is variable and related to the degree of immunosuppression.
- Exudative or rhegmatogenous retinal detachment.

T. Mathen, MD
Department of Ophthalmology, University of Texas Southwestern Medical Center,
5323 Harry Hines Boulevard, Dallas, TX 75390, USA
e-mail: tahiramathen@gmail.com

C.A. Medina et al. (eds.), *Manual of Retinal Diseases: A Guide to Diagnosis and Management*, DOI 10.1007/978-3-319-20460-4_105

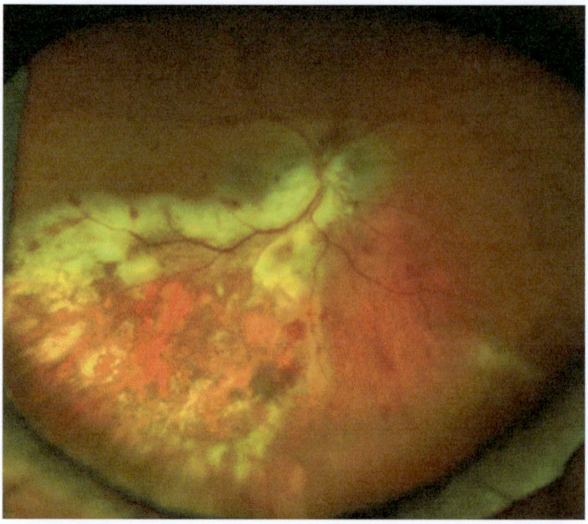

Fig. 105.1 Perivascular retinitis, retinal necrosis, and hemorrhage in active CMV

- CMV retinitis may resemble cotton-wool spots of HIV retinopathy early in the course of the disease.
- Other signs: fine keratic precipitates on the corneal endothelium or anterior uveitis, optic atrophy (late finding).

Congenital CMV

- Ocular: chorioretinitis, retinal scars, optic atrophy, and strabismus
- Systemic: microcephaly, seizures, thrombocytopenia, sensorineural hearing loss, hepatosplenomegaly, jaundice, petechiae, feeding difficulties, and abnormal brain imaging

105.4 Epidemiology

- Before the advent of HAART therapy, around 30 % of AIDS patients developed CMV retinitis.
- Since HAART therapy, incidence of new cases of CMV retinitis in patients with CD4 < 200 has declined to 1.8 %.
- CMV retinitis is less frequent in children with AIDS than in adults but has a higher incidence of bilateral disease and posterior pole disease at presentation.
- Congenital CMV by vertical transmission from an infected mother to fetus hematogenously, perinatal vaginal secretions, or through breast milk. Transmission is more likely to occur with primary rather than recurrent infection in the mother.
- 1 % of babies are born with congenital CMV infection; 90 % are asymptomatic.

105.5 Predisposing Conditions

- In HIV patients: CD4 < 50 is the most significant risk factor.

  High HIV RNA viral load (>100,000 copies/mL)
  CMV viremia
  History of prior opportunistic infection
  Steroid use
  Lack of HAART treatment

- In non-HIV patients: chemotherapy, immunosuppressive therapy, lupus, and transplant patients

105.6 Differential Diagnosis

- Necrotizing herpetic retinitis from herpes simplex or varicella zoster, toxoplasmosis, syphilis, candida, Behcet's disease, and HIV retinopathy

105.7 Etiology

- Cytomegalovirus is acquired through direct contact of body fluids such as saliva, blood, urine, semen, vaginal fluids, and breast milk. It has been reported after organ transplant and blood transfusion.
- CMV retinitis occurs by hematogenous spread of the virus to the eye.

105.8 Workup/Testing

Congenital

- Urine or saliva CMV viral culture
- Urine or serum CMV PCR

Adults

- Aqueous for CMV PCR when diagnosis is uncertain.
- Quantitative serum CMV PCR.
- Testing for CMV IgG is rarely helpful because >70 % of the population is seropositive for CMV and however may help rule out infection.

105.9 **Prognosis and Management** (Tables 105.1, 105.2, and 105.3)

- Retinitis progresses without treatment 10–21 days after presentation.
- Coordinate with patient's HIV specialist to start HAART.
- Check CBC twice a week during induction and once a week during maintenance to monitor for bone marrow suppression from valganciclovir and ganciclovir.
- Check creatinine monthly on valganciclovir or ganciclovir (monitor nephrotoxicity and adjust dose to renal function).
- May discontinue maintenance therapy after 3–6 months of therapy and CD4 > 100.
- Rhegmatogenous retinal detachment:

  Forty to fifty percent of patients with CMV retinitis develop retinal detachment within 1 year due to break in necrotic retina. Treat with pars plana vitrectomy, endolaser, and silicone oil, or less commonly, long-acting gas (C3F8) ± scleral buckling. Laser retinopexy alone may be performed for limited, extramacular detachments.

Table 105.1 Systemic treatment for CMV retinitis in adults

Drug	Route	Dose
Valganciclovir	PO	Induction: 900 mg BID for 3 weeks Maintenance: 900 mg daily
Ganciclovir	IV	Induction: 5 mg/kg BID for 2–3 weeks Maintenance: 5 mg/kg daily
Foscarnet	IV	Induction: 90 mg/kg BID for 2 weeks Maintenance: 120 mg/kg daily
Cidofovir	IV	Induction: 5 mg/kg weekly for 3 weeks Maintenance: 3–5 mg/kg every 2 weeks

To decrease involvement of other eye and extraocular CMV
PO valganciclovir has equal efficacy to IV ganciclovir and is therefore a first-line treatment

Table 105.2 Intravitreal treatment for CMV retinitis

Drug	Route	Dose
Foscarnet	Intravitreal	2.4 mg / 0.1 mL Induction: twice a week for 3 weeks Maintenance: once a week
Ganciclovir	Intravitreal	2.0 mg / 0.1 mL Induction: twice a week for 3 weeks Maintenance: once a week
Ganciclovir implant (Retisert)	Implant	No longer manufactured

For sight-threatening lesions : <1500 μm from the fovea or adjacent to the optic nerve head

Table 105.3 Systemic treatment for CMV retinitis in infants

Drug	Route	Dose
Valganciclovir	PO	16 mg/kg BID
Ganciclovir	IV	6 mg/kg BID

Immune recovery uveitis (IRU): 20 % of patients develop IRU (iritis, vitritis, macular edema, epiretinal membrane, cataract) once CD4 > 100, months to years after initiation of HAART. Rule out CMV reactivation or other infections. Treat with topical steroids; if periocular or intravitreal steroids are given, antiviral therapy should be restarted

105.10 Follow-Up

- Early CMV lesions may be difficult to differentiate from HIV retinopathy. Serial exams over 1–2 weeks and fundus photos demonstrating enlargement of the spots to >750 μm aid diagnosis.
- Wide-angle fundus photography to document progression and to monitor for reactivation.
- Relapse occurs at a rate of 0.03/person-year in patients with CD > 100; therefore lifetime follow-up is mandatory.

References and Suggested Reading

1. Benson CA, Kaplan JE, Masur H, Pau A, Holmes KK, CDC, National Institutes of Health, Infectious Diseases Society of America. Treating opportunistic infections among HIV-infected adults and adolescents: recommendations from CDC, the National Institutes of Health, and the HIV Medicine Association/Infectious Diseases Society of America. MMWR Recomm Rep. 2004;53(RR-15):1.
2. Demmler-Harrison G. Cytomegalovirus infection and disease in newborns, infants, children and adolescents. In: Post TW, editor. UpToDate. Waltham: UpToDate. Accessed Mar 2015.
3. Jabs DA, Enger C, Dunn JP, Forman M. Cytomegalovirus retinitis and viral resistance: ganciclovir resistance. CMV Retinitis and Viral Resistance Study Group. J Infect Dis. 1998;177(3):770.
4. Jacobson M. Pathogenesis, clinical manifestations, and diagnosis of AIDS-related cytomegalovirus retinitis. In: Post TW, editor. UpToDate. Waltham: UpToDate. Accessed Mar 2015.
5. Jacobson M. Treatment of AIDS-related cytomegalovirus retinitis. In: Post TW, editor. UpToDate. Waltham: UpToDate. Accessed Mar 2015.
6. Panel on Opportunistic Infections in HIV-Infected Adults and Adolescents. Guidelines for the prevention and treatment of opportunistic infections in HIV-infected adults and adolescents: Recommendations from the Centers for Disease Control and Prevention, the National Institutes of Health, and the HIV Medicine Association of the Infectious Diseases Society of America. http://aidsinfo.nih.gov.foyer.swmed.edu/contentfiles/lvguidelines/adult_oi.pdf.
7. Schwartz L, Chen MJ, Vittinghoff E, Hsu L, Schwartz S. Declining incidence of AIDS-defining opportunistic illnesses: results from 16 years of population-based AIDS surveillance. AIDS. 2013;27(4):597–605.
8. Smith BT, Regillo CD. How to treat cytomegalovirus retinitis. EyeNet. 2005. http://www.aao.org/publications/eyenet/200510/pearls.cfm.
9. Urban B, Bakunowicz-Łazarczyk A, Michalczuk M. Immune recovery uveitis: pathogenesis, clinical symptoms, and treatment. Mediators Inflamm. 2014;2014:971417.
10. Yust I, Fox Z, Burke M, Johnson A, Turner D, Mocroft A, Katlama C, Ledergerber B, Reiss P, Kirk O. Retinal and extraocular cytomegalovirus end-organ disease in HIV-infected patients in Europe: a EuroSIDA study, 1994–2001. Eur J Clin Microbiol Infect Dis. 2004;23(7):550.

Chapter 106
Diffuse Unilateral Subacute Neuroretinitis

Kevin Rosenberg and Anu S. Patel

106.1 Definitions

Diffuse unilateral subacute neuroretinitis (DUSN) is a unilateral, ocular infection of the retina and choroid caused by one of two as yet unidentified nematodes invading the subretinal space.

106.2 Symptoms

- Early: asymptomatic or mild, insidious vision loss in one eye including central or paracentral scotoma, photopsias, floaters, and ocular discomfort (rare)
- Late: dense central or paracentral scotoma with permanent vision loss

K. Rosenberg, MD
Kresge Eye Institute, Wayne State University,
Detroit, MI, USA

A.S. Patel, MD (✉)
Department of Ophthalmology, Kresge Eye Institute, Wayne State University,
4717 St. Antoine Street, Detroit, MI 48201, USA
e-mail: anpate@med.wayne.edu

C.A. Medina et al. (eds.), *Manual of Retinal Diseases: A Guide to Diagnosis and Management*, DOI 10.1007/978-3-319-20460-4_106

106.3 Signs

- Early: mild to moderate vitritis; optic disc edema; recurrent, multifocal, yellow-white, evanescent, outer retinal, and choroidal lesions which disappear in 1–2 weeks; new lesions typically arise in an area the worm has migrated to; and the anterior segment is usually quiet.
- Late: afferent papillary defect (APD), depigmentation of the retinal pigmentary epithelium (RPE), optic atrophy, retinal arteriole narrowing, and evidence of white-yellow subretinal tunnels.
- Note: the live worm can be seen in any stage of the disease.

106.4 Epidemiology

Most patients are children and young adults between 5 and 22 years of age in the Southeastern USA (smaller worm), the Northern-Midwestern USA (larger worm), the Caribbean, and Latin America (smaller worm). Males are more often affected.

106.5 Predisposing Conditions

- Outdoor activity
- History of cutaneous larval migrans
- Travel to South and Central America

106.6 Differential Diagnosis (Table 106.1)

Table 106.1 Differential diagnosis of DUSN

Early stages mimic:	Late stages mimic:
MEWDS	Occlusive vascular disease
AMPPE	Toxic retinopathy
MFC	Posttraumatic chorioretinopathy
Serpiginous choroiditis	Unilateral retinitis pigmentosa
Birdshot chorioretinopathy	Sarcoidosis
	Presumed ocular histoplasmosis syndrome

106.7 Etiology

Conclusive evidence pointing to specific nematodes responsible for DUSN has not yet been established. However, it is presumed that two nematodes are responsible for DUSN (Fig. 106.1). The smaller one (400–1000 μm) is thought to be *Ancylostoma caninum*, a hookworm of dogs, and the larger one (1500–2000 μm) is thought to be *Baylisascaris procyonis*, found in the intestinal tract of raccoons and squirrels. The pathogenesis most likely results from a local toxic tissue effect of the outer retina in response to toxic by-products released by the subretinal worm (Table 106.2).

106.8 Workup/Testing

- Careful search for the worm on dilated fundus exam.
- Check serology for *Toxocara* species, stool examination for ova and parasites, and CBC for eosinophilia (although labs often normal).

Fig. 106.1 Fundus photograph showing a nematode in the inferotemporal arcade (*left*), intraoperative fundus photograph where the nematode being aspirated through a cannula (*right*)

Table 106.2 Etiology of DUSN

Name	Size (μm)	Host	Location
Ancylostoma caninum	400–1000	Dog	Southeastern USA, Latin American
Baylisascaris procyonis	1500–2000	Raccoon, squirrel	Northern-Midwestern USA

- Fluorescein angiography (FA):

  Early disease—may show hypofluorescent active retinitis with late staining, leakage from optic disc capillaries, perivenous dye leakage
  Late disease—may show increased RPE pigment loss, with early hyperfluorescence from window defects and delay in retinal perfusion

- Indocyanine green (ICG): early hypofluorescent dark spots which either persist or become isofluorescent.
- Optical coherence tomography (OCT): diffuse retinal thinning and retinal nerve layer atrophy.
- Electroretinogram (ERG): usually reduced, with b-wave being more affected than the a-wave but is rarely completely extinguished.
- Visual fields: variable.

106.9 Prognosis and Management

- Definitive treatment: laser photocoagulation of live worm at any stage of the disease. The earlier in the disease process this is achieved, the more vision can be saved.
- Systemic therapy: antihelminthic drugs have mixed results (perhaps more effective with active vitritis and breakdown of blood-retinal barrier).

  Thiabendazole 22 mg/kg PO BID × 2–4 days (max of 3 g/d)
  Albendazole 200 mg PO BID × 30 days
  Diethylcarbamazine 100 mg PO TID × 21 days

106.10 Follow-Up

Close follow-up is paramount until the live worm is found and destroyed with laser photocoagulation or another diagnosis is made.

References and Suggested Reading

1. Avila M, Isaac D. Helminthic disease. In: Ryan SJ, Schachat AP, Wilkinson CP, Hinton DR, Sadda SR, Wiedemann P, editors. Retina; Elsevier Saunders, Philadelphia; 2012. p. 1506–13.
2. Barney NP. Diffuse unilateral subacute neuroretinitis. In: Foster SC, Vitale AT, editors. Diagnosis and treatment of uveitis. New Delhi: Jaypee Brothers Medical Publishers; 2013. p. 665–70.
3. Garcia CA, Sabrosa NA, Gomes AB, Segundo PS, Filho CA, Sabrosa AS. Diffuse unilateral subacute neuroretinitis – DUSN. Int Ophthalmol Clin. 2008;48(3):119–30.
4. Agarwal A. Infectious diseases of the retina and choroid. In: Agarwal A, editor. Gass' atlas of macular diseases. Elsevier Saunders, Philadelphia; 2012. p. 864–72.

Chapter 107
Syphilitic Chorioretinitis

Ella Leung

107.1 Definitions

Syphilitic involvement of the retina and choroid, usually presenting during or after the secondary stage of syphilis

107.2 Symptoms

Flashes, floaters, blurriness, pain, redness, and photophobia

107.3 Signs

- Uveitis: anterior (granulomatous, large keratic precipitates), intermediate, posterior, panuveitis, episcleritis/scleritis, and iris nodules
- Optic nerve: optic neuritis, optic neuropathy, and neuroretinitis

E. Leung, MD
Department of Ophthalmology, Bascom Palmer Eye Institute, University of Miami, 900 NW 17th Street, Miami, FL 33136, USA
e-mail: ehleung@med.miami.edu

C.A. Medina et al. (eds.), *Manual of Retinal Diseases: A Guide to Diagnosis and Management*, DOI 10.1007/978-3-319-20460-4_107

- Retina/choroid: posterior placoid chorioretinitis, ground-glass retinitis, superficial creamy punctate precipitates, and serous retinal detachments
- Vascular: iris roseolae (dilated iris vessels), retinal vasculitis, Kyrieleis plaques (nodular arteritis), and vascular occlusion
- Intraocular pressure: inflammatory ocular hypertension syndrome
- Other signs: interstitial keratitis, dacryocystitis, and Argyll Robertson pupil

107.4 Epidemiology

Incidence is 0.01/100 person-years and prevalence of 0.1 % in patients on HAART. Approximately 85 % with ocular syphilis have CNS disease.

107.5 Predisposing/Associated Conditions

- HIV/AIDS
- High-risk sexual behavior, history of other sexually transmitted diseases

107.6 Differential Diagnosis (Table 107.1)

Table 107.1 Differential diagnosis of syphilitic *chorioretinitis*

Infectious	Autoimmune	Neoplastic
Toxoplasmosis	JIA	Lymphoma
Toxocariasis	HLA-B27	Leukemia
ARN	Sarcoidosis	
PORN	VKH syndrome	
APMPPE	SLE	
Serpiginous choroidopathy	Posterior scleritis	

107.7 Etiology

Infectious infiltration of the retina and choroid by the syphilis spirochete with resultant inflammation.

107.8 Workup/Testing

- Enzyme immunoassay (EIA) and chemiluminescent immunoassay (CIA) to *Treponema pallidum* antibody → if positive: reflex testing with non-treponemal tests (RPR, VDRL) → confirm with treponemal tests (TP-PA).
- Lumbar puncture (LP): positive if >5 WBCs/mm^3, protein > 50 mg/dL, and +VDRL in CSF.
- Evaluate for other infectious diseases, like HIV, gonorrhea, and chlamydia.
- Consider aqueous or vitreous biopsy for PCR or darkfield microscopy.
- Fundus photos, optical coherence tomography, possible fluorescein angiography, or indocyanine green angiography.

107.9 Prognosis and Management

- Treat if initial labs are:

  1. FTA-ABS positive, VDRL negative, and no previous treatment (Fig. 107.1)
  2. FTA-ABS positive, VDRL ≥1:8

- Ocular involvement should be treated as neurosyphilis:

  Penicillin G 2–4 million units IV q 4 h ×10–14 days
  If penicillin allergy: consult infectious disease specialist

    Consider ceftriaxone 2 g IV/IM ×10–14 days.
    Tetracycline 500 mg PO 4 times a day ×30 days.
    Penicillin desensitization in the intensive care unit.

  Topical prednisolone acetate 1 % 4×/day and cyclopentolate 2 % TID

- Congenital syphilis: manage with pediatrician/infectious disease specialist.

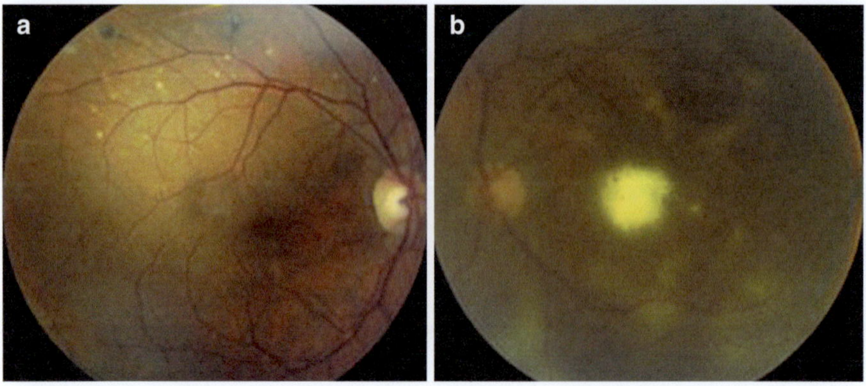

Fig. 107.1 Uveitis with subretinal macular lesion in the left eye. The patient was FTA-ABS positive. Patient also underwent panretinal photocoagulation for proliferative diabetic retinopathy in both eyes (**a**, right eye; **b**, left eye)

107.10 Follow-Up

- Lumbar puncture every 6 months for 2 years.
- VDRL at 3 and 6 months after treatment.
- Serum VDRL should decrease at least fourfold within 1 year and should be ≤1:4 within 1 year for primary syphilis, 2 years for secondary syphilis, and 5 years for tertiary syphilis.
- Retreat if repeat labs:
  1. Titers > 1:4 5 years after previous treatment.
  2. VDRL ≥1:8 and does not decrease fourfold after initial treatment.
  3. VDRL increases fourfold after treatment.
- Titers may be more difficult to follow in severely immunocompromised patients with AIDS.

References and Suggested Reading

1. Becker KN, Becker NM. Ocular manifestations seen in HIV. Dis Mon. 2014;60(6):268–75.
2. CDC. National Notifiable Disease Surveillance System. Syphilis (Treponema pallidum). Available at http://wwwn.cdc.gov/NNDSS/script/casedef.aspx?CondYrID=941&DatePub=1/1/2014%20 12:00:00%20AM.
3. Davis JL. Ocular syphilis. Curr Opin Ophthalmol. 2014;25(6):513–8.
4. Jabs DA, Van Natta ML, Holbrook JT, Kempen JH, Meinert CL, Davis MD, Studies of the Ocular Complications of AIDS Research Group. Longitudinal study of the ocular complications of AIDS: 1. Ocular diagnoses at enrollment. Ophthalmology. 2007;114(4):780–6.
5. Mathew RG, Goh BT, Westcott MC. British Ocular Syphilis Study (BOSS): 2-year national surveillance study of intraocular inflammation secondary to ocular syphilis. Invest Ophthalmol Vis Sci. 2014;55(8):5394–400.

Chapter 108
Neuroretinitis

Daniel S. Churgin, Blake Isernhagen, and Jack Stringham

108.1 Definitions

Inflammation of the optic nerve and retina

108.2 Symptoms

- Systemic symptoms: fever, chills, lymphadenopathy, and flu-like illness. A papule, vesicle, or pustule may form at the inoculation site.
- Ocular symptoms: Unilateral (rarely bilateral) acute painless loss of vision (mild to severe), decreased color vision, RAPD, central or centrocecal scotoma, or sometimes entirely asymptomatic.

108.3 Signs

Early development of disc edema and exudative peripapillary serous retinal detachment, followed by the development of a macular star 1–2 weeks later with improved disc edema (Fig. 108.1). Vitreous cells are typically present.

D.S. Churgin, MD (✉) • B. Isernhagen, MD
J. Stringham, MD
Bascom Palmer Eye Institute, University of Miami,
900 NW 17th Street, Miami, FL 33136, USA
e-mail: daniel.churgin@jhsmiami.org

C.A. Medina et al. (eds.), *Manual of Retinal Diseases: A Guide to Diagnosis and Management*, DOI 10.1007/978-3-319-20460-4_108

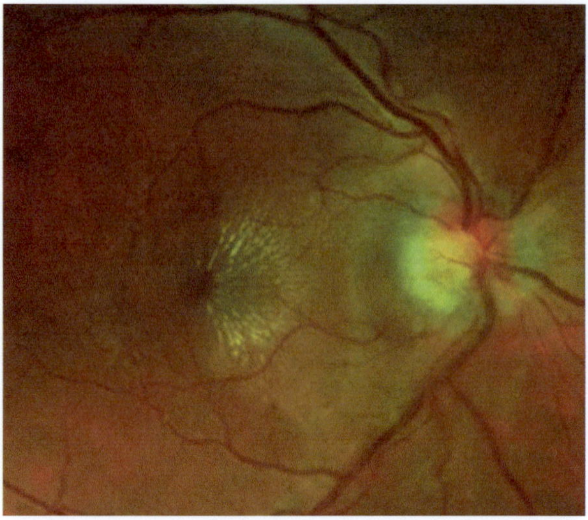

Fig. 108.1 Exudates in the macula appear as a star-shaped pattern due to radially oriented deposition in the outer plexiform layer

108.4 Epidemiology

Depends on etiology with the differential diagnosis for disc edema with macular star broad and includes many infectious and noninfectious entities. Between 1 and 64 % of patients who are seropositive for cat scratch disease present with neuroretinitis.

108.5 Predisposing Factors

- Exposure to cats (more risk with kittens)
- Immunosuppression
- HIV/AIDS
- Travel to endemic area
- Specific medication use

108.6 Differential Diagnosis (Table 108.1)

Table 108.1 Differential diagnosis of optic disc edema with macular star

Infectious	Noninfectious
Bacteria: Bartonella Rocky Mountain spotted fever Tuberculosis Salmonella Ehrlichiosis	*Inflammatory:* Sarcoidosis Inflammatory bowel disease Polyarteritis nodosa
Spirochetes and protozoa: Syphilis Lyme disease Leptospirosis Toxoplasmosis	*Vascular:* Diabetic papillitis Hypertensive retinopathy Anterior ischemic optic neuropathy
Virus: Herpes simplex Varicella Zoster	*CNS disease:* Papilledema Idiopathic intracranial hypertension
Nematode: *Toxocariasis*	*Neoplastic:* Leukemic infiltration of the optic nerve Optic disc and juxtapapillary tumors
	Toxic: Bis-chloroethyl-nitrosourea (BCNU chemotherapy) Procarbazine
	Idiopathic

108.7 Etiology

For cat scratch disease, direct invasion of the organism or an autoimmune reaction results in inflammation of the optic nerve head and optic nerve vasculature. Subsequently, there is fluid and lipid exudation into the surrounding retina.

108.8 Workup/Testing

Complete physical exam and thorough history are necessary in order to tailor further workup, as the differential diagnosis is broad.

- OCT; consider fluorescein angiography
- Bartonella titers (IgG and IgM)
- RPR and/or FTA-ABS

- PPD or QuantiFERON gold
- ESR/CRP/CBC if there is suspicion of giant cell arteritis.
- Not necessary for diagnosis but may show optic nerve enhancement on contrast-enhanced MRI

108.9 Prognosis and Management

- Up to 93 % of patients may achieve vision of 20/40 or greater in infectious neuroretinitis.
- Most patients have excellent visual recovery, with or without intervention.
- If the patient is immunocompromised or has profound vision loss, consider starting antibiotics while lab results are pending.
- Treatment options.

  Adults: azithromycin, erythromycin, ciprofloxacin, and doxycycline.
  Children: azithromycin and trimethoprim-sulfamethoxazole.
  Rifampin may be given as an adjunct therapy.
  Oral steroids if protracted or progressive course.

- Fundus findings.

  The exudates forming a macular star resolve over time with possible RPE defects. The optic nerve may return to baseline appearance or become pale within 8–12 weeks.

108.10 Follow-Up

Initially within a few days to ensure no unexpected progression or change in appearance. Once the patient begins to improve, follow-up can be extended to weekly and then monthly.

References and Suggested Reading

1. Bhatti M, Lee M. Should patients with bartonella neuroretinitis receive treatment? J Neuroophthalmol. 2014;34:412–6.
2. Ghauri R, Lee A. Optic disk edema with a macular star. Surv Ophthalmol. 1998;43(3):270–4.
3. Kitamei H, Suzuki Y, Takahashi M, Katsuta S, Kato H, Yokoi M, Kase M. Retinal angiography and optical coherence tomography disclose focal optic disc vascular leakage and lipid-rich fluid accumulation within the retina in a patient with Leber idiopathic stellate neuroretinitis. J Neuroophthalmol. 2009;29:203–7.
4. Purvin V, Sundaram S, Kawasaki A. Neuroretinitis: review of the literature and new observations. J Neuroophthalmol. 2011;31:58–68.
5. Suhler E, Lauer A, Rosenbaum J. Prevalence of serologic evidence of cat scratch disease in patients with neuroretinitis. Ophthalmology. 2000;107(5):871–6.

Section XVI
Endophthalmitis

Ajay E. Kuriyan

Chapter 109
Approach to Endophthalmitis

Ajay E. Kuriyan

109.1 Definitions

Endophthalmitis – intraocular inflammation affecting all intraocular cavities

- Infectious
  - Endogenous
  - Traumatic
  - Post-surgical (e.g., cataract, glaucoma drainage device, keratoplasty/keratoprosthesis, trabeculectomy, vitrectomy)
  - Post-intravitreal injection
  - Corneal ulcer-related
- Sterile
  - Post-intravitreal injection
  - Postsurgical
    - Toxic anterior segment syndrome
    - Retained lens fragments

A.E. Kuriyan, MD
Bascom Palmer Eye Institute, University of Miami,
900 NW 17th Street, Miami, FL 33136, USA
e-mail: akuriyan@med.miami.edu

C.A. Medina et al. (eds.), *Manual of Retinal Diseases: A Guide to Diagnosis and Management*, DOI 10.1007/978-3-319-20460-4_109

109.2 Symptoms/Signs

Symptoms include decreased vision, increased eye pain, conjunctival injection, and lid swelling. Exam findings include marked anterior chamber reaction, hypopyon, fibrin, and vitreous cell/membranes. Differentiating between infectious and sterile endophthalmitis is often difficult and the whole clinical picture and history needs to be evaluated.

109.3 Epidemiology

- Infectious
  - Endogenous: 0.05–0.4 %
  - Traumatic
    - All penetrating trauma: 4–13 %
    - Penetrating trauma with intraocular foreign body: 7–31 %
  - Postsurgical
    - Post-cataract: 0.7–0.13 %
    - Glaucoma drainage device: 1–6 %
    - Keratoplasty: 0.16–0.67 %
    - Keratoprosthesis: 7–12 %
    - Trabeculectomy: 0.2–9.6 %
    - Vitrectomy: 0.06–0.23 %
  - Post-intravitreal injection: 0.029–0.056 %
  - Corneal ulcer related: 0.5 %
- Sterile
  - Post-intravitreal injection: 0.09–1.1 %
  - Postsurgical
    - Toxic anterior segment syndrome: 0.1 %
    - Retained lens fragments: 0.007–0.01 %

109.4 Differential Diagnosis

Uveitis-glaucoma-hyphema (UGH) syndrome, noninfectious uveitis, ocular toxoplasmosis, and lymphoma

109.5 Etiology

- Infectious

  Endogenous: hematogenous spread of infection into the eye from the bloodstream
  Exogenous: spread of infection into the eye during ocular surgery or penetrating trauma

- Sterile – etiology unknown – thought to be inflammatory reaction to preservatives or other substances used during surgery.

109.6 Workup/Testing

- A thorough history to evaluate for risk factors associated with endogenous endophthalmitis, past ocular surgeries, or ocular trauma.
- Perform a CT scan to assess for any intraocular foreign bodies in patients with history of penetrating ocular trauma.
- Assess integrity of wounds in postoperative patients and blebs in patients with history of trabeculectomy using the Seidel test.
- Ultrasound: vitreous membrane formation is indicative of an infectious etiology but the lack thereof does not rule out infection.
- Obtain vitreous fluid for culture by vitreous paracentesis (appendix: "*Tap and Inject Principles and Technique*") or vitrectomy if suspicious for infectious endophthalmitis. Cataract surgery-associated endophthalmitis patients with vision of light perception at presentation had better visual outcomes with initial treatment with vitrectomy compared to tap and inject.

109.7 Prognosis and Management

Cases of sterile endophthalmitis can be managed with topical steroids and vision generally returns to baseline. After the vitreous sample is obtained in infectious endophthalmitis cases, broad-spectrum, empiric intravitreal antibiotics, such as vancomycin (1.0 mg/0.1 ml) and ceftazidime (2.25 mg/0.1 ml), should be used. Intravitreal amikacin (0.4 mg/0.1 ml) may be used instead of ceftazidime in patients with allergies. In cases in which fungal etiologies are suspected, intravitreal injection of voriconazole (100 mcg/0.1 ml) and/or amphotericin B (5–10 mcg/0.1 ml) is recommended. Intravitreal dexamethasone (0.4 mg/0.1 ml) may also be used when there is a low suspicion for fungal etiologies. Additionally, patients should be started on empiric fortified topical antibiotics, such as vancomycin (25 mg/ml) in combination with ceftazidime (50 mg/ml) or tobramycin (14 mg/ml) drops every hour. Topical steroids (q.i.d) and cycloplegics (t.i.d) should also be used to address the inflammation. Oral prednisone can be used in selected cases of bacterial endophthalmitis with severe inflammation. Systemic antibiotics are necessary in endogenous cases but are not necessary in exogenous cases. Prompt vitrectomy should be considered in culture-positive patients who do not improve after vitreous tap and injection.

The prognosis is largely dependent on the causative organisms. Coagulase-negative *Staphylococcus* has a more favorable prognosis than other organisms.

109.8 Follow-Up

Daily until improvement is noted.

References and Suggested Reading

1. Al-Torbak AA, Al-Shahwan S, Al-Jadaan I, Al-Hommadi A, Edward DP. Endophthalmitis associated with the Ahmed glaucoma valve implant. Br J Ophthalmol. 2005;89:454–8.
2. Chen JY, Jones MN, Srinivasan S, et al. Endophthalmitis after penetrating keratoplasty. Ophthalmology. 2015;122:25–30.
3. Dave VP, Pathengay A, Schwartz SG, Flynn Jr HW. Endophthalmitis following pars plana vitrectomy: a literature review of incidence, causative organisms, and treatment outcomes. Clin Ophthalmol. 2014;8:2183.
4. Eydelman MB, Tarver ME, Calogero D, Buchen SY, Alexander KY. The food and drug administration's proactive toxic anterior segment syndrome program. Ophthalmology. 2012;119: 1297–302.
5. Henry CR, Flynn HW, Miller D, Forster RK, Alfonso EC. Infectious keratitis progressing to endophthalmitis: a 15-year study of microbiology, associated factors, and clinical outcomes. Ophthalmology. 2012;119:2443–9.
6. Kangas TA, Greenfield DS, Flynn HW, Parrish RK, Palmberg P. Delayed-onset endophthalmitis associated with conjunctival filtering blebs. Ophthalmology. 1997;104:746–52.
7. Marticorena J, Romano V, Gomez-Ulla F. Sterile endophthalmitis after intravitreal injections. Mediators Inflamm. 2012. http://www.hindawi.com/journals/mi/2012/928123/abs/.
8. Ramchandran RS, DiLoreto DA, Chung MM, et al. Infectious endophthalmitis in adult eyes receiving Boston type I keratoprosthesis. Ophthalmology. 2012;119:674–81.
9. Results of the Endophthalmitis Vitrectomy Study. A randomized trial of immediate vitrectomy and of intravenous antibiotics for the treatment of postoperative bacterial endophthalmitis. Endophthalmitis Vitrectomy Study Group. Arch Ophthalmol. 1995;113(12):1479.
10. Reynolds DS, Flynn Jr HW. Endophthalmitis after penetrating ocular trauma. Curr Opin Ophthalmol. 1997;8:32–8.
11. Schwartz SG, Flynn Jr HW. Endophthalmitis associated with intravitreal anti-vascular endothelial growth factor injections. Curr Ophthalmol Rep. 2014;2:1–5.
12. Schwartz SG, Flynn Jr HW. Update on the prevention and treatment of endophthalmitis. Expert Rev Ophthalmol. 2014;9:425–30.
13. Taban M, Behrens A, Newcomb RL, et al. Acute endophthalmitis following cataract surgery: a systematic review of the literature. Arch Ophthalmol. 2005;123:613–20.

14. Vanner EA, Stewart MW. Meta-analysis comparing same-day versus delayed vitrectomy clinical outcomes for intravitreal retained lens fragments after age-related cataract surgery. Clin Ophthalmol. 2014;8:2261.
15. Vaziri K, Pershing S, Albini TA, Moshfeghi DM, Moshfeghi AA. Risk factors predictive of endogenous endophthalmitis among hospitalized patients with hematogenous infections in the United States. Am J Ophthalmol. 2015;153(3):498–504.

Chapter 110
Endophthalmitis Associated with Intravitreal Injections

Jack D. Stringham and Ajay E. Kuriyan

110.1 Definitions

- Postinjection infectious endophthalmitis
- Postinjection sterile endophthalmitis
  - Acute intraocular inflammation of the vitreous cavity that resolves without the need of intravitreal antibiotics and/or vitreoretinal surgery

110.2 Symptoms/Signs

Differentiating between infectious and sterile endophthalmitis is often difficult and no particular sign or symptom makes the diagnosis but rather the whole clinical picture must be considered (Table 110.1).

110.3 Epidemiology

- Infectious: 0.029–0.056 %
- Sterile: 0.09–1.1 %

J.D. Stringham, MD (✉) • A.E. Kuriyan, MD
Bascom Palmer Eye Institute, University of Miami,
900 NW 17th Street, Miami, FL 33136, USA
e-mail: jack.stringham@med.miami.edu

C.A. Medina et al. (eds.), *Manual of Retinal Diseases: A Guide to Diagnosis and Management*, DOI 10.1007/978-3-319-20460-4_110

Table 110.1 Symptoms and signs of infectious and sterile endophthalmitis

Symptoms/signs	Infectious endophthalmitis	Sterile endophthalmitis
Decreased vision	Generally dramatic	Mild-moderate
Pain	Generally painful	None to mild discomfort
Conjunctival injection	Very common	Mild if any
Fibrin	Always present	Rare
Hypopyon	Very common	Rare
Vitreous opacities	Moderate to dense	Mild to moderate

110.4 Minimizing Infection Risk

- Povidone iodine should be applied to the ocular surface as part of the preparation, its bactericidal effects are maximized when applied at least 1 min prior to injection, and it should be the last agent applied to the intended injection site.
- Reduce contamination from oral flora (*Streptococcus*) with either the use of surgical masks by all persons present in the treatment room or the instruction of all persons present to minimize speaking during the injection preparation and procedure.
- Avoid contamination of the needle and injection site by the eyelashes or the eyelid margins; this can be achieved with an eyelid speculum or manual retraction.

110.5 Differential Diagnosis

- Infectious endophthalmitis
- Sterile endophthalmitis
- Pseudo-endophthalmitis (following a triamcinolone injection, crystals migrate from vitreous into the anterior chamber)

110.6 Etiology

- Infectious

  - Forty-four percent coagulase-negative *Staphylococcus*
  - Twenty-four percent *Streptococcus* species (*Streptococcus* endophthalmitis rates are three times higher after injections than after cataract surgery. The source is thought to originate from oral flora, thus the recommendation for minimizing speaking or use of face masks during the preparation and procedure.)
- Sterile – etiology unknown

110.7 Workup/Testing

- A thorough history and exam to evaluate for features listed in Table 110.1 should be performed.
- Ultrasound, vitreous membrane formation, is indicative of an infectious etiology but the lack thereof does not rule out infection.
- Obtaining vitreous fluid for culture by vitreous paracentesis (see appendix for "Tap and Inject Principles and Technique") or vitrectomy if suspicious for infectious endophthalmitis.

110.8 Prognosis and Management

Cases of sterile endophthalmitis can be managed with topical steroids and vision generally returns to baseline. After the vitreous sample is obtained in infectious endophthalmitis cases, broad-spectrum and empiric intravitreal antibiotics, such as vancomycin (1.0 mg/0.1 ml) and ceftazidime (2.25 mg/0.1 ml) should be used. Intravitreal dexamethasone (0.4 mg/0.1 ml) may also be used when there is a low suspicion for fungal etiologies. Topical (± subconjunctival) antibiotics should be used as well. Additionally, topical prednisolone acetate 1 % and cycloplegics are often used as an adjunct to reduce inflammation.

The prognosis is largely dependent on the etiology; studies have found visual outcomes to be 20/400 or worse in 12 % of cases caused by coagulase-negative *Staphylococcus* compared to 95 % of cases caused by *Streptococcus*.

110.9 Follow-Up

Daily until improvement is noted.

References and Suggested Reading

1. Fileta JB, Scott IU, Flynn Jr HW. Meta-analysis of infectious endophthalmitis after intravitreal injection of anti-vascular endothelial growth factor agents. Ophthalmic Surg Lasers Imaging Retina. 2014;45(2):143–9.
2. Marticorena J, Romano V, Gómez-Ulla F. Erratum to "sterile endophthalmitis after intravitreal injections." Mediators Inflamm. 2013;2013:1–6.

Chapter 111
Post-Cataract Extraction Endophthalmitis

Wen-Shi Shieh and Ajay E. Kuriyan

111.1 Definitions

Postoperative endophthalmitis (POE)
Cataract extraction (CE)
Tap and injection (T&I)
Endophthalmitis vitrectomy study (EVS)
Pars plana vitrectomy (PPV)

111.2 Symptoms

Decreased vision, increased eye pain, conjunctival injection, and lid swelling

W.-S. Shieh, MD (✉)
Department of Ophthalmology, Wills Eye Hospital, 840 Walnut, Philadelphia, PA 19107, USA
e-mail: wshieh08@gmail.com

A.E. Kuriyan, MD
Bascom Palmer Eye Institute/Univ of Miami Miller School of Medicine, Miami FL, USA

C.A. Medina et al. (eds.), *Manual of Retinal Diseases: A Guide to Diagnosis and Management*, DOI 10.1007/978-3-319-20460-4_111

111.3 Signs

- *Acute (<6 weeks after surgery)*: marked anterior chamber reaction, hypopyon, fibrin, vitreous cell and membranes; severe infection, loss of red reflex and afferent pupillary defect.
- *Subacute*: recurrent granulomatous anterior uveitis, hypopyon, keratic precipitates, minimal conjunctival injection and/or pain, and white opacities on lens capsule.
  - *Note*: *rare findings on presentation include retinal vasculitis/periphlebitis or hemorrhages.*
- *Chronic (>6 weeks after surgery)*: as described above but usually indolent course, may demonstrate clinical improvement with topical corticosteroid and recur with tapering/discontinuation of steroid therapy.

111.4 Epidemiology

Incidence of infectious endophthalmitis after CE has steadily decreased as a result of improved surgical techniques. Current estimates range from 0.7 to 0.13 % [1, 2].

111.5 Predisposing Conditions: Table 111.1

Table 111.1 Risk factors for endophthalmitis after cataract surgery [4]

Preoperative	Intraoperative	Postoperative
Blepharitis Conjunctivitis Canaliculitis Immunosuppression	Inadequate disinfection of eyelid/conjunctiva Improper sterilization and/or handling of equipment Surgery duration >60 min Posterior capsule rupture Vitreous loss Silicone IOLs	Wound leak/dehiscence Vitreous to surgical wound Inadequately buried sutures Incomplete suture removal

111.6 Differential Diagnosis

Postoperative uveitis, toxic anterior segment syndrome (TASS), aseptic (sterile) endophthalmitis, retained lens material, and uveitis-glaucoma-hyphema (UGH) syndrome

111.7 Etiology

- Most common: *Staphylococcus epidermidis*
- Common: *Staphylococcus aureus*, *Streptococcus* species
- Less common: gram-negative bacteria, fungal organisms
- Most common cause of chronic infection: *Propionibacterium acnes*

111.8 Workup/Testing

A thorough history to assess the risk factors is listed above. A complete ophthalmic examination should be performed including Seidel test on the cataract wounds. If the view to the fundus is obscured, ultrasonography should be used to document any posterior pole findings. It is helpful to compare these findings (i.e., vitreous debris/membranes) to the contralateral eye. Vitreous fluid should be obtained via pars plana paracentesis or vitrectomy and cultured.

111.9 Prognosis and Management

- Vitreous Paracentesis and Injection of Intravitreal Antibiotics
  - See appendix for "Tap and Inject Principles and Technique."
- Vitrectomy and Injection of Intravitreal Antibiotics
  - The EVS found that acute, POE eyes with initial visual acuity of hand motion or better in patients had similar visual outcomes after initial treatment with PPV or T&I. However, patients with light perception vision had a threefold increased chance of achieving 20/40 vision after initial treatment with PPV compared to T&I.

- Antibiotic Selection
  - Mainstay antibiotics include vancomycin (1 mg/0.1 ml) to target gram-positive bacteria and ceftazidime (2.25 mg/0.1 ml), a third-generation cephalosporin with broad coverage for gram-negative and gram-positive organisms, which is favored over amikacin due to decreased risk of retinotoxicity.
  - Although controversial, intravitreal dexamethasone (0.4 mg/0.1 ml) may be beneficial for acute cases [3]. Topical (± subconjunctival) antibiotics should be used as well. Additionally, topical prednisolone acetate 1 % and cycloplegic agents are often used as an adjunct to reduce inflammation.
  - In the EVS, poor outcomes were associated with worse initial vision, small pupil size after maximal dilation, presence of rubeosis irides, and an absence of a red reflex [5]. Of these, initial visual acuity is the most useful predictive factor of visual outcome in acute bacterial POE. The causative organism also impacts the visual outcome.

111.10 Follow-Up

Daily until improvement is noted.

References and Suggested Reading

1. Mamalis N, Kearsley L, Brinton E. Postoperative endophthalmitis. Curr Opin Ophthalmol. 2002;13(1):14–8.
2. Nentwich M, Ta C, Kreutzer T, et al. Incidence of postoperative endophthalmitis from 1990 to 2009 using povidone-iodine but no intracameral antibiotics at a single academic institution. J Cataract Refract Surg. 2015;41(1):58–66.
3. Gan IM. Intravitreal dexamethasone as adjuvant in the treatment of postoperative endophthalmitis: a prospective randomized trial. Graefes Arch Clin Exp Ophthalmol. 2005;243(12):1200–5.
4. Kernt M, Kampik A. Endophthalmitis: pathogenesis, clinical presentation, management, and perspectives. Clin Ophthalmol. 2010;4:121–35.
5. Results of the Endophthalmitis Vitrectomy Study. A randomized trial of immediate vitrectomy and of intravenous antibiotics for the treatment of postoperative bacterial endophthalmitis. Endophthalmitis Vitrectomy Study Group. Arch Ophthalmol. 1995;113(12):1479–96.

Chapter 112
Bleb-Associated Endophthalmitis

Carlos A. Medina, Angelica G. Ortiz, and Ajay E. Kuriyan

112.1 Definitions

Bleb-associated infection can be subdivided:

- Blebitis: infection limited to in or around the filtering bleb. Although a mild to moderate anterior chamber reaction or even hypopyon may be present, no vitreous involvement is observed.
- Bleb-associated endophthalmitis (BAE): occurs when infectious or inflammatory material extends beyond the anterior chamber and into the vitreous.
  - Acute (≤6 weeks after surgery).
  - Delayed onset (>6 weeks after surgery).

112.2 Symptoms

Decreased vision, pain, and photophobia

C.A. Medina, MD (✉) • A.G. Ortiz • A.E. Kuriyan, MD
Department of Ophthalmology, Bascom Palmer Eye Institute,
University of Miami, 900 NW 17th Street, Miami, FL 33136, USA
e-mail: camedina2020@gmail.com

C.A. Medina et al. (eds.), *Manual of Retinal Diseases: A Guide to Diagnosis and Management*, DOI 10.1007/978-3-319-20460-4_112

112.3 Signs

Both blebitis and BAE can have hypotony, discharge, and sudden onset of hyperemic and injected conjunctiva with a white or opacified bleb (classic "white on red appearance"), anterior chamber cell and fibrin with or without hypopyon, and possible Seidel + bleb leak (Fig. 112.1). In BAE these signs can be more robust than those observed with blebitis alone. Additionally, BAE has vitreous inflammation seen on exam or on ultrasonography, which is the key finding to differentiate it from blebitis (Fig. 112.2).

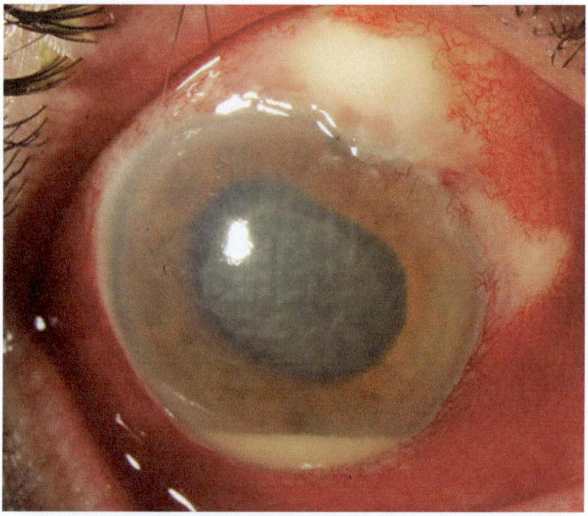

Fig. 112.1 Anterior segment photograph showing opacified bleb (with or without hypopyon)

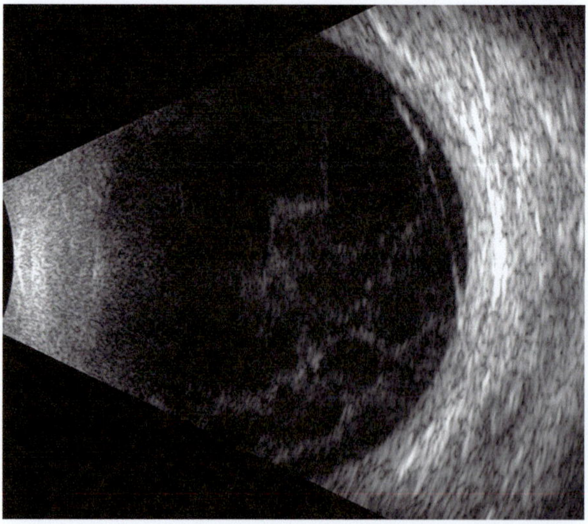

Fig. 112.2 Vitreous inflammation by ultrasonography (B scan)

112.4 Epidemiology

Reported incidence ranges from 0.2 to 9.6 %.

112.5 Predisposing Conditions

Use of intraoperative antimetabolites, inferior location of the bleb, thin bleb, history of bleb infection (blebitis), bleb leakage, or postoperative complications (such as flat AC or suprachoroidal hemorrhage). Patients with blepharitis, conjunctivitis, prior infection, axial myopia, diabetes, young age, black race, absence of a posterior lens capsule, nasolacrimal duct obstruction, history of bleb needling, laser suture lysis, contact lens use, and chronic antibiotic use may also be at higher risk.

112.6 Differential Diagnosis

In the acute postoperative phase, retained lens fragments and toxic anterior segment syndrome should be considered. In the absence of bleb involvement, endogenous endophthalmitis, endophthalmitis associated with other ocular surgical procedures, and noninfectious uveitis should be considered.

112.7 Etiology

Similar to acute-onset endophthalmitis after cataract surgery, *Staphylococcus epidermidis* is the most common causative organism associated with early-onset BAE. In delayed-onset BAE, *Streptococcus* species are the most common organisms followed by gram-negative bacteria such as *Haemophilus influenzae*.

112.8 Workup/Testing

A complete ophthalmic examination should be performed including a Seidel test to detect bleb leak. Microhypopyon can be detected on gonioscopy. If the view to the fundus is poor or inexistent, ultrasonography should be used to document any posterior pole findings. It is sometimes helpful to compare these findings (i.e., vitreous debris/membranes) to the contralateral eye. Vitreous cultures via pars plana paracentesis or vitrectomy should be performed if the diagnosis is suspected (Appendix: "Tap and Inject Principles and Technique."). Additionally, conjunctival swabs (including purulent material from the bleb, if present) and anterior chamber fluid should be cultured.

112.9 Prognosis and Management

Unlike blebitis where the visual outcome is usually much better than endophthalmitis, BAE carries a poor visual prognosis even with aggressive medical and surgical intervention.

Early diagnosis and prompt intensive treatment are critical. Because of the lack of prospective randomized clinical studies, a wide variation exists in the management of BAE, and standard treatment regimen does not currently exist at. After vitreous, anterior chamber, and conjunctival cultures are obtained, the patient should be treated with empiric intravitreal antibiotics, such as vancomycin (1.0 mg/0. 1 ml) and ceftazidime (2.25 mg/0.1 ml). Amikacin (0.4 mg/0.1 ml) may be used instead of ceftazidime. Intravitreal dexamethasone (0.4 mg/0.1 ml) may also be used when there is a low suspicion for fungal etiologies. Additionally, patients should be started on empiric fortified topical antibiotics, such as vancomycin (25 mg/ml) in combination with ceftazidime (50 mg/ml) or tobramycin (14 mg/ml) drops every hour. Topical steroids (q.i.d) and cycloplegics (t.i.d) should also be used to address the inflammation. Systemic antibiotics are usually not recommended, but oral fluoroquinolones may be considered in eyes with marked inflammation, LP vision, or rapid onset. Prompt vitrectomy should be considered in culture-positive patients who do not improve after vitreous tap and injection.

112.10 Follow-Up

Daily until improvement is noted.

References and Suggested Reading

1. Busbee BG, Recchia FM, Kaiser R, Nagra P, Rosenblatt B, Pearlman RB. Bleb-associated endophthalmitis: clinical characteristics and visual outcomes. Ophthalmology. 2004;111(8): 1495–503; discussion 503.
2. Chiam PJ, Arashvand K, Shaikh A, James B. Management of blebitis in the United Kingdom: a survey. Br J Ophthalmol. 2012;96(1):38–41.
3. Jacobs DJ, Pathengay A, Flynn Jr HW, Leng T, Miller D, Shi W. Intravitreal dexamethasone in the management of delayed-onset bleb-associated endophthalmitis. Int J Inflam. 2012; 2012:503912.
4. Jampel HD, Quigley HA, Kerrigan-Baumrind LA, Melia BM, Friedman D, Barron Y. Risk factors for late-onset infection following glaucoma filtration surgery. Arch Ophthalmol. 2001;119(7):1001–8.
5. Lehmann OJ, Bunce C, Matheson MM, Maurino V, Khaw PT, Wormald R, et al. Risk factors for development of post-trabeculectomy endophthalmitis. Br J Ophthalmol. 2000;84(12): 1349–53.
6. Leng T, Miller D, Flynn Jr HW, Jacobs DJ, Gedde SJ. Delayed-onset bleb-associated endophthalmitis (1996–2008): causative organisms and visual acuity outcomes. Retina. 2011;31(2):344–52.
7. Poulsen EJ, Allingham RR. Characteristics and risk factors of infections after glaucoma filtering surgery. J Glaucoma. 2000;9(6):438–43.

Chapter 113
Endophthalmitis Associated with Glaucoma Drainage Implants

Carlos A. Medina, Ajay E. Kuriyan, William E. Smiddy, and Justin H. Townsend

113.1 Definitions

Glaucoma drainage implant (GDI)

113.2 Symptoms

Decreased vision, pain, and photophobia

113.3 Signs

Exposed glaucoma drainage implant (tube or plaque) by conjunctival breakdown. Hypotony, shallow anterior chamber, hyphema, corneal edema, as well as typical signs of endophthalmitis such as redness, hypopyon, fibrin, and vitreous debris/strands are observed. Chronic anterior chamber cell and flare (iridocyclitis) should raise the suspicion of a chronic low-grade or atypical infection.

C.A. Medina, MD (✉) • A.E. Kuriyan, MD • W.E. Smiddy, MD • J.H. Townsend, MD
Department of Ophthalmology, Bascom Palmer Eye Institute,
University of Miami, 900 NW 17th Street, Miami, FL 33136, USA
e-mail: camedina2020@gmail.com

C.A. Medina et al. (eds.), *Manual of Retinal Diseases: A Guide to Diagnosis and Management*, DOI 10.1007/978-3-319-20460-4_113

113.4 Epidemiology

Previous studies estimate the incidence of endophthalmitis after GDI surgery to be between 1 and 6 %.

113.5 Predisposing Conditions

Trabeculectomy and glaucoma drainage implant (GDI) are the two most frequently performed incisional glaucoma surgeries.

113.6 Differential Diagnosis

Iritis from tube cornea/iris touch and postoperative inflammation (if acute)

113.7 Etiology

Exposed hardware is the greatest risk factor in the development of endophthalmitis, and conjunctival breakdown is seen in approximately half the cases.

113.8 Workup/Testing

A complete ophthalmic examination should be performed, including a Seidel test. If the view to the fundus is poor or nonexistent, ultrasonography should be used to evaluate for any posterior pole findings including vitreous debris or membranes and retinal or choroidal detachment. It is sometimes helpful to compare these findings (i.e., vitreous debris/membranes) to the contralateral eye. Vitreous cultures via pars plana paracentesis or vitrectomy should be performed if the diagnosis is suspected (appendix: "Tap and Inject Principles and Technique").

113.9 Prognosis and Management

If exposure of the GDI is observed, revision or removal should be strongly considered. Even in the absence of tube exposure, some have suggested removing the GDI to resolve the active infection or remove encapsulated infectious material to prevent

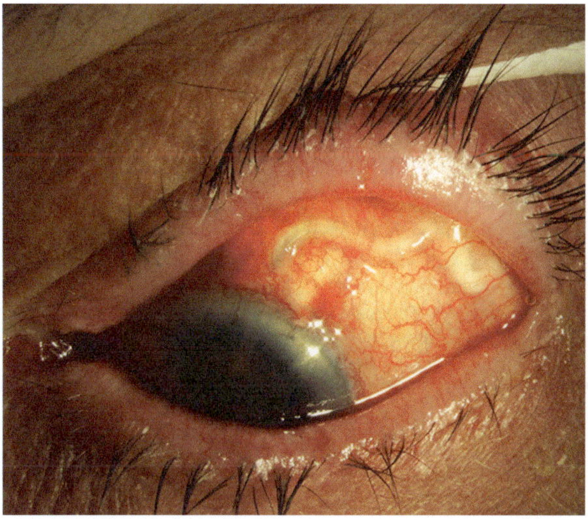

Fig. 113.1 Slit lamp photograph demonstrating a superotemporal tube shunt with exposure from conjunctival breakdown just posterior to the sclerotomy site

recurrence; however other sources indicated removal is unnecessary if proper antibiotic treatment is initiated. After vitreous and GDI cultures (if exposure is present) are obtained, the patient is treated with empiric intravitreal antibiotics, such as vancomycin (1.0 mg/0.1 ml) and ceftazidime (2.25 mg/0.1 ml). Intravitreal dexamethasone (0.4 mg/0.1 ml) may also be used when there is a low suspicion for fungal etiologies. Additionally, patients should be started on empiric fortified topical antibiotics, such as vancomycin (25 mg/ml) in combination with ceftazidime (50 mg/ml) or tobramycin (14 mg/ml) drops every hour while awake. Topical steroids (q.i.d) and cycloplegics (t.i.d) should also be used to address the inflammation. Systemic antibiotics are usually not recommended but oral fluoroquinolones may be considered in eyes with marked inflammation, LP vision, or rapid onset. The predominance of highly virulent species as the causative organisms (*Staphylococcus* and *Streptococcus*) coupled with the typically advanced glaucomatous changes may explain the very poor visual outcomes of these patients (Fig. 113.1).

113.10 Follow-Up

Daily until improvement is noted.

References and Suggested Reading

1. Munoz M, Tomey KF, Traverso C, Day SH, Senft SH. Clinical experience with the Molteno implant in advanced infantile glaucoma. J Pediatr Ophthalmol Strabismus. 1991;28(2):68–72.

2. Hill RA, Heuer DK, Baerveldt G, Minckler DS, Martone JF. Molteno implantation for glaucoma in young patients. Ophthalmology. 1991;98(7):1042–6.
3. Chihara E, Kubota H, Takanashi T, Nao-i N. Outcome of white pump shunt surgery for neovascular glaucoma in Asians. Ophthalmic Surg. 1992;23(10):666–71.
4. Krupin eye valve with disk for filtration surgery. The Krupin Eye Valve Filtering Surgery Study Group. Ophthalmology. 1994;101(4):651–8.
5. Lloyd MA, Baerveldt G, Fellenbaum PS, Sidoti PA, Minckler DS, Martone JF, et al. Intermediate-term results of a randomized clinical trial of the 350- versus the 500-mm2 Baerveldt implant. Ophthalmology. 1994;101(8):1456–63; discussion 63–4.
6. Perkins TW, Cardakli UF, Eisele JR, Kaufman PL, Heatley GA. Adjunctive mitomycin C in Molteno implant surgery. Ophthalmology. 1995;102(1):91–7.
7. Nguyen QH, Budenz DL, Parrish 2nd RK. Complications of Baerveldt glaucoma drainage implants. Arch Ophthalmol. 1998;116(5):571–5.
8. Krishna R, Godfrey DG, Budenz DL, Escalona-Camaano E, Gedde SJ, Greenfield DS, et al. Intermediate-term outcomes of 350-mm(2) Baerveldt glaucoma implants. Ophthalmology. 2001;108(3):621–6.
9. Gedde SJ, Scott IU, Tabandeh H, Luu KK, Budenz DL, Greenfield DS, et al. Late endophthalmitis associated with glaucoma drainage implants. Ophthalmology. 2001;108(7):1323–7.
10. Perkins TW. Endophthalmitis after placement of a Molteno implant. Ophthalmic Surg. 1990;21(10):733–4.
11. Krebs DB, Liebmann JM, Ritch R, Speaker M. Late infectious endophthalmitis from exposed glaucoma setons. Arch Ophthalmol. 1992;110(2):174–5.
12. Ellis BD, Varley GA, Kalenak JW, Meisler DM, Huang SS. Bacterial endophthalmitis following cataract surgery in an eye with a preexisting Molteno implant. Ophthalmic Surg. 1993; 24(2):117–8.
13. Jacobs DJ, Pathengay A, Flynn Jr HW, Leng T, Miller D, Shi W. Intravitreal dexamethasone in the management of delayed-onset bleb-associated endophthalmitis. Int J Inflam. 2012;2012: 503912.

Chapter 114
Endogenous Endophthalmitis

Nadim Rayess and Jayanth Sridhar

114.1 Definitions

Endogenous endophthalmitis: endophthalmitis due to hematogenous spread from a systemic source

114.2 Symptoms

Decreased vision, pain, red eye, and lid swelling. Systemic symptoms may include fever, lethargy, and symptoms dependent on the source of infection.

114.3 Signs

Lid swelling, corneal edema, anterior chamber cell, fibrin, hypopyon, posterior synechia, vitritis, vitreous opacities, and chorioretinitis

N. Rayess, MD • J. Sridhar, MD (✉)
Mid-Atlantic Retina, Wills Eye Hospital,
840 Walnut Street Suite 1020, Philadelphia, PA 19106, USA
e-mail: nmrayess@gmail.com; jsridhar119@gmail.com

C.A. Medina et al. (eds.), *Manual of Retinal Diseases: A Guide to Diagnosis and Management*, DOI 10.1007/978-3-319-20460-4_114

114.4 Epidemiology

- Represents 2–8 % of endophthalmitis cases.
- Liver abscess is the most common source of infection, more common in Asia.
- Other sources: pneumonia, endocarditis, and soft tissue infections.

114.5 Predisposing Conditions

Recent surgery, pharmacologic immunosuppression, diabetes, intravenous drug user, HIV, cardiac disease (e.g., valve abnormalities, endocarditis), systemic malignancy, indwelling catheters, and kidney or liver disease

114.6 Differential Diagnosis

Exogenous endophthalmitis, viral retinitis, ocular toxoplasmosis, noninfectious uveitis, and lymphoma

114.7 Etiology

Results from hematogenous spread of infection from a systemic source into the eye. The most common etiology is fungal (*Candida albicans*) endogenous endophthalmitis, followed by bacterial endogenous endophthalmitis (primarily gram-positive *Streptococci* and *Staphylococci*). In the neonatal population, the most common etiology is fungal (*Candida albicans*), and the second most common is *Pseudomonas aeruginosa.*

114.8 Workup/Testing

Past medical history, including querying prior hospitalizations, prior non-ocular surgery, indwelling lines, diabetes mellitus, intravenous drug use, immunosuppression, total parenteral nutrition, and steroid use, is essential to identify a possible source of systemic infection.

Symptoms of bacteremia or fungemia, including fevers, chills, night sweats, and weight loss, should be assessed. Once endogenous endophthalmitis is diagnosed, vitreous cultures should be obtained via a vitreous tap and injection. Especially in suspected fungal cases, vitrectomy may provide a higher rate of positive culture results than needle paracentesis. Systemic sources, including blood and urine, should be cultured and inpatient admission and consultation with an infectious disease specialist should be performed. Further systemic workup, including transthoracic and/or transesophageal echocardiogram, should be obtained based on the patient's risk factors and other medical history.

114.9 Prognosis and Management

- Regardless of cause management rests on finding the source of the infection and treating the underlying disease with appropriate systemic intravenous antibacterial or antifungal agents.
- Bacterial endogenous endophthalmitis: Intravitreal broad-spectrum antibiotics (e.g., vancomycin (1 mg/0.1 ml) and ceftazidime (2.25 mg/0.1 ml) should be injected at the time of vitreous sampling. Injections are typically not repeated unless there is non-response or recurrence of infection. Prognosis is generally poor; final visual acuity was found to worse than 20/400 in 78 % of cases in one series.
- Fungal endogenous endophthalmitis: With minimal vitreous inflammation and sparing of the macula and optic nerve, systemic antifungal therapy may be sufficient initially. Otherwise, intravitreal injection of antifungals is recommended at the time of vitreous sampling. Voriconazole (100 mcg/0.1 ml) and amphotericin B (5–10 mcg/0.1 ml) are commonly used. Injections may be repeated in cases of non-response or progression. Prognosis is better than bacterial cases with 65 % of eyes in one series achieving 20/400 vision or better. Yeast (*Candida albicans*) cases typically have better outcomes than mold (*Aspergillus* species) cases.
- Indications for vitrectomy are not well defined for endogenous endophthalmitis. In general, vitrectomy should be considered in patients not responding to a combination of systemic and intravitreal therapy. Vitrectomy has been shown to improve outcomes in cases of yeast endogenous endophthalmitis when performed within a week of diagnosis. Possible advantages of vitrectomy include removal of vitreous debris, obtaining a larger sample for diagnosis in cases of persistent negative cultures, and if necessary, debride subretinal microabscesses. The patient's general medical status must be also taken into account when considering vitrectomy surgery.

114.10 Follow-Up

Daily until improvement is noted. Additional intervention may be required.

References

1. Essman TF, Flynn Jr HW, Smiddy WE, et al. Treatment outcomes in a 10-year study of endogenous fungal endophthalmitis. Ophthalmic Surg Lasers. 1997;28:185–94.
2. Jackson TL, Eykyn SJ, Graham EM, Stanford MR. Endogenous bacterial endophthalmitis: a 17-year prospective series and review of 267 reported cases. Surv Ophthalmol. 2003;48:403–23.
3. Lemley CA, Han DP. Endophthalmitis: a review of current evaluation and management. Retina. 2007;27(6):662–80.
4. Soheilian M, Rafati N, Peyman GA. Prophylaxis of acute posttraumatic bacterial endophthalmitis with or without combined intraocular antibiotics: a prospective, double-masked randomized pilot study. Int Ophthalmol. 2001;24:323–30.

Chapter 115
Fungal Endophthalmitis

Alia Durrani and Jayanth Sridhar

115.1 Definitions

Exogenous or endogenous endophthalmitis due to yeasts or molds

115.2 Symptoms

Decrease in vision, redness, pain, and/or floaters. May be asymptomatic

115.3 Signs

Both endogenous and exogenous patients may have hypotony, discharge, conjunctival injection, anterior chamber cell, and fibrin with or without hypopyon.

Endogenous: focal, yellow or white retinal, or choroidal lesions and "string of pearls" vitreous opacities (Fig. 115.1).

A. Durrani, MD
Wills Eye Hospital, 840 Walnut Street Suite 1020,
Philadelphia, PA 19106, USA
e-mail: alia.k.durrani@gmail.com

J. Sridhar, MD (✉)
Mid-Atlantic Retina, Wills Eye Hospital,
840 Walnut Street Suite 1020, Philadelphia, PA 19106, USA
e-mail: jsridhar119@gmail.com

C.A. Medina et al. (eds.), *Manual of Retinal Diseases: A Guide to Diagnosis and Management*, DOI 10.1007/978-3-319-20460-4_115

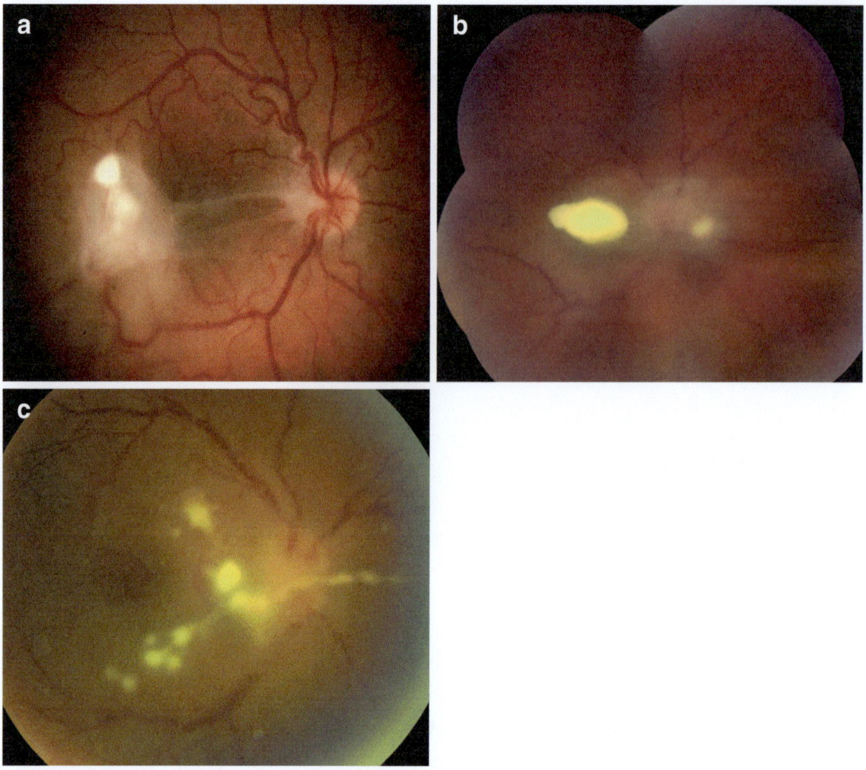

Fig. 115.1 Fundus features of endogenous endophthalmitis. Focal, yellow retinochoroidal lesions (**a**, **b**) and "string of pearls" vitreous opacities (**c**)

Exogenous: may initially present with anterior segment findings and progressively develop posterior segment findings. Look for signs of associated penetrating trauma (Seidel positive), corneal ulcer, or ocular surgery (check all surgical wounds for Seidel positivity).

115.4 Epidemiology

Endogenous: *Candida albicans* most common, followed by *Aspergillus* species, *Fusarium* species, *Candida tropicalis*, and *Cryptococcus neoformans*

Exogenous: *Fusarium* species, *Aspergillus* species, less likely *Candida* species

115.5 Risk Factors

Endogenous: prior or current hospitalization, prior non-ocular surgery, indwelling lines, diabetes mellitus, intravenous drug use, immunosuppression, total parenteral nutrition, broad-spectrum antibiotic use, or steroid use

Exogenous: prior fungal keratitis, intraocular surgery, or trauma

115.6 Differential Diagnosis

Non-infectious uveitis, bacterial endophthalmitis, ocular toxoplasmosis, and viral retinitis

115.7 Etiology

- Endogenous: hematogenous seeding of the choroid and retina from blood-borne infection
- Exogenous: spread from penetrating trauma, corneal ulcer, or prior intraocular surgery

115.8 Workup/Testing

Endogenous: If not already admitted, admission and systemic workup are warranted for diagnosis and treatment, including blood cultures and infectious disease consultation. Vitreous sampling should be completed via vitreous paracentesis (see appendix for "*Tap and Inject Principles and Technique*") or vitrectomy, with both fungal culture and smear along with bacterial culture and gram stain ordered. Vitrectomy has been noted to provide a higher rate of positive culture results as compared to vitreous or aqueous paracentesis.

Exogenous: Vitreous sampling should be completed either via vitreous paracentesis or vitrectomy.

115.9 Prognosis and Management

Systemic agents include oral or intravenous voriconazole, intravenous amphotericin B, and oral fluconazole.

Endogenous endophthalmitis: With extramacular lesions and minimal to no vitritis, systemic antifungal therapy may be sufficient initial therapy with frequent ophthalmologic monitoring for progression. With the presence of vitritis or macular/macula-threatening/optic nerve-threatening lesions, intravitreal injection of antifungals is recommended with voriconazole (100 mcg/0.1 ml) or amphotericin B (5–10 mcg/0.1 ml) commonly used. Injections may be repeated if there is evidence of nonresponse or progression. Vitrectomy along with intravitreal injection of either voriconazole or amphotericin B may be necessary in cases of moderate to severe vitritis and may improve visual acuity outcomes when performed within a week of diagnosis. Retinal detachment is a common complication. Outcomes are typically better in yeast than in mold cases, with the latter carrying a higher risk of enucleation.

Exogenous endophthalmitis: Intravitreal injection of antifungals is recommended.

Topical therapy in the form of voriconazole 1 % or amphotericin B 0.15 % should be administered as adjunct therapy if fungal keratitis is present. In post-cataract surgery cases, surgical removal of the intraocular lens and lens capsule may be necessary to eliminate a persistent nidus of infection. Visual outcomes vary according to causative organism with high rates of enucleation, especially in trauma.

115.10 Follow-Up

Daily until improvement is noted. Additional intervention may be required.

References and Suggested Reading

1. Lingappan A, Wykoff CC, Albini TA, et al. Endogenous fungal endophthalmitis: causative organisms, management strategies, and visual acuity outcomes. Am J Ophthalmol. 2012;153(1):162–6.
2. McDonnell PJ, McDonnell JM, Brown RH, Green WR. Ocular involvement in patients with fungal infections. Ophthalmology. 1985;92(5):706–9.
3. Silva RA, Sridhar J, Miller D, Wykoff CC, Flynn Jr HW. Exogenous fungal endophthalmitis: an analysis of isolates and susceptibilities to antifungal agents over a 20-Year Period (1990–2010). Am J Ophthal. 2015;159(2):257–64.
4. Wykoff CC, Flynn Jr HW, Miller D, Scott IU, Alfonso EC. Exogenous fungal endophthalmitis: microbiology and clinical outcomes. Ophthalmology. 2008;115(9):1501–7.

Section XVII
Systemic Disease and Associated Retinal Disease

Marco A. Gonzalez

Chapter 116
Vision Changes in a Pregnant Woman

Thalmon R. Campagnoli and William E. Smiddy

116.1 Definitions

Pregnancy is responsible for multiple hormonal, metabolic, hematologic, cardiovascular, and immunologic changes believed to increase the risk of manifesting variable forms of retinopathy. Normal pregnancies are usually not accompanied by notable ocular changes. However, a number of conditions may arise or worsen during this period; in rare occasions permanent vision loss may ensue (Table 116.1).

116.2 Symptoms

Decreased vision, scotomas, photopsias, floaters, diplopia, blindness.

116.3 Signs

- *Preeclampsia/eclampsia*: Focal or generalized arteriolar narrowing is the earliest and most common finding; choroidopathy leading to serous retinal detachments or yellow retinal pigment epithelium (RPE) lesions occur in severe cases; retinal and optic nerve ischemia may occur. These changes are often bilateral.
- *Central serous chorioretinopathy (CSC)*: Central subretinal edema containing typical *whitish* exudate (90 % whitish exudate in pregnant vs. 10 % in men and nonpregnant women) is unique in this setting. Usually this is unilateral.

T.R. Campagnoli, MD • W.E. Smiddy, MD (✉)
Department of Ophthalmology, University of Miami, Bascom Palmer Eye Institute, 900 NW 17th St., Miami, FL 33136, USA
e-mail: wsmiddy@med.miami.edu

C.A. Medina et al. (eds.), *Manual of Retinal Diseases: A Guide to Diagnosis and Management*, DOI 10.1007/978-3-319-20460-4_116

Table 116.1 Pregnancy-related diseases

Arising in pregnancy	Preeclampsia/eclampsia retinopathy and choroidopathy
	Central serous chorioretinopathy
	Occlusive vascular disorders (retinal artery and vein occlusion, DIC, TTP)
	Amniotic fluid embolism
	Uveal melanoma
Preexisting	Diabetic retinopathy
	Toxoplasma retinochoroiditis
	Noninfectious uveitis (VKH, Behçet, idiopathic)

DIC disseminated intravascular coagulopathy, *TTP* thrombotic thrombocytopenic purpura, *VKH* Vogt-Koyanagi-Harada

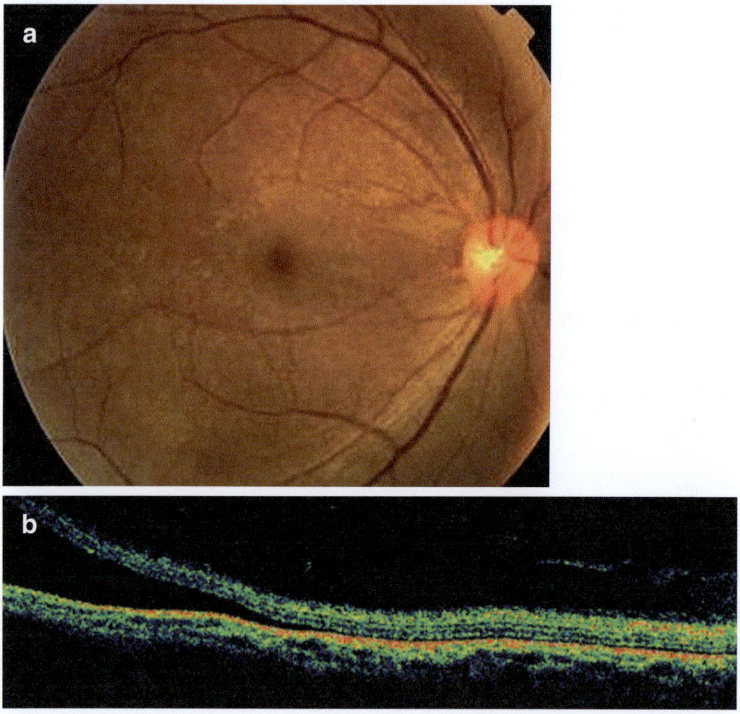

Fig. 116.1 Disseminated intravascular coagulopathy: yellow RPE lesions (**a**) and bilateral serous detachment (**b**)

- *Disseminated intravascular coagulopathy* (*DIC*)/*thrombotic thrombocytopenic purpura* (*TTP*): Findings may include bilateral serous detachment or yellow RPE lesions (Fig. 116.1).
- *Retinal artery occlusion*: Retinal ischemic whitening with focal or diffuse arteriolar narrowing and possible optic disc pallor; central macula cherry red spot

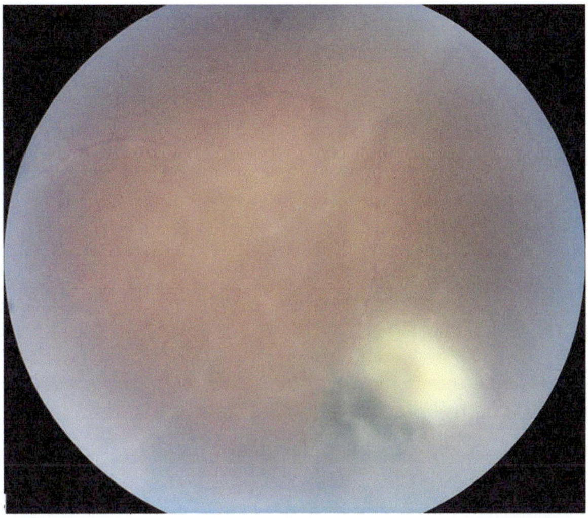

Fig. 116.2 Toxoplasmic retinochoroiditis: characterized by whitish focal necrotizing retinochoroiditis satellite lesion adjacent to hyperpigmented focal scars surrounded by vitreous opacities

and afferent pupillary defect can be findings in central artery occlusion. This is usually unilateral, unless associated with systemic disease.
- *Amniotic fluid embolism*: A characteristic appearance is multiple branch arteriolar occlusions, which may be uni- or bilateral.
- *Retinal vein occlusion* (*RVO*): This is characterized by segmented or diffuse intraretinal hemorrhages, cotton wool spots, capillary nonperfusion areas, retinal edema, and increased vessel tortuosity. It may be uni- or bilateral and is extremely rare.
- *Uveal melanoma*: This appears as a variably pigmented (or nonpigmented) choroidal mass associated with RPE changes, drusen, subretinal fluid, and/or orange pigments, and may display rapid growth; whereas orange-red choroidal mass with margins that blend with the surrounding choroid are characteristic of circumscribed *choroidal hemangioma*. These are usually unilateral.
- *Diabetic retinopathy* (*DR*): Microaneurysms, intraretinal hemorrhages, hard exudates, cotton wool spots, venous beading, capillary nonperfusion areas, IRMAs (intraretinal microvascular abnormalities), macular edema, neovascularization. Bilateral.
- *Toxoplasmic retinochoroiditis*: Characterized by whitish focal necrotizing retinochoroiditis satellite lesion adjacent to hyperpigmented focal scars surrounded by vitreous opacities. This is most commonly unilateral (Fig. 116.2).

116.4 Predisposing Conditions

- Preexisting systemic hypertension
- Uncontrolled hypertension/glycemia
- Coagulopathies
- Immunosuppression
- Pregnancy stage (e.g., third trimester – CSC, DIC)

116.5 Differential Diagnosis

Retinal pathologies that may be similar to the conditions aforementioned are age-related macular degeneration (AMD), choroidal nevus, retinal macroaneurysm, and perifoveal retinal telangiectasis. Necrotizing retinitis due to CMV, HSV, VZV, syphilis, and tuberculosis are other diagnoses to exclude.
Systemic events (stroke, migraine) should also be considered.

116.6 Etiology

The main etiologic factors contributing to vision changes in pregnancy include:

- Retinal and choroidal blood flow changes or ischemia (preeclampsia/eclampsia, DIC, arterial or venous occlusion, diabetic retinopathy)
- Localized RPE dysfunction (CSC)
- Hormonal response or immune modulation (uveal melanomas, diabetic retinopathy, toxoplasmic retinochoroiditis, uveitis)

116.7 Workup/Testing

The most useful tests for diagnosis and/or follow-up:

- Dilated fundus examination.
- Fundus photography; recommended for documentation, especially at baseline.
- Ultrasound (USG, A-scan and B-scan); posterior segment changes (retinal traction, detachment) in the presence of media opacities, choroidal tumors evaluation.
- Fluorescein angiography (FA); evaluates retinal vascular diseases as well as choroidal tumors. Fluorescein crosses the placenta. Its use in pregnancy should be considered only if the disease assessment wouldn't be possible through any other method and the results would change the management of a vision-threatening pathology. Appropriate informed consent should always be obtained (pregnancy category C).
- Indocyanine green angiography (ICGA); useful in choroidal vascular lesions and tumors. Although indocyanine does not cross the placental barrier, the same considerations for fluorescein angiography use during pregnancy should take place regarding ICGA use.
- Spectral domain OCT (SD-OCT); definitive test for retinal edema and evaluation of RPE and ellipsoid layers abnormalities.
- Fundus autofluorescence (FAF); helps detecting mild RPE changes.
- Multifocal electroretinogram (m-ERG).

Medical investigation/management of systemic diseases (cardiovascular, neoplasia, immune-related) is indicated in some instances.

116.8 Prognosis and Management

Overall, vision changes occurring during pregnancy are transient, carrying good prognosis, and most can be managed after delivery if persistent.

Severe visual loss may occur when serous retinal detachment and RPE lesions caused by preeclampsia/eclampsia, DIC, and TTP takes place. However, complete visual recovery usually returns postpartum without need for treatment. Optic atrophy and cortical blindness, although rare, may occur in severe preeclampsia and eclampsia cases.

CSC can cause moderate visual loss, but commonly resolves within weeks to few months after delivery without treatment. It may recur in subsequent pregnancies.

Retinal artery occlusion typically presents within 24 h of delivery and final visual acuity may range from 20/20 to 4/200 depending on the vessel occluded and timing of intervention. Branch retinal artery occlusion carries a much better prognosis than central retinal artery occlusion. Treatment is recommended within the first 24 h of symptom onset and options include ocular massage, lowering IOP medications, and anterior chamber paracentesis. Laser photocoagulation should be used in the treatment of neovascularization. Enzymatic thrombolysis is contraindicated. The visual deficit due to an artery occlusion is usually permanent.

The prognosis of uveal melanoma in pregnant women does not appear to differ from the general population, although faster tumor growth has been reported in some patients (debatable). Treatment with plaque radiotherapy or brachytherapy can be offered during pregnancy, although safer if applied towards the end or after delivery.

Diabetic retinopathy, including diabetic macular edema, may worsen during pregnancy; these changes may regress postpartum. Proliferative complications often require treatment. Duration and degree of diabetic retinopathy at the onset of pregnancy are the major determinants of progression; therefore, tight HbA1C control is strongly advisable in diabetic women who may become pregnant. Treatment with laser photocoagulation is recommended according to guidelines established for the general population. Fundus examination should be performed at the first trimester and repeated each 1–3 months in case of severe NPDR or PDR.

Toxoplasmic retinochoroiditis in pregnancy does not differ in severity, duration, or outcomes compared to nonpregnant women, but recurrences characteristically can be precipitated by pregnancy. Treatment should be considered if vision-threatening disease occurs. Spiramycin, azithromycin, clindamycin, and atovaquone are safe to use during pregnancy and breast-feeding period. Sulfadiazine is contraindicated in the third trimester while pyrimethamine and thrimethoprim/sulfamethoxazole are contraindicated in the first trimester of pregnancy, besides all being contraindicated during breast-feeding. Irreversible visual deficit may occur even with treatment.

116.9 Follow Up

The follow up regimen is determined by the pathology and severity of the ocular findings, the pregnancy stage, and the therapeutic options available.

References and Suggested Reading

1. American Academy of Ophthalmology Retina/Vitreous Panel. Preferred Practice Pattern® Guidelines. Diabetic retinopathy. San Francisco: American Academy of Ophthalmology; 2014. Available at: www.aao.org/ppp.
2. Kump LI, Androudi SN, Foster CS. Ocular toxoplasmosis in pregnancy. Semin Exp Ophthalmol. 2005;33(5):455–60.
3. Moshiri A, Brown JC, Sunness JS. Pregnancy-related diseases. In: Ryan SJ, editor. Retina. 5th ed. Philadelphia: Elsevier Saunders; 2013. p. 1571–82.

Chapter 117
Ocular Albinism

Marco A. Gonzalez and Nisreen Ezuddin

117.1 Definitions

A group of genetic abnormalities caused by a reduction or absence of melanin synthesis that results in reduced pigmentation compared to others of the same racial background. There are two main types that manifest in ocular conditions:

1. Oculocutaneous albinism: An autosomal recessive (AR) condition that results in hypopigmentation of the hair, skin, and eye.
2. Ocular albinism: An X-linked recessive (XLR) disorder where only ocular hypopigmentation is apparent. Female carriers may demonstrate mosaicism, resulting from X-inactivation.

117.2 Symptoms

Decreased vision, reduced stereopsis, photophobia, nystagmus, and minimal pigmentation of the skin/hair/iris

M.A. Gonzalez, MD (✉) • N. Ezuddin
Department of Ophthalmology, University of Miami, Bascom Palmer Eye Institute, 900 NW 17th St., Miami, FL 33136, USA
e-mail: mgonzalez6@med.miami.edu

C.A. Medina et al. (eds.), *Manual of Retinal Diseases: A Guide to Diagnosis and Management*, DOI 10.1007/978-3-319-20460-4_117

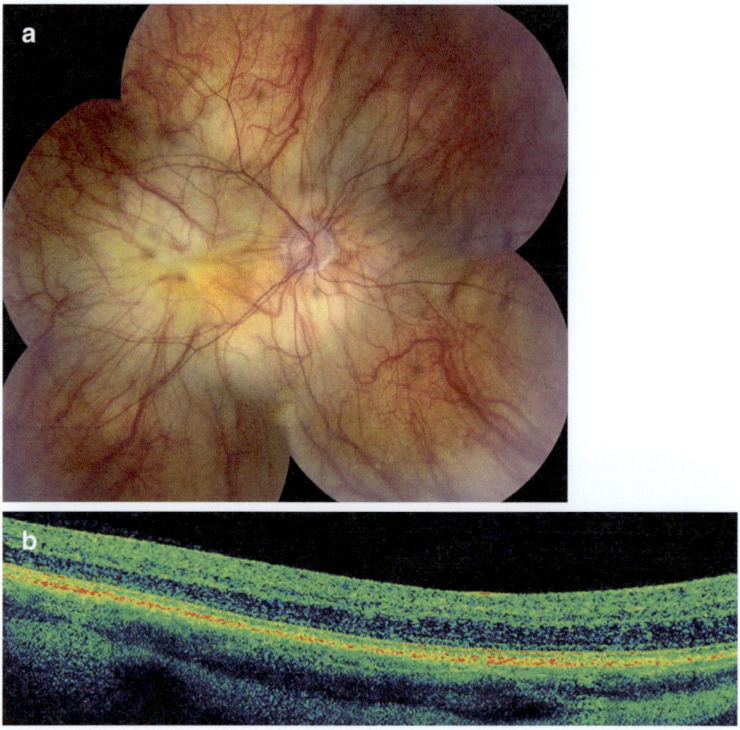

Fig. 117.1 Albinism. Note fundus hypopigmentation with highly visible choroidal vasculature (**a**). The absence of a foveal contour by OCT (**b**)

117.3 Signs

Fundus hypopigmentation with highly visible choroidal vasculature, iris transillumination, and foveal hypoplasia (Fig. 117.1).
Others: high refractive error, strabismus, and amblyopia

117.4 Epidemiology

Worldwide prevalence ranges from 1 in 5,000 to 1 in 40,000.

117.5 Differential Diagnosis

Retinal pathologies that present with depigmentation of retinal pigment epithelium and/or foveal hypoplasia are chronic Vogt-Koyanagi-Harada (VKH) syndrome, sympathetic ophthalmia, achromatopsia, and retinopathy of prematurity.

Several syndromic forms of albinism have been described and are important to exclude:

A. *Chédiak-Higashi syndrome*: An autosomal recessive (AR) disorder that affects white blood cell function, resulting in an increased susceptibility to infections and that may lead to death.
B. *Hermansky-Pudlak syndrome*: An autosomal recessive (AR) condition where defective platelets cause easy bruising and bleeding, more common in patients of Puerto Rican descent.
C. *Waardenburg syndrome*: An autosomal dominant (AD) disorder caused by abnormal distribution of melanocytes during embryogenesis. It manifests with patchy skin hypopigmentation and deafness in 20 % of affected individuals.

117.6 Etiology

Albinism is a group of hereditary diseases associated with mutations in several enzymes or membrane proteins that contribute to melanin synthesis. The phenotype arises from a defect in melanocyte differentiation that renders synthesis and/or transport of melanin dysfunctional within cells. Melanin synthesis is responsible for retinal pigment epithelial pigmentation. Lack of appropriate retinal pigment epithelial pigmentation leads to foveal underdevelopment during embryogenesis.

117.7 Workup/Testing

Optical coherence tomography can be used to evaluate for the absence of a foveal contour. Referral to primary care provider is necessary if there is concern for syndromic manifestations of albinism. Genetic testing and family counseling may be appropriate in some cases.

117.8 Prognosis and Management

No medical or surgical therapy has proven effective in the treatment of fundus hypopigmentation and macular hypoplasia resulting from albinism. Visual prognosis is guarded and current treatment is aimed at minimizing the development of amblyopia.

References and Suggested Readings

1. Gerstenblith Adam T, Rabinowitz Michael P. The Wills Eye manual: office and emergency room diagnosis and treatment of eye disease. Baltimore: Lippincott, Williams and Wilkins; 2012.
2. King RA, Jackson IJ, Oetting WS. Human albinism and mouse models. In: Wright AF, Jay B, editors. Molecular genetics of inherited eye disorders. Chur: Harwood Academic; 1994. p. 89–122.

3. Oetting W, editor. The albinism database website. Human genome variation society. Available at http://albinismdb.med.umn.edu/. Last updated September 21, 2009. Accessed 16 Jan 2015.
4. Schubert HD. Basic and clinical science course, Section 12: retina and vitreous. American Academy of Ophthalmology, San Francisco, CA 2014–15. p. 10–11.
5. Summers CG. Albinism: classification, clinical characteristics, and recent findings. Optom Vis Sci. 2009;86(6):659–62.
6. Traboulsi EI, Green WR. Duane's ophthalmology; Ch. 38 An overview of albinism and its visual system manifestations. Lippincott Williams & Wilkins, Philadelphia; 2006.

Chapter 118
Vitamin A Deficiency

Thalmon R. Campagnoli and William E. Smiddy

118.1 Definitions

Vitamin A deficiency is the leading cause of blindness in children from developing countries. Ocular findings are part of a larger syndrome of vitamin A deficiency that includes anemia, growth retardation, immune suppression, and malnutrition, potentially leading to death. Early ophthalmic diagnosis allows prevention of definitive visual loss and, ultimately, death.

118.2 Symptoms

Most patients with mild vitamin A deficiency present no ocular symptoms. Nyctalopia (earliest and most common manifestation; reversible with vitamin A replacement), visual field abnormalities, decreased vision, itching, and burning of ocular surface.

T.R. Campagnoli, MD • W.E. Smiddy, MD (✉)
Department of Ophthalmology, University of Miami, Bascom Palmer Eye Institute,
900 NW 17th St., Miami, FL 33136, USA
e-mail: wsmiddy@med.miami.edu

C.A. Medina et al. (eds.), *Manual of Retinal Diseases: A Guide to Diagnosis and Management*, DOI 10.1007/978-3-319-20460-4_118

118.3 Signs

Earlier phases:

- Conjunctival dryness and roughness (xerosis) usually occur in association with night blindness symptoms. Reversible.
- Bitot's spot: well-demarcated region of keratinized, squamous metaplasia in the bulbar conjunctiva. Pathognomonic of vitamin A deficiency. Usually reversible but may be irreversible if longstanding.

Later phases:

- Corneal xerosis; may be reversible with vitamin A replacement depending on the extension of the disease
- Corneal ulceration/keratomalacia; usually irreversible
- Corneal scar

Xerophthalmic fundus is the typical retinal finding in hypovitaminosis A. It is characterized by fine white, cream-colored, or grayish dot-like, oval, or linear opacities in the retina (Fig. 118.1). It may occur in association with any of the ocular signs listed above, and the lesions may regress or may not regress completely after vitamin A replacement.

118.4 Epidemiology

Vitamin A deficiency in childhood is associated with extreme poverty, malnutrition, and a history of child mortality in the mother or household in developing countries. Around 20,000–100,000 cases of blindness worldwide per year are thought to be

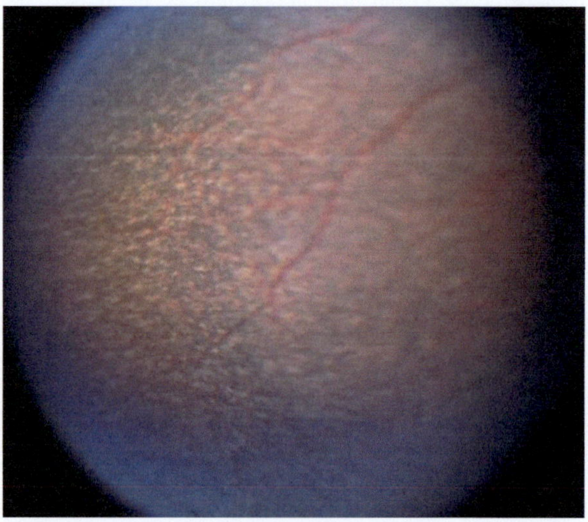

Fig. 118.1 Xerophthalmic fundus. Typical retinal finding of fine white, cream-colored, or grayish dot-like, oval, or linear opacities in the retina

related to vitamin A deficiency. Mortality of children presenting with keratomalacia may reach 90 % if not treated. Most cases of vitamin A deficiency in developed countries occur as a result of conditions in which metabolism or storage of vitamin A is deranged (chronic alcoholism, cirrhosis, bowel surgery) and/or conditions of fat malabsorption (pancreatitis, cystic fibrosis).

118.5 Predisposing Conditions

- Malnutrition
- Respiratory or diarrheal disease
- Inadequate breast-feeding
- Malabsorption syndrome
- Liver disorders
- Long-term parenteral nutrition
- Pregnancy

118.6 Differential Diagnosis

Conjunctivitis, infectious keratitis, dry eye syndrome, retinitis pigmentosa, albinism, gyrate atrophy, and congenital stationary night blindness are some of the diseases that can simulate some of the vitamin A deficiency's findings.

118.7 Etiology

Ocular metabolic changes responsible for the visual impairment of vitamin A deficiency include:

- Deficit on initiation of neural impulses from the photoreceptors
- Decreased photoreceptor outer segment turnover and phagocytosis of outer segment material
- Abnormal conjunctival epithelial cell RNA and glycoprotein synthesis, leading to keratinization of mucosal surfaces and loss of goblet cells

118.8 Workup/Testing

Diagnosis is based on clinical signs and symptoms at ocular examination. Symptoms of night blindness and the presence of Bitot's spots are the most common clinical determinants of vitamin A deficiency.

Some tests are helpful to assess vitamin A status:

- Serum retinol concentration (deficiency if <0.35 μmol/L).
- Breast milk retinol concentration.
- Ocular tests may also add in the diagnosis:
- Dark adaptation
- Electroretinogram (ERG)
- Visual field

118.9 Prognosis and Management

Night blindness symptoms, conjunctival xerosis, and Bitot's spots are reversible with vitamin A replacement. Treatment dose recommendation is according to the age and should be given *immediately* on diagnosis:

- <6 months of age = 50,000 IU
- 6–12 months of age = 100,000 IU
- >12 months of age = 200,000 IU

The same doses should be repeated on the next day *and* at least 2 weeks later. Women of reproductive age presenting night blindness or Bitot's spots should be treated with 10,000 IU/day for 2 weeks or 25,000 IU/week for 4 weeks; if presenting acute corneal lesions (xerosis, ulceration, keratomalacia), they should be treated according to the general recommendations abovementioned. Aggressive corneal lubrication with artificial tears and ointment is needed in case of advanced xerosis, ulceration, or keratomalacia.

118.10 Follow-Up

Patients should receive follow-up according to the severity of the ocular findings. Close follow-up is essential to confirm the absence of progression of corneal thinning to perforation. Once initially treated and stabilized, reevaluation every 4–6 months is advisable, and administration of vitamin A is considered for the prevention of new episodes.

References and Suggested Reading

1. American Academy of Ophthalmology International Panel. Middle East/North Africa. Vitamin A deficiency. San Francisco: American Academy of Ophthalmology; 2013. Available at: http://one.aao.org/topic-detail/vitamin-deficiency--middle-eastnorth-africa.
2. Semba RD. Nutritional blindness. In: Albert DM, Miller JW, editors. Albert and Jakobiec's principles and practice of ophthalmology. 3rd ed. Philadelphia: Elsevier Saunders; 2008. p. 4579–85.

Chapter 119
Hematologic Disorders

Christine L. Bokman and Marco A. Gonzalez

119.1 Definitions

Blood dyscrasia – A pathologic condition in which any of the constituents of blood (red blood cells, white blood cells, platelets) are abnormal in structure, function, or quality. As a result, fundus manifestations are a direct manifestation of ineffective nutrient delivery to a highly metabolic end organ.

119.2 Anemia

119.2.1 Symptoms

Usually asymptomatic; visual acuity loss occurs later in disease. May also present with central or cecocentral scotoma.

119.2.2 Signs

NFL hemorrhages and infarcts, cotton wool spots, macular edema, dilated arteriolar vessels, increased vessel tortuosity, neovascularization, VH, and bilateral optic neuropathy.

C.L. Bokman, BA (✉) • M.A. Gonzalez, MD
Department of Ophthalmology, Bascom Palmer Eye Institute, University of Miami, 900 NW 17th St., Miami, FL 33136, USA
e-mail: clbokman@med.miami.edu; mgonzalez6@med.miami.edu

C.A. Medina et al. (eds.), *Manual of Retinal Diseases: A Guide to Diagnosis and Management*, DOI 10.1007/978-3-319-20460-4_119

119.2.3 Differential Diagnosis

- Diabetic retinopathy
- Hypertensive retinopathy
- Collagen vascular disease
- Plasma cell dyscrasia
- Central retinal vein occlusion (CRVO)
- Branch retinal vein occlusion (BRVO)

119.2.4 Etiology

Decrease in red blood cell mass increases the incidence of hemorrhage in the retina.

119.2.5 Workup/Testing

- Anemia workup: to investigate blood loss, hemolysis, and decreased red blood cell production
- Dilated fundus examination

119.2.6 Management/Prognosis

Medical management of anemia may result in good visual recovery.

119.2.7 Complications

Persistent VH, RD, and optic nerve atrophy

119.3 Polycythemia

119.3.1 Symptoms

Asymptomatic until advanced or rapidly progressive disease, visual loss, painless loss of vision if venous occlusion occurs.

119.3.2 Signs

NFL hemorrhages, cotton wool spots, macular edema, neovascularization, VH, and retinal venous occlusion. Milder polycythemia is associated with subtler changes, i.e., venous tortuosity and microaneurysms.

119.3.3 Differential Diagnosis

- Diabetic retinopathy
- Hypertensive retinopathy
- Collagen vascular disease
- Plasma cell dyscrasia
- CRVO or BRVO

119.3.4 Etiology

Increase in red blood cell mass leads to hyperviscosity and decreased blood flow, damaging blood vessel endothelium and causing ischemia that may lead to neovascularization and vitrous hemorrhage.

119.3.5 Workup/Testing

- Polycythemia workup: to investigate if increase in red blood cell mass is primary (polycythemia rubra vera) or secondary (due to hypoxemic response).
- Dilated fundus examination
- Fluorescein angiography

119.3.6 Management/Prognosis

Medical management of polycythemia. If corrected early in the course of the disease, visual function may improve. Persistence of secondary complications related to neovascularization may be managed at the discretion of the treating ophthalmologist.

119.3.7 Follow-Up

Medical monitoring of polycythemia recurrence and relapse. If neovascularization present, regular follow-up with dilated fundus exam.

119.3.8 Complications

VH, extensive neovascularization, traction RD, and CRVO/BRVO

119.4 Multiple Myeloma (MM) and Waldenström's Macroglobulinemia (WM)

119.4.1 Symptoms

Decreased visual acuity, sudden, painless loss of vision more common in WM than MM secondary to hyperviscosity syndrome, and proptosis with plasmacytoma development associated with MM.

119.4.2 Signs

Flame-shaped hemorrhages, cotton wool spots, NFL infarcts, and microaneurysms. Signs more commonly associated with WM than MM include more frequent and severe retinal hemorrhages, vessel dilation and tortuosity, CRVO/BRVO, neovascularization, and VH (Fig. 119.1).

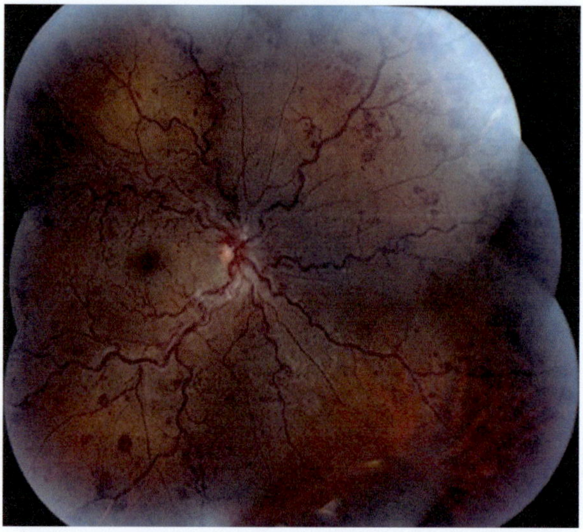

Fig. 119.1 Multiple myeloma and Waldenström's macroglobulinemia. Retinal hemorrhages and vessel dilation and tortuosity are typical findings

119.4.3 Differential Diagnosis

- Anemia/polycythemia
- Thrombocytopenia
- Hypertensive retinopathy
- Diabetic retinopathy
- Hypercoagulable states

119.4.4 Etiology

Secondary anemia from MM leads to small vessel leakage, while in WM, hyperviscosity plays a more significant role with direct damage to vessel endothelium, leading to more severe hemorrhage and pathological changes (3).

119.4.5 Workup/Testing

- MM/WM workup: to investigate extent of disease, which includes CBC, serum, and urine protein electrophoresis
- B-scan ophthalmic ultrasonography: to visualize potential retrobulbar plasmacytoma associated with MM
- Head CT scan with coronal imaging: to visualize extent of disease and ocular involvement
- Dilated fundus examination

119.4.6 Management/Prognosis

Medical management of MM/WM is the mainstay of therapy (i.e., plasmapheresis, chemotherapy). Systemic treatment of MM/WM may improve retinopathy. More frequent follow-up with full eye examination should occur if more severe retinal changes are present at the time medical treatment is initiated.

119.4.7 Complications

Exudative RD, CRVO/BRVO, persistent or recurrent VH, papilledema secondary to intracranial plasmacytomas, and secondary retinal changes from chemotherapy treatment for MM/WM.

119.5 Acute Lymphoblastic Leukemia (ALL)/Acute Myeloblastic Leukemia (AML)

119.5.1 Symptoms

Typically asymptomatic until disease is advanced, decreased visual acuity, rarely sudden vision loss secondary to VH, CRVO

119.5.2 Signs

- Primary leukemic infiltrate represented by white nodules with surrounding hemorrhage and optic nerve head infiltration causing pale gray swelling of nerve (Fig. 119.2)
- Secondary signs: Intraretinal hemorrhage, cotton wool spots, vessel attenuation and tortuosity, and rarely, peripheral neovascularization. Intraretinal hemorrhage, cotton wool spots, and vessel tortuosity are more common in AML than ALL.

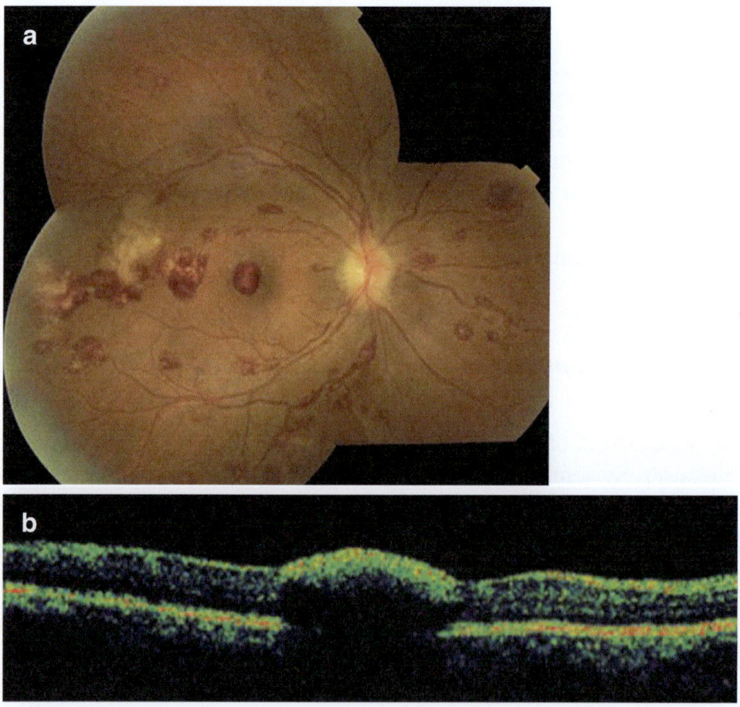

Fig. 119.2 Acute lymphoblastic/myeloblastic leukemia. Leukemic infiltrates appear as white nodules with surrounding hemorrhage (**a**). OCT appearance (**b**)

119.5.3 Differential Diagnosis

- Hypertensive retinopathy
- Hyperviscosity syndromes (polycythemia, factor V Leiden)
- Systemic emboli
- Infections (HIV, CMV, endocarditis)
- Autoimmune disorders
- Anterior ischemic optic neuropathy

119.5.4 Etiology

Direct infiltration of leukemia causes retinal changes while increased white blood cell count results secondarily in hyperviscosity and damage to vascular endothelium of the retina.

119.5.5 Workup/Testing

- ALL/AML workup: to investigate extent of neoplastic process; in some cases, ophthalmic manifestations are the first signs of ALL/AML
- Dilated fundus examination
- Fluorescein angiography

119.5.6 Management/Prognosis

Medical treatment of ALL/AML with chemotherapy and radiation. Because this is an acute neoplastic process, the prognosis is poor, especially in adults. In children, treatment may result in recovery of visual function with resolution of disease.

119.5.7 Complications

VH, RD (exudative, traction), CRVO/BRVO, and secondary complications from ALL/AML treatment side effects.

119.6 Idiopathic Thrombocytopenic Purpura (ITP)/ Thrombotic Thrombocytopenic Purpura (TTP)

119.6.1 Symptoms

In ITP, usually asymptomatic unless platelet count is so low that severe hemorrhage results and causes decreased visual acuity and/or sudden, painless loss of vision. TTP also results in decreased visual acuity but is also associated with extraocular muscle palsies and visual field defects secondary to brain involvement.

119.6.2 Signs

- ITP: intraretinal hemorrhage, subretinal hemorrhage, and VH
- TTP: intraretinal hemorrhage, retinal vascular occlusion, serous RD, and papilledema

119.6.3 Differential Diagnosis

- Vascular occlusive disease
- Purtscher's retinopathy
- DIC (serous RD)
- Hypertensive retinopathy
- Radiation retinopathy
- Graves' disease
- Anemia

119.6.4 Etiology

ITP is the immune-mediated destruction of platelets. TTP is the nonimmunologic destruction of platelets of unknown etiology that results in the pentad: thrombocytopenia, microangiopathic hemolytic anemia, fever, CNS dysfunction, and renal disease. In ITP, low platelet count leads to spontaneous intraretinal hemorrhage, and the lower the platelet count, the worse the hemorrhage. In TTP, serous RD results from occlusion of the choriocapillaris, causing damage to the retinal pigment epithelium and blood-retinal barrier disruption.

119.6.5 Workup/Testing

- ITP/TTP workup: including platelet count and coagulation studies to distinguish from DIC in the presence of serous RD
- Dilated fundus examination
- Spectral-domain OCT: to visualize serous RD
- Fluorescein angiography: shows focal nonperfusion of choriocapillaris and late leakage into subretinal space

119.6.6 Management/Prognosis

Medical management of ITP/TTP. For ITP, prednisone and IVIG for short-term use; splenectomy cures a majority of patients. TTP is treated with plasmapheresis and corticosteroids. Management also includes treatment of secondary ophthalmic complications. ITP has a better prognosis for visual outcomes than does TTP; however, even severe complications of TTP (serous RD) can result in a favorable outcome with proper management.

119.6.7 Complications

- CRVO/BRVO, persistent VH, serous RD, and RPE changes

119.7 Disseminated Intravascular Coagulation (*DIC*)

119.7.1 Symptoms

Asymptomatic, loss of visual acuity, flashing lights, sudden vision loss, and secondary to serous RD.

119.7.2 Signs

Classic ocular finding is serous RD; also intraretinal hemorrhage, VH

119.7.3 Differential Diagnosis

- TTP
- Vascular occlusive disease
- Systemic emboli
- Vogt-Koyanagi-Harada (VKH) disease
- Choroidal inflammatory disease
- Malignant hypertension
- Toxemia of pregnancy
- Coats's disease

119.7.4 Etiology

See TTP.

119.7.5 Workup/Testing

- DIC workup: including coagulation studies to distinguish from TTP and initiate proper management
- Dilated fundus examination
- Spectral-domain OCT: to visualize serous RD
- Fluorescein angiography

119.7.6 Management/Prognosis

Medical management of DIC – i.e., mainly supportive therapy and plasmapheresis. For serous RD, reversal of detachment; however, prognosis of complete visual resolution is poor.

119.7.7 Complications

VH, serous RD, RPE necrosis, and fibrinoid necrosis of choriocapillaris

References and Suggested Reading

1. Holt JM, Gordon-Smith EC. Retinal abnormalities in disease of the blood. Br J Ophthalmol. 1969;53(3):145–60.
2. Knapp AJ, Gartner S, Henkind P. Multiple myeloma and its ocular manifestations. Surv Ophthalmol. 1987;31(5):343–51.
3. Mansour AM, Lee JW, Yahng SA, et al. Ocular manifestations of idiopathic aplastic anemia: retrospective study and literature review. Clin Ophthalmol. 2014;17(8):777–87.
4. Rothstein T. Bilateral central retinal vein closure as the initial manifestation of polycythemia. Am J Ophthalmol. 1972;74(2):256–60.
5. Schachat AP, Markowitz JA, Guyer DR, et al. Ophthalmic manifestations of leukemia. Arch Ophthalmol. 1989;107(5):697–700.
6. Lambert SR, High KA, Cotlier R, et al. Serous retinal detachments in thrombotic thrombocytopenic purpura. Arch Ophthalmol. 1985;103(8):1172–4.

Chapter 120
Hypertensive Retinopathy

Christine L. Bokman and Marco A. Gonzalez

120.1 Definition

Hypertension (HTN): Systolic readings greater than or equal to 140 mmHg or diastolic readings greater than or equal to 90 mmHg.

120.2 Symptoms

In chronic HTN, asymptomatic early in disease, decreased visual acuity late in disease. In malignant (acute) HTN, symptoms include headache, eye pain, reduced visual acuity, and diplopia.

120.3 Signs

- Chronic HTN: Narrowing of retinal arterioles, almost always bilateral. Classification based on the Keith Wagener Barker (KWB) grading scale from grade 1 (mild) to grade 4 (severe) (Table 120.1).
- Malignant HTN: Papilledema, hard exudates often forming a ring around the macula ("macular star"), and grade 4 hypertensive retinopathy

C.L. Bokman, BA (✉) • M.A. Gonzalez, MD
Department of Ophthalmology, Bascom Palmer Eye Institute, University of Miami,
900 NW 17th St., Miami, FL 33136, USA
e-mail: clbokman@med.miami.edu; mgonzalez6@med.miami.edu

C.A. Medina et al. (eds.), *Manual of Retinal Diseases: A Guide to Diagnosis and Management*, DOI 10.1007/978-3-319-20460-4_120

Table 120.1 Hypertensive retinopathy: Keith Wagener Barker (KWB) grading scale

Grade 1: Arteriolar narrowing, vessel tortuosity
Grade 2: Grade 1 plus more severe vessel changes including copper wiring, silver wiring, and AV nicking
Grade 3: Grade 2 plus flame hemorrhages, cotton wool spots, microaneurysms, or hard exudates
Grade 4: Grade 3 plus papilledema or macular star

120.4 Differential Diagnosis

- Diabetic retinopathy
- Radiation retinopathy
- Central retinal vein occlusion or branch retinal vein occlusion
- Anemia
- Autoimmune disease

120.5 Etiology

Acutely, HTN causes vasospasm and increased vascular tone. Chronically, HTN causes damage and necrosis of vascular endothelial cells, leading to intimal thickening and sclerosis, media wall hyperplasia, and hyaline degeneration of arterioles.

120.6 Workup/Testing

- History: duration and control of HTN and comorbidities, i.e., diabetes and radiation
- Blood pressure measurement
- Dilated fundus exam detects early changes (Fig. 120.1)
- Spectral-domain OCT
- Fluorescein angiography (wide field preferably as this may demonstrate extensive peripheral nonperfusion)

120.7 Management and Prognosis

Therapy focuses on blood pressure control with a goal of <140/90 [1]. Full clinical eye exam including dilated fundus exam should occur every 6–12 months. Retinopathy due to chronic hypertension is irreversible, while acute HTN changes (malignant HTN, grade 4 signs) are reversible with medical treatment of acute HTN [2, 3, 4].

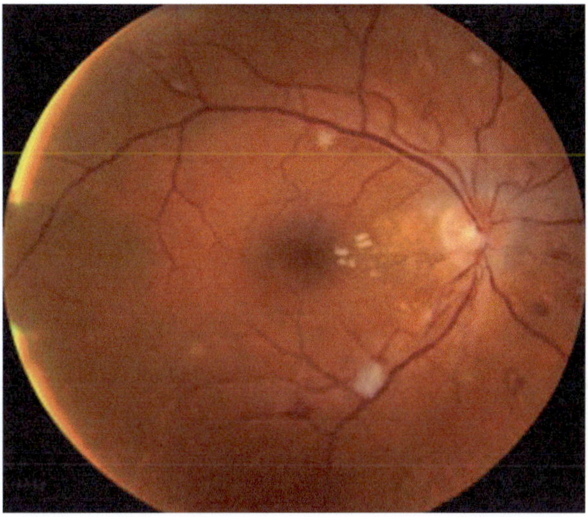

Fig. 120.1 Grade 3 hypertensive retinopathy. Characteristic findings include AV nicking, flame hemorrhages, cotton wool spots, and hard exudates

120.8 Complications

Central or branch retinal artery or vein occlusion, retinal arterial macroaneurysms. Ischemia can lead to neovascularization, vitreous hemorrhage, epiretinal membrane formation, traction retinal detachment, and progression of diabetic retinopathy.

References and Suggested Reading

1. James PA, Oparil SO, Carter BL, et al. 2014 Evidence-based guidelines for the management of high blood pressure in adults: Report from the panel members appointed to the eighth joint national committee (JNC 8). JAMA. 2014;311(5):507–20.
2. Wong TY, Klein R, Nieto FJ, et al. Retinal microvascular abnormalities and ten-year cardiovascular mortality. A population-based case-control study. Ophthalmology. 2003;110(5):933–40.
3. Wong TY, Klein R, Couper DJ, et al. Retinal microvascular abnormalities and incident clinical strokes. The Atherosclerosis Risk in the Communities Study. Lancet. 2001;358(9288): 1134–40.
4. Wong TY, McIntosh R. Hypertensive retinopathy signs as risk indicators of cardiovascular morbidity and mortality. Br Med Bull. 2005;73–74(1):57–70.

Appendix: Drugs and Doses

Route	Class	Agent	Dose/volume
Topical	Antibiotic (fortified)	Vancomycin	25 mg/ml
		Ceftazidime	50 mg/ml
Periocular (subconjunctival)	Antibiotic	Vancomycin	25 mg
		Ceftazidime	100 mg
	Steroid	Dexamethasone	12–24 mg
Intravitreal	Antibiotic	Vancomycin	1 mg/0.1 ml
		Ceftazidime	2.25 mg/0.1 ml
		Amikacin	0.4 mg/0.1 ml
		Clindamycin	1 mg/0.1 ml
	Antifungal	Amphotericin	0.005 mg/0.1 ml
		Voriconazole	0.1 mg/0.2 ml
	Antiviral	Foscarnet	2.4 mg/0.1 ml
		Ganciclovir	2 mg/0.05 ml
	Steroid	Dexamethasone	0.4 mg/0.1 ml
		Triamcinolone	4 mg/0.1 ml
	Antiangiogenic	Bevacizumab	1.25 mg/0.05 ml
		Ranibizumab	0.5 mg/0.05 ml
		Aflibercept	2 mg/0.05 ml
	Antineoplastic	Methotrexate	0.4 mg/0.1 ml
		Rituximab	1 mg/0.1 ml

C.A. Medina et al. (eds.), *Manual of Retinal Diseases: A Guide to Diagnosis and Management*, DOI 10.1007/978-3-319-20460-4

Route	Class	Agent	Dose/volume
Oral	Antifungal	Voriconazole	200 mg BID
		Fluconazole	200 mg BID
		Itraconazole	200 mg BID
		Ketoconazole	200 mg BID
	Antiviral	Acyclovir	800 mg five times daily
		Valacyclovir	1000 mg–2000 mg TID
		Famciclovir	500 mg TID
		Valganciclovir	Induction 900 mg BID × 3 weeks Maintenance: 900 mg QD
Intravenous	Antibiotic	Vancomycin	1 g IV q 12 h
		Ceftazidime	1 g IV q 12 h
	Antifungal	Amphotericin B	0.25–1.0 mg/kg
	Antiviral	Ganciclovir	Induction 5 mg/kg BID for 2–3 weeks Maintenance: 5 mg/kg daily
		Foscarnet	Induction 90 mg/kg BID for 2 weeks Maintenance: 120 mg/kg daily
		Cidofovir	Induction 5 mg/kg weekly for 3 weeks Maintenance: 3–5 mg/kg every 2 weeks

The dose, duration, and route of administration may vary with severity of ocular disease, immunocompetence status, renal function, liver disease, presence of systemic infection, and other factors. Consultation with infectious disease specialist is recommended

QD once daily, *BID* two time daily, *TID* three times daily

MIX
Papier aus verantwortungsvollen Quellen
Paper from responsible sources
FSC® C105338

If you have any concerns about our products,
you can contact us on
ProductSafety@springernature.com

In case Publisher is established outside the EU,
the EU authorized representative is:
Springer Nature Customer Service Center GmbH
Europaplatz 3, 69115 Heidelberg, Germany

Printed by Libri Plureos GmbH
in Hamburg, Germany